EXERCISE AND HEALTH

Exercise and Health

The Evidence and the Implications

Gregory S. Thomas
Philip R. Lee
Pat Franks
Ralph S. Paffenbarger, Jr.

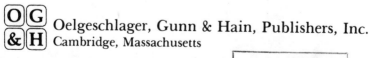 Oelgeschlager, Gunn & Hain, Publishers, Inc.
Cambridge, Massachusetts

Copyright © 1981 by Oelgeschlager, Gunn & Hain, Publishers, Inc.
All rights reserved. No part of this publication may be reproduced, stored
in a retrieval system, or transmitted in any form or by any means—electronic
mechanical photocopy, recording, or otherwise—without
the prior written consent of the publisher.

International Standard Book Number: 0-89946-048-8

Library of Congress Catalog Card Number: 80-23376

Printed in the United States of America

Library of Congress Cataloging in Publication Data

Main entry under title:

Exercise and health.

Includes bibliographical references and index.
1. Exercise. 2. Exercise—Physiological aspects. 3. Physical fitness—United
States. 4. Physical education and training—United States. 5. Medical policy—
United States. I. Thomas, Gregory S.
RA784.E95   613.7   80-23376
ISBN 0-89946-048-8

This book is dedicated to Joanne Thomas; Bill and Dianne Thomas; Dorothy, Paul, Amy, Margie, and Ted Lee; Duskie Gelfand; Erica and Mark Johnson; Robert T. Hyde and Alvin L. Wing; and the Health Policy Program runners, swimmers, soccer players, tennis players, cyclists, and skiers—Ruth Weiller, Joan Trauner, Suzanne Stenmark, David Sobel, Sharon Solkowitz, Jon Showstack, Dennis Seely, Steve Schroeder, Lois Myers, Peggy McManus, Susan Maerki, Lauren LeRoy, Cathy Kulka, Barbara Johnson, Chris Herman, Helen Gonzales, Ernestine Florence, Phyllis Fetto, Eunice Chee, Connie Celum, Lew Butler, Peter Budetti, and Nancy Brown Ramsay.

Contents

Contents

Foreword

Personal fitness is increasingly recognized as often more important to one's health than drug therapy or other medical technologies. Exercise can occupy a central role in achieving fitness. What one may and may not expect in benefits from exercise and what one can do to enhance the influence of exercise on health are treated objectively and realistically in this book.

Health *is* more than absence of disease or infirmity, as the World Health Organization (WHO) has long affirmed. Yet, society still invests far more in disease, its prevention and treatment, than it does in health. Not only does exercise have the potential to be used in the prevention of some diseases and in the treatment of others, but it can, as well, increase the positive enjoyment of life that is implicit in the WHO statement. The authors' major task in this book is to put the potential of exercise in perspective, to make clear what may be accomplished with exercise without indulging in exaggerated expectations.

Since 1940, therapeutic strategies for managing disease have advanced almost exponentially. Critical physicians recognize, however, that these advances appy to relatively few of the diseases and disabilities that afflict mankind. For the majority of these ills, we still depend in the long run on the body's magnificent capacity for self-restoration, whatever "treatment" may or may not be used. Here is where the principle of general support, which often means watchful waiting rather that specific action, does more to help than chemical or herbal concoctions or other interventions.

One aspect of general support, long known but sometimes forgotten, is the interaction between mind and body. Contact with exotic "systems" of medicine—China has been a fascinating example—has reemphasized the profound effect that mind–body interaction has on the onset of illness as well as on recovery and rehabilitation. Unfortunately, our knowledge of the dimensions and characteristics of this interaction is still primitive. There is a good reason to believe, however, that what makes a person feel good helps make him or her "healthier." Where we are lacking is in our knowledge of how to promote more of this good feeling among the infinite variety of human beings. What helps one person may not help another. Almost 2000 years ago, Galen, in one of the oldest texts on health promotion and disease prevention—*De Sanitate Tuenda*—outlined regimens for living that still have validity. Galen recognized, however, as we often do not today, that just telling a person what is "good" for him or her may have little effect or even a countereffect.

One observation bears underlining. Any lifestyle change that a person undertakes because it is prescribed has far less chance of attaining permanence than something that has grown up as a personal desire. Adults who derive real pleasure from physical activity, with or without enjoying the stress of competition, have uniformly had a positive early experience. The reverse is often true. Is it too much to ask that society help parents provide, in the preschool and school years, an atmosphere in which exercise can be a joyful experience and not one that is too often viewed as the drudgery of routine calisthenics? Those of us in our senior years who still thoroughly enjoy voluntarily induced physical exhaustion appreciate the futility of trying to change the lifetime habits of a sedentary colleague. There is more to be gained in investing time and effort so that all who can benefit from exercise will have both a positive early experience and a continued opportunity to repeat it. Exercise is not necessarily good for everyone, but it is unfair not to give everyone the best chance to see whether he or she enjoys it.

This sensible book on exercise is a welcome addition to our resources. It emphasizes a practical approach and outlines for practicing physicians the demonstrated possibilities for exercise prescription, including indications and contraindications, as well as the adverse effects of exercise. The book also provides for public health specialists plans of action to promote exercise in the community.

Exercise is not a panacea, but it ought to be fun. If this book can help make exercise both meaningful and enjoyable, it will have accomplished its purpose.

Myron E. Wegman, M.D.
Dean Emeritus
School of Public Health
University of Michigan

Acknowledgments

The authors wish to acknowledge public and private agencies whose support has made possible this exploration of the relationship between exercise and health. Policy research and analysis conducted by Dr. Lee, Ms. Franks, and Dr. Thomas in the general area of health promotion and disease prevention, and in the specific area of exercise and health, have been supported by the Stern Fund, New York, New York; The Max and Anna Levinson Foundation, Springfield, Massachusetts; The Robert Wood Johnson Foundation, Princeton, New Jersey; the National Center for Health Services Research, U.S. Department of Health and Human Services (Grant No. HS 02975); and the University of California, San Francisco. Dr. Paffenbarger's research on physical activity, work assignment, and cardiovascular disease in San Francisco longshoremen was supported initially by a U.S. Public Health Service research grant from the National Institute of Neurological Diseases and Stroke (Grant No. NB06818) and a contract from the National Institute for Occupational Safety and Health (Contract No. HSM99-7258). His studies of factors predisposing to chronic disease in Harvard and University of Pennsylvania students and alumni have been supported by the National Institute of Mental Health (Contract No. PH 43-67-1450); the National Heart, Lung, and Blood Institute (Grant Nos. HL 19839 and HL 24133); the National Institute of Child Health and Human Development (Grant No. HD04753); and the National Institute on Aging (Grant No. AG00309).

The authors also wish to thank several people who played a special role in the preparation of this book. Sharon Solkowitz performed literature searches and aided us in many other ways in preparing the final manuscript. David Sobel, M.D., Stephen Havas, M.D., Myron Wegman, M.D., Peggy McManus, Suzanne Stenmark, Jon Showstack, Lauren LeRoy, and Lois Myers acted as reviewers of the manuscript. Their thoughtful criticism and comments have helped us write a better book. Danita Kulp and Lee Glickstein typed the many drafts of the manuscript; Cathy Kulka helped to proofread them. Eunice Chee coordinated production of the book.

Introduction

Why another book on exercise? Our purpose in writing this book is to lay out the evidence on exercise and health and to explore the implications of this evidence—for physicians; public health professionals; students in the health professions; policymakers and program managers at the federal, state, and local levels of government; decision-makers in business and industry; leaders of community organizations; and individual Americans. Books of all kinds advocate exercise programs—from jogging to jumping rope—for people of all ages and from all walks of life. Rather than relying on advocates of one approach or another, we felt that it would be useful to examine both clinical and epidemiological evidence related to exercise and health, and then to look at the implications from both a clinical and a community point of view. Also, we wanted to link the world of policy with the worlds of community and clinical medicine.

Both health professionals, including primary care physicians and public health specialists, and public policymakers are faced with a number of questions about exercise and health. What are the patterns of exercise among the American population? Are we a sedentary population or a physically active one? Is there a relationship between lack of physical activity and risk of coronary heart disease? Does regular, vigorous exercise have any protective effect against coronary heart disease? Does exercise have any benefit in relation to other major health problems? Do the health benefits of regular vigorous exercise warrant the prescription of exercise for individual patients? Is the evidence on exercise and health sufficient to warrant the development of public policies and large-scale community-based programs to promote exercise, with the expectation that increasing the number of individuals who exercise regularly will help improve health status in the United States?

In attempting to answer these questions, we begin by assessing present levels of exercise and changing patterns of exercise in the U.S. population. Next we describe different types of exercise and discuss how physical fitness is related to the type, intensity, duration, and frequency of exercise performed. We then look at the evidence on

1

exercise in relation to coronary heart disease, hypertension, obesity, diabetes mellitus, anxiety, depression, and asthma. Here our focus is on evidence related to dynamic aerobic exercise in primary and secondary prevention, especially of coronary heart disease, and on the usefulness of exercise in treatment and rehabilitation. Using this evidence as a base, we discuss the prescription of exercise by physicians, including indications and contraindications for a prescription of dynamic aerobic exercise as well as risks and complications of exercise. Next we examine the place of exercise in broader strategies to promote health and to prevent disease at federal, state, and local levels of government, and we develop a community prescription for exercise—plans of action to promote exercise in the workplace, at home, in schools, and in the community itself.

Chapter 1 shows that patterns of exercise in the United States are changing, but that the great majority of Americans still engage in little regular physical activity. Public polls reveal that the percentage of people who report that they exercise regularly has increased greatly during the past twenty years. However, only from a third to a half of the population exercises regularly. The elderly, the poor, nonwhites, and women are underrepresented in the exercising population. There also has been a decrease or leveling off in recent years in the percentage of children and teens who exercise. More than half of all Americans believe that they get enough exercise. The question is, do they get enough exercise, and does the exercise that they get provide any health benefits?

Chapter 2 describes different types of exercise—dynamic aerobic exercise, low-intensity exercise, isometric and isotonic exercise, relaxation exercise, and therapeutic exercise. This book is primarily about dynamic aerobic exercise, that is, exercise that helps condition the heart and lungs. Aerobic exercise is exercise in which the energy needed is supplied by inspired oxygen. Dynamic aerobic exercise involves the repetitive use of large muscle masses. When large muscle groups are activated, an increased demand for oxygen is created. This demand is met by an increase in heart rate, stroke volume, and respiratory rate, and by a reduction in peripheral vascular resistance. When oxygen demand does not exceed oxygen supply, a state of oxygen balance is achieved, and exercise can be performed for long periods. When dynamic aerobic exercise is performed at a level of intensity sufficient to produce a heart rate that is 70 percent of an individual's maximum heart rate for 20 minutes three times per week, a "training effect" is produced. This "training effect" is manifested in improved physical fitness—increased stamina and physical work capacity. Other changes that occur with regular, sustained dynamic aerobic exercise may produce other health benefits.

Chapter 3 points out the growing importance of epidemiology as a tool in identifying multiple risk factors associated with coronary heart disease and in clarifying the role of dynamic aerobic exercise in primary and secondary prevention of the disease. We regard the findings of long-term studies of physical activity at work in San Francisco longshoremen as some of the strongest evidence of a protective effect of exercise against heart attack. Studies of leisure-time physical activity of Harvard alumni over nearly a twenty-year span show that exercise habits correlate with risk of some health problems, heart attack in particular. The benefits of regular vigorous exercise seem to be great, but these benefits appear to fade if people do not remain physically active. New findings are presented here to shed further light on the importance of exercise in the secondary prevention of heart attack. The optimum standards for frequency, duration, type, and intensity of exercise are yet to be firmly established, but the importance of exercise in primary prevention of coronary heart disease is no longer in question.

In Chapter 4 our main interest is in the value of dynamic aerobic exercise in the prevention of other major health problems as well as in the treatment and rehabilitation of patients with these problems. The prevalence of five problems—hypertension, obesity, diabetes mellitus, anxiety, and depression—and their impact on individuals as well as on the health care system merit consideration of the value of exercise in managing these problems. We also consider exercise in asthma because of conflicting evidence relating to the usefulness of exercise in this condition.

Chapter 5 indicates that, despite evidence of the beneficial effects of exercise, physicians rarely prescribe exercise for patients who are considered to be healthy. Even patients with cardiovascular disease, including those recovering from acute myocardial infarction, are only occasionally given specific exercise prescriptions or placed in organized programs of exercise as part of a cardiac rehabilitation program. Exercise prescription is designed to promote beneficial clinical effects. Dynamic aerobic exercise has many beneficial effects: physical, physiological, biochemical, and psychological. Exercise increases maximal oxygen uptake, slows the resting heart rate, lowers elevated blood pressure, improves the efficiency of cardiac action, increases cardiac output, and enhances physical work capacity. Exercise alters the blood lipid profile favorably, as it does fibrinolytic activity, platelet aggregation, and carbohydrate metabolism. Exercise also can improve sleep patterns, enhance self-confidence, and heighten the sense of well-being. To promote these beneficial effects through exercise prescriptions for patients, physicians need to be familiar with different types of exercise, particularly dynamic aerobic exercise. A key factor in any exercise prescription is the intensity of the activity. Also important are the frequency and duration of activity to be prescribed. Indications and contraindications for different types of exercise as well as tools for self-assessment and medical assessment of exercise and fitness status are presented for healthy people in different age groups, for patients with cardiovascular risk factors, and for patients with coronary heart disease. The problem of exercise dropouts—those who do not comply with exercise prescriptions—is confronted, and reasons for both noncompliance and compliance are examined.

Chapter 6 focuses on the diagnosis, prevention, and treatment of adverse effects of exercise, including both cardiac and noncardiac complications. We devote most of out attention to common musculoskeletal problems associated with exercise. Although exercise produces many positive effects on the musculoskeletal system, sometimes the component parts of the system are subjected to overuse. The result is acute or chronic musculoskeletal overload. The concept of overload is defined, and such factors as age, inherent differences in connective tissue, degenerative changes, and conditioning are discussed. The consequences of the overload syndrome can be prevented or minimized through proper conditioning exercises—stretching, strengthening, warming up—and proper protective equipment. If an orthopedic malady, temporary or permanent, forces a person to curtail or stop a specific exercise or sport, there is usually an alternative path to follow.

Chapter 7 broadens the perspective on exercise and health as we look at the place of exercise in federal, state, and local strategies to improve the health of Americans. To understand how exercise fits into broader strategies to improve health, we examine the context in which public policies on health are emerging, the evolution of new health promotion and disease prevention strategies in the United States, and the role of specific federal, state, and local government agencies in promoting exercise.

In Chapter 8 we lay out a framework for community action to promote exercise and present case studies of some plans turned into action—in the workplace, in homes, in schools, and in the community. Basically, we try to answer these questions: What can be done to promote exercise? How can it be done? Who can help do it? Who stands to benefit from it? Can the benefits be measured? Our framework for community action includes defining the range of potential actions: (1) exercise information and education; (2) exercise services, programs, and events; (3) exercise and recreation facility development; (4) legislative and regulatory measures; and (5) economic measures. In addition, the framework includes cataloging community resources, targeting population groups, choosing a setting or locale, devising a plan of action, searching for funding sources, setting the plan into action, and attempting to evaluate the results.

We see exercise as a behavioral factor in health that touches everyone, regardless of age, sex, race, heredity, education, income, or other personal characteristics. We believe that, if more people become more vigorously active through dynamic aerobic exercise and sports, there is some promise of reducing heart attack rates. We also believe that this type of exercise has other benefits in relation to other health problems. However, we believe also that to talk about exercise as if only sustained dynamic aerobic activity "qualifies" as beneficial exercise not only is scientifically and medically inaccurate, but also may be extremely discouraging to people who want to exercise. Some people do not want to—or are not able to—run several miles per day or swim laps on a regular basis. We believe that many of the benefits of exercise are not strictly health related, and that the value of exercise for a person is largely defined by the person. As one of our colleagues, Jon Showstack, noted in his review of this book:

> The value of exercise may be less in what one does or how much one does than in the fact that one does it at all. The half hour or so a day that I run is the only time all day that I have to myself. That, in itself, is very valuable to me. Other people may not find exercise valuable—it will not make them live healthier or happier lives. This is exactly the reason government policy should never be directed toward telling people that exercise is "good" for them. Policy should be responsive to the needs and desires of both exercisers and non-exercisers. Exercise is not competition, fashion, health, or heart rate. Exercise is not a question of "yes" or "no" but rather a continuum from less to more. At its most basic level, exercise is simply part of being alive.

In short, you must choose and conduct your own program to alter your own lifestyle. You must do your own jogging or swimming and live with the beating of your own heart. Exercise, after all, is mostly a one-person show. You have to do it yourself.

Chapter 1

Patterns of Exercise in the American Population

Throughout most of human evolution, human survival depended on the capacity to engage in sustained physical activity. Strength, speed, stamina, and agility were an advantage to nomads, hunter-gatherers, and early farmers. In fact, vigorous physical activity was central to the lives of men, women, and children from the time of earliest human development until the Industrial Revolution. Since that time, more and more people in industrialized nations, including the United States, have come to lead sedentary lives. A century ago, a third of the energy used in U.S. workshops and factories and on farms was supplied by human muscles; today only 1 percent of this energy is supplied by human labor.[1] For the great majority of adults and children, neither work nor school activities provide sufficient opportunities for exercise. There is some evidence, however, that leisure-time exercise patterns are beginning to change in the United States.

Foundations for this change appear to have been laid in the 1950s.[2] After President Eisenhower's myocardial infarction in 1955, Dr. Paul Dudley White, a Boston cardiologist and senior medical consultant to the president, expressed his views on the benefits of exercise in cardiac rehabilitation not only to the president but also to the American public. Dr. White also advocated exercise as a first line of defense against heart attacks. He opposed cigarette smoking and cited overeating as inviting trouble, but he became best known for his trademark of the bicycle, emblematic of his prescription for adequate exercise.[3] (A bicycle path named in honor of the late Dr. White, who lived a long and active life, now winds along Boston's Charles River.) President Eisenhower followed Dr. White's advice about exercise and returned to an active life. He played golf regularly, was able to win reelection, and served a second term as president. On July 16, 1956, President Eisenhower created by Executive Order the President's

Council on Youth Fitness (now the President's Council on Physical Fitness and Sports).[4] The advent of the Kennedy administration brought an emphasis on youth and fitness; highlights of the Kennedy family's touch football games were seen around the nation on the evening news. President Kennedy, who observed, "We are under-exercised as a nation; we look instead of play; we ride instead of walk,"[5] initiated several pilot fitness programs for school children. During the 1960s, there also was a growing public interest in the environment and in outdoor recreational activities. By the late 1960s, public participation in exercise programs and activities had already begun to grow. Membership records of the YMCA show that 740,000 men aged thirty and over joined the "Y" in 1963, with figures rising to 870,000 in 1967, and to 1,744,000 by 1969.[6] Aggregate enrollments in YWCA athletic programs parallel these figures, with 605,000 women enrolled in 1963, 804,000 in 1968, and 1,070,000 in 1972.[7] Membership in the Sierra Club, which is best known for its environmental protection activities, but is, in fact, largely composed of people who like to walk or hike, has grown steadily, from 18,000 in 1962, to 45,000 in 1967, to 178,000 in 1977.[8]

Since the late 1960s, public interest in exercise has been stimulated by a number of developments.[9] Books, magazines, newspapers, radio, and television began to devote increasing attention to sports, recreation, exercise, and physical fitness. Several industries, including sports and recreation equipment and apparel manufacturers, began to sponsor events and to launch extensive advertising campaigns to promote exercise—along with their products. Voluntary and professional health associations, including the American Heart Association and the American Medical Association, began to promote exercise through public service announcements. Health and life insurance companies began to feature reminders about the importance of exercise as part of their advertising campaigns. More businesses and industries began to offer employee fitness programs, often as a result of the encouragement of sports-minded executives and of the President's Council on Physical Fitness and Sports. More recently, other government agencies have begun to promote exercise as part of initiatives to promote health and to prevent disease.

During the 1970s, various sports and fitness activities have dominated media attention—and public attention—tennis, bicycling, downhill and cross-country skiing, soccer, racquetball, platform tennis, jogging, and swimming among them. Tennis and bicycling were popular during the early 1970s. Jogging or running, which has grown steadily in popularity since the mid-1970s, seems to be the current symbol of a national exercise movement. Interest in jogging or running (no distinction will be drawn in this book between these two terms) has been spurred by a number of books. In 1967, University of Oregon track coach William J. Bowerman and Dr. W. E. Harris wrote the book *Jogging*.[10] Dr. Kenneth Cooper's popular and influential book *Aerobics*[11] appeared in 1968, and it was followed by three more Cooper bestsellers.[12] A spate of successful books by Henderson,[13] Ullyot,[14] Sheehan,[15] and others was climaxed by Fixx's *The Complete Book of Running*,[16] which topped bestseller lists for months in 1978. Fixx's book was on *The New York Times* bestseller list for almost two years—91 weeks (second only to *Games People Play*, which ran for 114 weeks in the 1960s)[17]—and sold over 750,000 hardcover copies.[18] This book helped running books pass sex manuals on the "how-to" bestseller charts in 1978.[19] *Jim Fixx's Second Book of Running*,[20] published in 1980, appears to be rivaling the success of Fixx's earlier book. Other new books on running include Ullyot's *Running Free: A Book for Women Runners and Their Friends*[21] and Wood's *Run To Health*.[22] Surveys conducted in the late 1970s of the number of Americans jogging yielded estimates ranging from 6 million[23] to 40 million.[24]

The great increase in interest in running can be demonstrated in a number of ways. In 1964 the annual San Francisco Bay–to–Breakers running race attracted 124 runners, mostly high school and college athletes;[25] in 1980, 24,000 runners of all descriptions, filling five city blocks at the start, ran the 7.6 miles between the San Francisco Bay and the Pacific Ocean.[26] Until 1966, there were never more than 12 marathon races (26-plus miles) each year in the United States.[27] There are now upward of 350 marathon races held each year, and more than 50,000 Americans have successfully completed at least one marathon. Interest in running is not limited to the United States. In Australia, Sydney's annual city-to-surf race drew more than 21,000 competitors in 1979.[28] The Stramilano 21-kilometer run (approximately 13 miles) in Milan, Italy, attracted 50,000 runners in 1978.[29] In Denmark and in the Federal Republic of Germany, running is attracting increasing numbers of enthusiasts. In the Federal Republic of Germany, there are now over 400 *volkslauf* ("people's races") per year, which attracted more than 500,000 participants in 1975.[30]

Swimming is perhaps even more popular than running. According to a 1979 Harris poll, 26 million adults swim on a regular basis, while only about 17 million run regularly.[31] Swimming, particularly for adults of all ages, received a great boost in the early 1970s when the Amateur Athletic Union adopted the suggestion of Dr. Ransom S. Arthur and began to sponsor masters swimming meets. More than 6000 swimmers are now in masters competition; the oldest known competitor is 88 years old, and many competitors are in their sixties and seventies.[32] There are now masters swim clubs in every major region in the country. Competition and fitness swimming is promoted by other organizations, such as the National Collegiate Athletic Association, the YMCA, and the Red Cross, as well as by city and county recreation departments and myriad private or community clubs. Despite its popularity, swimming is a sport not easily pursued by everyone. Statistics show that there are over 1.1 million residential swimming pools in the United States, but only 55,000 pools in private clubs and 46,000 public recreation pools.[33] Low-income residents of inner cities and rural residents often have inadequate access to swimming facilities. Swimming has not attracted the attention of mass media that running has, and until recently there have not been books for swimmers or potential swimmers comparable to those on running. A number of new books, however, have been written about fitness swimming, including *Swim for Fitness* by Brems[34] and *Total Swimming* by Wiener.[35] In addition, national journals, such as *Swim Swim*, devoted to fitness swimming, and *Swim Masters*, devoted to competitive swimming, also provide information for swimmers.

Women are joining the exercise ranks in ever-increasing numbers, spurred on by the women's movement and Title IX of the Educational Act Amendments of 1972. Girls are playing Little League Baseball and participating in high school sports in growing numbers. More than 1 million girls were playing soccer in 1980; virtually no girls were involved in this sport a decade ago. The number of high school girls participating in interscholastic sports increased sixfold between the academic years 1968–1969 (294,000) and 1976–1977 (1.6 million).[36] Females have yet to reach parity, however: in the 1978–1979 academic year there were 2 million girl athletes, compared with 4.2 million boys; males still accounted for two-thirds of all high school athletes.[37] In contrast to the growing participation of girls in high school athletics, over 30 percent nationwide, the National Organization of Women found that in Alabama girls still make up only 15 percent of high school athletes.[38] The growing interest and participation of women in sports is evident in a number of sports. For example, since 1970 the number of women tennis players reportedly has jumped from 3 million to 11 million, the number of golfers from 500,000 to more than 5 million, the number of joggers from only a few thousand to at least 6 million.[39] A study by an advertising agency in 1979 revealed that 49 percent of all tennis players, 44 percent of downhill skiers, 39 percent of backpackers, and 36 percent of squash players are women.[40]

Many surveys have been undertaken in an attempt to assess patterns of exercise in the U.S. population. Although a number of these surveys is very informative, they often do not include exercise associated with the ordinary activities of daily living. Another common problem is that when persons interviewed are asked if they participate in a certain activity, they are rarely asked how often or how long they actually engage in the activity. If a person owns a racquetball racquet and knows how to play racquetball, for example, does this person qualify as a racquetball player? And, if not, how often does the person need to play to be called a racquetball player? These inadequacies and other problems associated with surveys of exercisers result in the great variation in the estimated number of joggers in the United States. Estimates of the two most prominent American polls, which included a count of persons who jog three or more times per week, diverge widely. A 1979 Harris poll estimated that the nation had 17.7 million joggers.[41] A Gallup organization poll in 1977 estimated that 24 million Americans jog; 14 percent claim to jog three miles; 23 percent, two miles; 37 percent, one mile; and 23 percent, less than one mile.[42]

The Gallup poll also documented a great overall increase in the number of people exercising.[43] In 1977, Gallup pollsters estimated that 47 percent of adults aged 18 and older participated in some form of exercise daily—nearly twice the 24 percent reported in a poll in 1961. The most popular form of exercise appears to be walking. In the Health Interview Survey conducted by the National Center for Health Statistics in 1975, seven out of ten people who reported exercising regularly said that they walked for exercise.[44] Calisthenics ranked next in popularity, followed by swimming, bicycling, jogging, and weight lifting.

Perhaps the most comprehensive of surveys on exercise is another Harris poll, this one commissioned by the Pacific Mutual Insurance Company in 1978.[45] In this survey, the Harris organization found that 37 percent of American adults were currently involved in a regular exercise (Table 1.1). Indicative of the recent increase in exercise participants, 38 percent of these exercisers reported that they began exercising regularly within the preceding year and 22 percent in the year prior to that. Only half of those exercising had done so regularly for five years or more. The elderly, the poor, nonwhites, and women were underrepresented in the exercising population. Only 30 percent of persons aged 50 or over exercised, compared with 51 percent of those 18 to 29 years of age. Of adults in households with an income of under $7000 per year, only 24 percent exercised, while 56 percent of those with incomes over $25,000 exercised. Only 25 percent of the nonwhite population exercised; 40 percent of the white population reported exercising. Forty percent of the men interviewed were found to exercise regularly, while only 34 percent of the women did so. This difference in the number of exercisers between the sexes is not as striking as the substantial differences between the young and the aged, the well-off and the poor, and the white and nonwhite. These differences were borne out when exercise habits were examined in relation to health insurance coverage.

People covered by Medicaid or Medicare (31 percent) and those without health insurance (30 percent) were less likely to exercise than those covered by either individual (36 percent) or group (41 percent) insurance or those who belong to a health maintenance organization (44 percent).

Harris poll findings on social class, income, and exercise are consistent with the findings of a recent survey of physical activities performed at least once in a two-week period by a random sample of Massachusetts physicians and lawyers.[46] The median family income of the physicians surveyed was $55,000; of the lawyers, $42,000. Over 70 percent of both groups engaged in some physical activity at least once a week. The most popular activities were gardening (over 50 percent), jogging (over 30 percent), calisthenics (24 percent for physicians, 32 percent for lawyers), racquetball, golf, and bicycling. Demographic differences among exercisers also were revealed in a 1977 Gallup poll,[47] in the 1975 Health Interview Survey conducted by the National Center for Health Statistics,[48] and in a study of the participants in the 1977 New York Marathon.[49] Among New York Marathon runners, Milvy reported finding an inverse relationship between occupational and leisure-time activity. Commenting on white-collar middle-class workers, he observed, "We push pencils all day, and are more physically active off the job."[50] Although it may not necessarily prove true for all types of exercise, running has been found to be more common in urban than in rural areas. For example, the District of Columbia[51] and Hawaii[52] have more runners per capita than any area of the country; South Dakota, North Dakota, and Arkansas are at the bottom of the scale.[53]

Examining the Harris poll data in a different light, we find that while 37 percent of the population exercises regularly, 63 percent of the population still does not exercise regularly. Also, while only 37 percent of the population exercises, 58 percent of the population believes that they get enough exercise (Table 1.2). Of these people who believe they get enough exercise, over half are not involved in regular exercise at all.[54] Ironically, 62 percent of all respondents in this same poll indicated that they believe that lack of exercise increases their chance of heart disease or heart attack.[55] Twenty-four percent of those polled reported that they exercise to strengthen the heart and/or lungs, 41 percent to lose weight, 24 percent to become more healthy, and 45 percent to stay healthy. Only 17 percent of adults surveyed exercise because their doctor recommended it. The most important reason for exercising is the desire to feel better in general; more than half of those interviewed in the Harris poll indicated that this is why they exercise.[56]

Poor health was cited as the reason for not exercising by 11 percent of the general population, but by 24 percent of those 50 years of age and older. Lack of time (42 percent) and the discipline required (24 percent) were the primary reasons that more adults did not exercise regularly. Only 10 percent of those interviewed stated that they were not interested in exercising. In spite of this encouraging statistic, only 16 percent of those who did not exercise reported it "very likely" that they would become involved in some form of regular exercise in the future; 56 percent considered it "hardly likely at all." For those aged 50 and over, only 7 percent considered regular exercise "very likely," and 79 percent considered it "hardly likely at all."[57]

Although 80 percent of the parents of school-aged children consider it "very important" that their children participate in exercise programs in school and another 16 percent consider it "somewhat important,"[58] there is growing evidence that such programs are either not available or that children are not participating in them regularly. Only one child in three now participates in a daily program of physical education at school.[59]

One of the consequences of the sedentary lifestyle of most people in the United States is being overweight. Obesity is related to physical inactivity as well as to eating habits (see Chapter 4). Also, most physically inactive people are unfit, and many Americans, even young adults and children, appear to be unfit. In comparing young American soldiers (U.S. Air Force recruits and permanently assigned airmen) with Austrian Army recruits, Cooper found that the Americans performed well below the Austrians on a standard fitness test.[60] A government study reportedly found that between 1965 and 1975 the physical fitness of boys and girls aged 10 to 17 showed no improvement.[61] Perhaps not coincidental are the results of a recent ten-state survey, in which 39 percent of boys and 33 percent of girls aged 11 to 18 were found to be overweight.[62]

Lack of regular vigorous physical activity is a factor contributing not only to overweight and obesity and to low levels of physical fitness, but also to increased risk factors in cardiovascular disease and to greater risk of coronary heart disease. A number of trends related to patterns of exercise in the United States have significant implications for physicians and other health professionals, for policymakers and decisionmakers in the public and private sectors, and for the American people: (1) The number of adults in the United States who report that they exercise regularly has increased significantly during the past twenty years. (2) The majority of American adults, however, still do not exercise regularly, and only one in three children now participates in a daily program of school physical education. (3) The elderly, low-income populations, minorities, and women are underrepresented among the exercising population. (4) Many people who do exercise regularly probably do not achieve levels of activity that might promote physical fitness or condition the heart and lungs. Walking is the most common form of exercise. For many millions of

Americans neither their jobs nor their work in or around their homes provides sufficient opportunities for exercise. Common leisure-time activities (e.g., watching television, viewing spectator sports) also involve little or no physical activity.

In the next three chapters, we will describe different types of exercise and how they are related to physical fitness and health, and we will examine evidence of the benefits of regular vigorous exercise—in coronary heart disease, hypertension, obesity, diabetes mellitus, anxiety, depression, and asthma—to establish a rationale for clinical and community prescriptions for exercise.

Table 1.1. Are You Involved in Any Regular Exercise Activities at the Present Time?

	(Number of Respondents)	Involved in Regular Exercise (%)	Not Involved in Regular Exercise (%)	Not Sure, It Depends, etc. (%)
Total Public	(1515)	37	62	1
Age				
18-29	(477)	51	48	*
30-49	(524)	33	66	1
50 and over	(511)	30	69	1
Income				
Under $7000	(302)	24	75	1
$7000-$14,999	(501)	34	65	1
$15,000-$24,999	(475)	42	58	*
$25,000 and over	(182)	56	43	1
Race				
White	(1307)	40	60	1
Nonwhite	(201)	25	74	1
Sex				
Male	(753)	41	58	1
Female	(762)	34	66	1
Business Leaders	(175)	75	25	—
Union Leaders	(35)	51	49	—
Public Insurance Coverage				
Medicaid/Medicare		31	68	2
Individual		36	64	—
Group		41	58	1
HMO		44	56	—
No coverage		30	69	1

Source: Health Maintenance, a survey commissioned by Pacific Mutual Insurance Company and conducted by Louis Harris and Associates, Inc. (San Francisco: Pacific Mutual Insurance Company, November 1978), p. 24.
   *Less than 0.5 percent.

Table 1.2. Would You Say That You Get Enough Exercise at the Present Time?

	(Number of Respondents)	*Get Enough Exercise (%)*	*Do Not Get Enough Exercise (%)*	*Not Sure (%)*
Total Public	(1516)	58	41	1
Age				
18–29	(477)	56	43	1
30–49	(523)	50	49	1
50 and over	(513)	68	31	1
Regular Exercise				
Involved	(582)	67	32	1
Not involved	(932)	53	46	1
Business Leaders	(176)	40	60	—
Union Leaders	(35)	31	66	3

Source: Health Maintenance, a survey commissioned by Pacific Mutual Insurance Company and conducted by Louis Harris and Associates, Inc. (San Francisco: Pacific Mutual Insurance Company, November 1978), p. 26.

Chapter 2

Exercise, Physical Fitness, and Health

Exercise produces a wide range of physical, physiological, biochemical, and psychological changes. The nature and magnitude of these changes are determined by the type, intensity, duration, and frequency of the exercise performed. Different types of exercise may be performed for different reasons: (1) to improve stamina and to condition the heart and lungs; (2) to increase flexibility or to improve muscular quality or quantity; (3) to relax; or (4) to restore normal function to a part of the body damaged by disease or injury. In this chapter, we will describe six types of exercise—dynamic aerobic exercise, low-intensity exercise, isometric and isotonic exercise, relaxation exercise, and therapeutic exercise.

One of the problems causing confusion in relation to exercise and health has been the variety of terms used to describe the type of exercise most likely to enhance physical fitness and to reduce the risk of coronary heart disease. Terms such as physical conditioning, cardiovascular conditioning, vigorous exertion, aerobic performance, aerobic power, endurance exercise or endurance sports, rhythmic endurance exercise, physical training, exercise conditioning, intensive exercise, rhythmic or dynamic exercise, physical activity intervention, and brisk, sustained, and regular exercise have been used to describe this type of physical activity. The lack of any consistent definition often makes comparative analysis of different exercise studies difficult.

DYNAMIC AEROBIC EXERCISE

Our main focus in this book is dynamic aerobic exercise.[1] Aerobic exercise is exercise in which the energy needed is supplied by inspired oxygen. Dynamic aerobic exercise involves the repetitive use of large muscle masses. When large muscle groups are activated, an increased demand for oxygen is created, which is normally met by an increase in heart rate, in stroke volume, and in respiratory rate, a reduction in peripheral vascular resistance, and a widening of systemic arteriovenous oxygen differences. The extent of these changes depends primarily on the intensity and duration of the exercise performed. When a steady state is reached, there is a balance between oxygen supply and oxygen utilization by skeletal muscles. An individual's aerobic exercise capacity is limited by the failure of oxygen supply to increase in proportion to workload. As maximum capacity is approached, anaerobic glycolysis in skeletal muscle can compensate for a brief period for the deficit in oxygen and meet the body's energy requirements. This compensation results, however, in the rapid accumulation of lactic acid and in oxygen debt (the amount of oxygen needed to metabolize the lactic acid), which induces pain and causes a person to reach the point of exhaustion quickly.

Dynamic aerobic exercise, utilizing a state of oxygen balance, can be performed for long periods. When this type of exercise is performed at a level of intensity sufficient to produce a heart rate that is 70 percent of a person's maximum heart rate (calculated by subtracting the individual's age from 220) for at least 20 minutes three times per week, a "training effect" is produced. This "training effect" is manifested in improved physical fitness.

Studies of long-term physiological adaptations to systematic physical activity in normal young adults, sedentary middle-aged adults, and patients with coronary artery disease have demonstrated improved cardiovascular functioning.[2] Data are limited on hemodynamic responses after training at maximal exercise levels in normal, middle-aged men, but data are available on younger men who have undergone endurance training. In three studies, maximal oxygen consumption increased by a mean of 15.4 percent, arteriovenous oxygen differences by 7.6 percent, cardiac output by 7.9 percent, and stroke volume by 10.9 percent above control levels, while heart rate decreased by a mean of 3.1 percent below control levels.[3] In a two-year follow-up study comparing changes in cardiovascular fitness of patients randomly allocated to a high-intensity exercise program and to a low-intensity exercise program, Cunningham, Ingram, and Rechnitzer found significant improvement in cardiovascular fitness in the high-intensity exercise group.[4]

Participation in a properly designed exercise program by healthy individuals, particularly those who have been sedentary, as well as by many patients with coronary artery disease, will increase the ability to perform sustained physical activity. A well-trained, physically fit individual will be able to perform any given exercise with a slower heart rate and a greater stroke volume with each heart beat. The tissues will extract more oxygen from the blood pumped to them. Circulating blood volume, primarily plasma volume, will increase. As the workload of an exercise increases, an untrained individual will reach his or her maximum capacity and be forced by fatigue to stop at a lower workload than a trained person. When the trained individual reaches maximum capacity and workload can no longer be increased, he or she will be taking in and using much more oxygen than an untrained individual. The oxygen uptake achieved during an all-out physical effort, the best measure of a person's fitness, is called the maximum oxygen uptake ($\dot{V}O_2$ max). The greater a person's $\dot{V}O_2$ max, the easier it is for that person to cover a given distance by running, swimming, or pedaling. At a given workload, a trained individual will have a lower blood lactic acid level as well as a lower myocardial oxygen demand and a lower myocardial blood flow relative to total capacity, and thus a greater reserve, than an untrained individual.[5] A trained individual will also manifest better neuromuscular coordination, which reduces the body's energy requirement for a given activity, and altered body composition, generally involving an increase in muscle mass and a decrease in adipose tissue. Training also improves exercise tolerance in patients with coronary artery disease, including those with angina pectoris[6] and those who have recovered from a myocardial infarction.[7] As Clausen observed in an article written in 1976, "As judged from the results obtained in exercise tests, training and nitroglycerin seem almost equally potent in alleviating or preventing angina pectoris on exertion. Beta-receptor blockade may be somewhat less efficient, whereas aortocoronary bypass surgery, where practicable, may be the most efficient treatment of exertional angina available today."[8]

Important metabolic or biochemical responses also occur both during exercise and after exercise training. Muscle glycogen, blood glucose, and free fatty acids are the main sources of energy during exercise. During the first five to ten minutes of exercise, muscle glycogen is the main source of energy. As exercise continues, muscle glycogen stores become depleted and the blood-borne substrates, glucose and free fatty acids, become increasingly important. If exercise is continued beyond 40 to 60 minutes, blood glucose levels begin to fall, and the oxidation of free fatty acids gradually increases. Exercise also causes a decrease in plasma insulin, and a rise in the level of plasma glucagon, catecholamines, and cortisol. Trained individuals demonstrate a lower respiratory exchange ratio and a smaller rise in lactic acid levels with exercise than do untrained subjects. They are thus better able to maintain a normal level of blood sugar. Trained individuals also have higher rates of free fatty acid uptake, which may decrease carbohydrate utilization in muscles. Finally, during prolonged exercise, a fall in insulin binding is observed in well-trained individuals in contrast to a rise in insulin binding in untrained subjects.[9] Not only does physical training through dynamic aerobic exercise have beneficial physical effects, such as improved work capacity and stamina, but it may increase the capacity to cope with stress and tension and heighten the sense of well-being.[10]

Activities such as tennis, jogging, running in place, jumping rope, racquetball, handball, squash, bicycling, aerobic dancing, cross-country skiing, hiking, rowing, soccer, swimming, walking, and stair climbing can become dynamic aerobic exercise if performed with enough vigor over a long enough period. As Havas notes, "Exercises that improve the condition of your heart and lungs . . . have three characteristics. These activities must be: (1) brisk—raising heart and breathing rates; (2) sustained—done at least 15 to 30 minutes without interruption; and (3) regular—repeated at least three times per week."[11] It is this type of exercise—dynamic aerobic exercise—that has benefits in relation to coronary heart disease, hypertension, and diabetes mellitus. Conditions such as obesity, anxiety, and depression also are apparently improved by dynamic aerobic exericise and possibly by other types of exercise as well.

LOW-INTENSITY EXERCISE

Low-intensity exercise includes all exercise that is either not vigorous enough or not prolonged enough to produce a "training effect." Stretching exercises designed to increase flexibility, such as calisthenics, and strengthening exercises, such as weight lifting, designed to increase muscular strength, as well as low-intensity physical activities of daily living are included in this category. For instance, most of the walking that we do falls into this category. Brisk walking (at a pace of about four miles per hour) is an aerobic exercise. The walking that we usually do (at a pace of about two miles per hour) will not produce a "training effect" except in the elderly, who reach their capacity with lower levels of exertion. While low-intensity exercise may help someone become limber, strong, and better able to carry out daily tasks, this type of exercise has rather limited cardiovascular benefit and should usually be regarded as supplemental to dynamic aerobic exercise. Most stretching exercises are low-intensity and impose little stress on the cardiovascular system. These exercises are safe for patients with coronary heart disease, hypertension, or other disorders limiting cardiovascular response. Low-intensity exercise also may benefit patients with peripheral vascular disease and osteoporosis, and those who are anxious, depressed, or obese.

Isometric exercises, which are conducted by contracting muscles against a resistance without motion occurring, are not an efficient way to build muscles, but they are effective in preventing some muscle atrophy.

Isotonic exercises, the most common means of strengthening muscles, are carried out by contracting muscles against a resistance and with motion. Push-ups and pull-ups are examples of isotonic exercise, as is working out with dumbbells.

RELAXATION EXERCISE

Exercise—either dynamic aerobic exercise or low-intensity exercise—may be performed for relaxation rather than for a "training effect," stretching, or strengthening. The relaxation sought through exercise may occur during or after exercise, while walking through a park or after sprinting along a running path. Whether a specific exercise is placed in the relaxation category obviously will differ from person to person and from time to time. Relaxation exercise may be of benefit in combating anxiety and depression as well as hypertension.

THERAPEUTIC EXERCISE

Therapeutic exercises often are prescribed by physicians and performed under the direction of a physical therapist or an occupational therapist. These exercises, which may include any of the types of exercise described above, are designed to correct alterations in the body's anatomy or physiology that result in a loss of normal function. Objectives include increased power and endurance, improved coordination, extended range of motion, and increased speed. In this book, we are concerned basically with therapeutic exercises designed to improve cardiovascular fitness.

Physical fitness achieved through exercise is not synonymous with health. However, some of the changes that occur during exercise, especially during dynamic aerobic exercise, may be the mechanisms by which specific health benefits are produced. Exercise also has benefits that are not strictly health related. Many people exercise simply for the pleasure that it brings them. Others exercise because it puts them in touch with other people, or on the other hand, gives them an opportunity to be alone. As we noted earlier, the ultimate value of exercise for an individual is determined largely by the individual, rather than by the type or amount of exercise.

Chapter 3

Exercise and Coronary Heart Disease

Coronary heart disease is the number-one cause of death and a leading cause of disability in the American population. Although our understanding of this disease is still far from complete, clinical and epidemiological studies conducted during the last few decades have helped to reveal the natural history of the disease and to suggest ways to intervene in its course. Epidemiology has been used as a tool to determine the frequency and distribution of the disease in populations, to search for and to identify causal factors in the disease and to estimate the risk associated with these factors, and to assess strategies for altering the natural course of the disease.

Multiple risk factors have been implicated in the development of coronary heart disease. Among them are hypertension, blood lipid abnormalities, cigarette smoking, carbohydrate intolerance, physical inactivity, overweight and obesity, diet, heredity, personality and behavior patterns, disorders in blood coagulation, elevation in blood uric acid levels, electrocardiographic abnormalities, and pulmonary function abnormalities.[1] No cause-and-effect relationship has been established unequivocally between any of these factors and coronary heart disease. Many of the factors are interrelated, and it has been difficult, if not impossible, to assess the relative importance of any single factor in comparison to other factors, especially for a single individual. It has been even more difficult to demonstrate the impact of modification of a specific risk factor on coronary heart disease incidence or mortality. However, we have learned one valuable piece of information: the risk of a coronary event increases exponentially as the number of risk factors increases.[2] The more risk factors an individual has, the greater the chance of a coronary event. The present tack in prevention is to reduce or to eliminate risk factors that are subject to modification with the hope that these multiple interventions will lead to a reduction in individual risk of coronary heart disease as well as to a reduction in coronary heart disease incidence and mortality in the population.

Physical inactivity is a risk factor in coronary heart disease that can be modified. More importantly, regular vigorous exercise appears to offer some degree of protection against heart attack and to have a favorable impact on a number of other risk factors—hypertension, obesity, and diabetes mellitus, among them. Evidence from carefully designed epidemiological studies of the relationship between exercise habits and the rate and risk of heart attack in study populations has implications both for those with a clinical view and for those with a community view of health. Findings from these studies, together with those from clinical studies, can help the physician to assess the risks of sedentary habits versus the risks of exercise in individual patients and to decide what benefits a given program of physical activity may have for a given patient. Results from epidemiological studies can provide for the health policymaker or the program manager an estimate of the risks associated with low levels of physical activity in the general population, or in a particular segment of the population, as well as an estimate of what health benefits might accrue if these levels of physical activity were increased. For example, if studies show that regular vigorous exercise is associated with a 40-percent reduction in heart attack risk, and that only one in three individuals in the population is exercising sufficiently to qualify for this advantage, then doubling the number of people who exercise regularly and vigorously might be expected to reduce considerably the number of heart attacks in the population.

In this chapter, we will look at coronary heart disease from an epidemiological perspective, focusing on evidence of the role of occupational and leisure-time exercise in primary and secondary prevention. Preventing or deferring the onset of a condition, such as the first clinical attack of coronary heart disease (i.e., a fatal or nonfatal heart attack), is generally called primary prevention. Delaying or preventing recurrence of heart attack is called secondary prevention. In the next chapter, Chapter 4, we will examine both clinical and epidemiological evidence related to primary and secondary prevention of hypertension, obesity, diabetes mellitus, and other health problems.

THE EPIDEMIOLOGICAL PERSPECTIVE

Epidemiology is, in a literal sense, the study of what "comes upon" groups of people (from the Greek *epi*, upon; *demos*, people; *logos*, study).[3] Epidemiologists are concerned typically with patterns of health and disease in populations, particularly the distributions, determinants, and deterrents of disease. Epidemiology is used descriptively, analytically, and experimentally. In our discussion of exercise and specific health problems throughout this book, we draw on results of all three types of epidemiological studies.

Descriptive epidemiology is used to determine how much disease is occurring in a population and how the disease is distributed with respect to time, place, and personal characteristics (e.g., age, sex, race, occupation, education, and economic status). Through descriptive epidemiology, we have learned that coronary heart disease deaths in the United States and in other Western industrialized nations increased rapidly during the period from 1915 to the 1960s, especially since the 1940s. Since the late 1960s, between 1968 and 1977 to be exact, the death rate from heart disease has fallen by 22 percent in the United States.[4] Despite this sharp decline, coronary heart disease remains the leading cause of death in this country. Finland, however, has the highest death rate from coronary disease in the world. In the 1970s, rates for whites in the United States ranked fourth behind rates for Finland, Scotland, and Northern Ireland, and just ahead of rates for Australia, England and Wales, Norway, and Denmark; the rates in Italy and Switzerland were less than half the rate in the United States.[5] Coronary heart disease is distributed differently not only over time and place,but also according to age, sex, race, and other personal characteristics.[6] Coronary heart disease is the leading cause of death for men aged 45 and older and for women aged 65 and older. It is the second leading cause of death for women aged 45 to 64 (cancer is first). Even between the ages of 25 and 44, heart disease ranks as the second leading cause of death for men and the third leading cause for women/Rates for white and black males are about equal, but the rate for black females is significantly higher than for white females.[7] It has been estimated that over 1 million people experience a heart attack each year. In one of five of these heart attacks, sudden death is the first—and only—coronary event.[8] One-third to one-half of all first heart attacks are fatal with or without delay, even though special emergency services appear to be saving some lives. Coronary heart disease not only kills; it also disables. It is the foremost cause of permanent disability claims among workers under 65, and it is responsible for more days of hospitalization than any other single disorder.[9] Heart disease is also the single most important cause of activity limitation among noninstitutionalized individuals. Over 4.7 million of these individuals report activity limitation due to heart disease, while 4.4 million are disabled by arthritis and rheumatism and almost 2 million by hypertension without heart involvement.[10] This attempt to answer three basic epidemiological questions about a disease—who, where, and when—frequently provides the basis, along with clinical and laboratory observations, for hypotheses regarding causal factors in the disease and specific mechanisms of action in the development of the disease.

Analytical or determinative epidemiology is used to test these hypotheses, to search for and to identify causal factors in disease (e.g., cigarette smoking in lung cancer, physical inactivity in coronary heart disease), and to estimate the risk associated with these factors. To assemble evidence to test a hypothesis, epidemiologists must often look for natural circumstances that mimic an experiment. As MacMahon and Pugh pont out, ". . . a human experiment to test the hypothesis that cigarette smoking causes lung cancer is impracticable, but advantage can be taken of the fact that, without any encouragement from epidemiologists, people have separated themselves into groups of smokers and nonsmokers. This at least allows determination of whether the two categories of things (smoking and lung cancer) are statistically associated and investigation of the characteristics of the association."[11] This circumstance is also true with respect to exercisers and nonexercisers—or vigorous and less vigorous exercisers—and coronary heart disease.

Epidemiologists test a hypothesis in two basic ways: directly through cohort (prospective) studies, and indirectly through case-control (retrospective) studies. In a cohort study, an investigator selects a group or groups of individuals (a cohort or cohorts) that can be defined in terms of certain characteristics and observes this population over a period of time to determine the frequency of a disease, usually the number of new cases of the disease (incidence) or the number of deaths from the disease (mortality) in the various cohorts in relation to these character-istics. In a case-control study, the investigator selects a study population consisting of a group of individuals with a disease (the cases) and a group of individuals without the disease (the controls) and then attempts to identify and compare the frequency of certain characteristics in the two groups.

Cohort studies may be either historical or contemporary. A historical cohort study is designed to analyze past data or past events—both the "cause" and the "effect" under investigation have already occurred, and the investigator looks back over time to analyze the "cause" in terms of the "effect." A contemporary cohort study is designed to analyze current and future data—information on the "cause" is recorded in advance of information on the "effect." The Framingham Heart Disease and Epidemiology Study is an example of a contemporary cohort study.[12] In 1949 a random sample of approximately 5000 people between 30 and 62 years of age was selected from the population of Framingham, Massachusetts, to be followed for twenty years to determine the relation of personal characteristics and living habits to the development of cardiovascular disease, including coronary heart disease. This population was selected for good reasons. The population allowed investigators to observe individuals before they entered and as they entered the years of highest cardiovascular disease incidence; the population was large enough and stable enough to provide reliable data on the frequency of cardiovascular disease over the twenty-year period; and the population included people of different socioeconomic, occupational, racial, and ethnic backgrounds. Individuals were categorized according to their personal characteristics (i.e., body weight, serum cholesterol levels, blood pressure levels, smoking and dietary habits) and other information obtained at entry to the study. Physical examinations and laboratory tests, which were conducted every two years, provided additional information on these characteristics as well as follow-up data on the incidence of cardiovascular disease. The Framingham Study has provided invaluable information about the natural history of cardiovascular diseases, including coronary heart disease, and about major risk factors—cigarette smoking, hypertension, and hypercholesterolemia—and estimates of risk associated with these factors. Physical inactivity also was identified as a risk factor, although the study gathered only limited data on exercise habits.[13]

Both historical and contemporary cohort studies, described in detail later in this chapter, have helped clarify the relationship between exercise habits and coronary heart disease. One major study, the study of work exercise in San Francisco longshoremen, is an example of a contemporary cohort study. The other major study, a study of leisure-time exercise in Harvard University alumni, is an example of both a historical and a contemporary cohort study, incorporating data from college life as well as adult life. A study of this type offers unusual opportunities for follow-up and analysis because it can "telescope" both time and experience.

In both cohort studies and case-control studies, investigators are faced with the problem of assessing risk. There are two common measures of risk—relative risk and attributable risk. Relative risk is the ratio of the rate of the disease, usually the incidence of the disease or mortality from the disease, among those who have a certain characteristic (or who have been exposed to a certain factor) and among those who do not have this characteristic (or who have not been exposed to this factor).[14] Attributable risk is the rate of disese in those who have a certain characteristic (or who have been exposed to a certain factor) that can be attributed to this factor.[15] Population-attributable risk may be used to provide an estimate of the amount by which a particular disease rate might be reduced in a population if a particular characteristic or exposure were removed.[16] In cohort studies, measures of risk can be computed directly from disease rates; in case-control studies, estimates of risk are usually calculated indirectly.

Analytical studies in epidemiology—cohort and case-control studies—are designed to detect a statistical association between two categories of things, usually a disease and some characteristic shared (or not shared) by groups of individuals, and to determine whether this association is causal. When a causal association cannot be determined by a direct experiment, and when a number of characteristics or confounding variables are to be considered, evaluating the causal nature of an association is not easy. Indeed, it may be impossible for a single investigator, or even a number of investigators, to establish a causal association unequivocally. Also, such associations established for groups of individuals do not necessarily hold true for the single individual. Despite these caveats, as MacMahon and Pugh note, ". . . there comes a point in the accumulation of evidence when it is more prudent to act on the basis that the association is causal rather than await further evidence."[17] While some epidemiological investigations may not resemble the neat structure of controlled clinical trials, they can approach the practical realities of a life situation that extends far beyond the limitations of an artificial research design. With the help of computerized records and data procesing, epidemiologists have begun to study complex data that, without such methods, would be too cumbersome to investigate. Access to larger populations, more sophisticated statistical methods, and better communication are making important information available. All these developments are influencing, too, the contributions of experimental epidemiology.

Experimental epidemiology is used to assess strategies for altering the natural history of disease. Three strategies are commonly applied: intervention trials to reduce risk factors (e.g., the Multiple Risk Factor Intervention Trial[18] and the Stanford Three Community Study[19]), clinical trials of treatment modalities (e.g., the prevention trial of the Lipid Research Clinic Program[20] of the National Heart, Lung, and Blood Institute), and screening for risk factors and early detection of disease (e.g., the National High Blood Pressure Education Progam). These experiments to assess ways to reduce risk factors and to prevent or delay the onset of cardiovascular disease in study populations drawn from the community are providing practical information that can aid both clinicians and policymakers. As experience is gained in this and other types of epidemiological research, more confidence may be justified in the validity, usefulness, and importance of epidemiological findings.

Coronary heart disease death rates, as previously noted, are declining in the United States. The reasons for this decline have been the focus of much speculation. It seems likely that a combination of factors, including a reduction in cigarette smoking among men, changes in diet, improvements in medical care—particularly in the detection and treatment of hypertension—and increased exercise have all played a role. Our interest is in the potential of exercise to contribute further to the decline in deaths from coronary heart disease.

THE EPIDEMIOLOGICAL EVIDENCE: EXERCISE IN PRIMARY PREVENTION OF CORONARY HEART DISEASE

Controversy continues to surround interpretation of epidemiological studies of the relationship between physical activity and coronary heart disease. In a recent literature survey, Froelicher listed 13 prospective studies that have examined the relationship between physical activity and the incidence of coronary heart disease.[21] Eight of these studies showed varying reduced rates of coronary heart disease with increased physical activity, four showed little difference in rates, and one study showed increased rates among blue-collar (high-activity) workers in comparison to white-collar (low-activity) workers. There have been a number of other recent reviews of the extensive epidemiological literature on exercise and coronary heart disease and on the effect on coronary risk factors.[22] All reviewers face similar problems in interpreting results of these studies. The studies differ in design; in the age range and other characteristics of populations selected for study; in the type, amount, and range of physical activity assessed; in the methods of measurement of physical activity; and in the disease rates evaluated (incidence of coronary heart disease, deaths from coronary heart disease, first heart attack rate, fatal heart attack rate). Rather than review these studies again in detail, we will consider selected studies of occupational exercise and leisure-time exercise that characterize the variety and scope—as well as some of the inherent problems—of investigations that have been made. Evidence from these studies should help guide the thinking of practitioners and health policymakers concerned with the problem of coronary heart disease and its primary and secondary prevention.

Occupational Exercise

J. N. Morris's studies in England of both vocational and leisure-time physical activity in relation to cardiovascular fitness and heart attack risk are regarded as pioneering. More than twenty-five years ago, Morris found that highly active conductors on London buses were at less risk of heart attack than were bus drivers who merely worked sitting at the wheel.[23] He reached similar findings when he reviewed the leisure-time exercise patterns of thousands of civil servants and assessed their heart attack risk during a follow-up period.[24] Morris's studies were not designed to discount confounding variables such as self-selection or different degrees of psychic stress, but they did attract wide attention to the probable importance of exercise and the need for further investigation. In general, his conclusions were that a moderate amount of physical activity, whether on or off the job, could reduce risk of heart attack significantly, especially if some strenuous exercise were included. He did take note of variables such as cigarette smoking and body types, but his data focused mainly on contemporary exercise habits and did not consider hereditary or other familial aspects of heart attack risk.

Other investigations of heart disease rates and occupational physical activity in Washington, D.C., letter carriers and postal clerks,[25] North Dakota farmers and nonfarmers,[26] Israeli kibbutzim workers in various jobs,[27] railroad workmen and clerks,[28] and San Francisco longshoremen[29] show lower heart disease risk with higher exercise levels. These studies, however, did not address all questions of diet, heredity, stress, smoking, and other confounding factors.

Some investigators have failed to find differences in heart disease risks between groups of civil service workers[30] and industrial workers,[31] perhaps because differences in physical activity in their jobs were insufficient or because other influences such as leisure-time exercise were not taken into account.[32] A 10-year follow-up of 12,763 men initially aged 40-59 comprising 16 culturally varied cohorts in seven countries produced confused results, apparently because of difficulties in defining or assessing physical activity levels in diverse international settings that complicated comparisons within or among groups.[33] The investigators decided that on a global scale the relationships of coronary heart disease and its risk factors were more complex than had been supposed. A further comment might be that lifestyles must be more carefully characterized and more closely studied if valid conclusions are to be drawn concerning them.

The study of work activity and fatal heart attack in San Francisco longshoremen[34] is interesting for several reasons. The study population of nearly 4000 cargo handlers and dockworkers included workers from 35 to 74 years of age, whose tasks ranged from supervisory and light machine work to lifting, toting, shoving, and stacking. These workers were given a multiphasic screening examination when they entered the study in 1951 to assess five personal characteristics: cigarette smoking, systolic blood pressure, diagnosed heart disease, weight for height, and glucose metabolism. (Serum cholesterol levels were measured in 1961.) Job classifications of the longshoremen were obtained from records maintained by the International Longshoremen's and Warehousemen's Union, and energy expenditures required for work tasks were calculated by measuring oxygen consumption of longshoremen as they performed actual work tasks. Low-energy workers were designated as those who expended fewer than 8500 kilocalories (Kcal) per week on the job, and high-energy workers as those who expended 8500 or more Kcal per week. (Leisure-time exercise was considered minimal for these men.) Job assignments were checked annually for job transfers that would have affected the level of energy expended at work. The longshoremen were then followed over a 22-year period to determine the rate and risk of fatal heart attack in low-energy and high-energy workers. Fatal heart attacks were classified as sudden or delayed deaths. Fatal heart attack rates and relative risks were computed in terms of man-years of work. Relative risks represent rates for low-energy longshoremen divided by rates for high-energy longshoremen.

Results of this long-term contemporary cohort study of work activity and fatal heart attack in San Francisco longshoremen can be summarized as follows: (1) High-energy and low-energy workers differed little in personal characteristics assessed at multiphasic screening at the outset of the study in 1951. High-energy and low-energy workers were alike in sharing recognized coronary risk factors. (2) About 10 percent of the longshoremen died of heart attack during the 22-year period. (3) Men who had expended 8500 or more Kcal per week had significantly less risk of fatal heart attack, particularly sudden death from heart attack, than did men whose jobs required less energy output. (4) Risk of fatal heart attack was reduced for high-energy workers even when account was taken of job transfers and of personal characteristics known to increase risk of fatal heart attack. With higher energy output, heart attack risk was lower both in the presence and in the absence of heavy cigarette smoking, hypertension, prior coronary heart disease, obesity, abnormal glucose metabolism, and high serum cholesterol levels. (5) If all longshoremen had worked at a level of 8500 or more Kcal per week, the death rate from heart attack might have been reduced by about 49 percent. (6) If all longshoremen had worked at high-energy levels, smoked less than a pack of cigarettes per day or not smoked at all, and had had systolic blood pressures lower than average for longshoremen of their age, the total reduction in heart attack death rate would have been approximately 88 percent.

We regard the findings of the San Francisco longshoremen study as some of the strongest evidence of a protective effect of exercise against heart attack. Even these findings must be interpreted with caution, however. We take the opportunity here to explore questions that might arise in interpreting the data, and we include graphic and tabular material at the end of this chapter for those interested in a more detailed presentation of the data (see Figures 3.1 to 3.5 and Table 3.1).

In deriving implications from a study such as this epidemiological survey of longshoremen, it is important to keep in mind that the analyses are relative. That is, comparisons are being made within a particular population in which energy expenditure in both high and low categories is considerable by almost any standard. Office workers, for example, would hardly be expected to approach the work output of any of the longshoremen doing jobs on the wharves, to say nothing of the output of highly active cargo handlers in the shipholds. When the longshoring work activity and fatal heart attack data were first published, medical reviewers demanded to know whether such high-energy output levels were to be considered necessary for everyone who wished to achieve cardiovascular fitness and to lessen risk of heart attack. Studies of more sedentary populations, which will be discussed later in this chapter, appear to indicate that the answer to the question is "no." However, these analyses are again relative. Much work remains to be done to determine optimum exercise patterns for different types of people.

Another question that arises is whether the longshoremen resemble either the marathoners or the sprinters of the exercise world. Analysis of the job activities of cargo handlers, the most active workers, suggests that many of these men worked in sustained, repeated bursts of extreme energy output, with rest periods or moments of less exertion between these peaks of effort. However, systems of work/rest relationships for holdgangs of eight men varied. For example, all men worked for 45 minutes and then rested for 15 minutes of each hour, or six men worked for an hour while two rested for half an hour. These work patterns approximate the intensive exercise now often recommended to achieve cardiovascular conditioning and, perhaps, protection from coronary heart disease. Some hypotheses hold that the work patterns also imply that high-energy workers may have crossed a threshold to a plateau of protection from coronary heart disease, whereas their low-energy counterparts did not. In the critical-threshold concept, the near approach to peak effort is more meaningful than total output at some lesser intensity of effort. For example, 20 to 30 minutes of physically stressful work or exercise is thought to produce a beneficial training effect on the cardiovascular system. Although more study is needed, it appears to be a safe assumption that both duration and vigor of exercise—total output and peak output—are important. This point should be considered in evaluating the health benefits of both occupational and leisure-time exercise activities.

The longshoremen data also support the view that continuing or contemporary exercise is important. High-energy work output was associated with reduced risk of heart attack at all ages, and many of the longshoremen continued working at high-energy levels for years. The longshoremen tended to be a stable work force who entered the industry in youth and remained active in it for many years. By union rules, the longshoremen routinely began their career in heavy work and continued in this work for a minimum of five years. (Workers actually remained in this heavy work category for an average of 13 years before transferring to less strenuous assignments.) The advantage of exercise fades if exercise is not maintained. Therefore, "lifetime" exercise habits, programs, and facilities are important, and this point should be a key concept in exercise-related policies and in advice provided to patients by their physicians.

The chief question that remains to be answered about the longshoremen study is the question of "protection versus selection." Did the high-energy-output longshoremen have lower rates of fatal heart attack because they were endowed with stronger cardiovascular systems from birth and gravitated toward more active work throughout life? Did the low-energy workers have inherently weaker cardiovascular systems and therefore move into less active work? Should the relationship of physical activity to risk of fatal heart attack be regarded as an increased risk through inactivity or a reduced risk through high-energy expenditure (i.e., a protective effect)? Although the selection of a longshoring career may imply the inheritance of a strong constitution, including a strong cardiovascular system, the union rules, as we pointed out earlier, required that all longshoremen work in physically demanding jobs as cargo handlers for at least their first five years of service, and some workers continued this heavy work for many more years. These work regulations and records argue against hereditary cardiovascular differences as an explanation for differences in heart attack rates observed when longshoremen were grouped into high-energy and low-energy output levels during the follow-up period. Also, if any favorable—or unfavorable—influences of physical activity on the cardiovascular system were to be identified, the levels of exertion displayed by the longshoremen should guarantee that the effects would show up in this study population. However, the rates and relative risks of fatal heart attack in the longshoremen study were similar whether or not account was taken of changes in work assignment during the 22-year follow-up, an indication that few job shifts to lighter work were made for health reasons. The low rate of sudden deaths among high-energy workers suggests that exercise may indeed have a further protective effect—highly active men may be better able to withstand initial heart attacks and may be less likely to die suddenly. This advantage appeared to be particularly important in younger age groups. This finding has implications for policies and programs aimed at reducing fatal heart attacks among young and middle-aged workers.

In sum, evidence from the San Francisco longshoremen study shows that work energy expenditure is strongly associated with risk of fatal heart attack. Although we are unable to determine to what extent high-energy output decreases risk, and low-energy output increases risk, we believe that the process is probably a two-way street. Exercise may strengthen or condition the cardiovascular system; physical inactivity may weaken it. The optimum standards for frequency, duration, type, intensity, amount, and timing of exercise are yet to be established, but the importance of exercise is no longer in question.

Leisure-Time Exercise

Some epidemiological studies have dealt with leisure-time activities or a blend of both occupational and leisure-time activities, and some have attempted to explore exercise patterns in more general populations. Morris's survey of 16,882 British male office workers has been mentioned earlier. In a two- to four-year follow-up, coronary heart disease developed in 26 percent of men who had reported no vigorous leisure-time exercise, but in only 11 percent of men who did have a habit of vigorous exertion. Four years later this advantage was still evident.[35] A community study of social classes in Evans County, Georgia, related heart disease levels to differences in physical activity occupationally or otherwise associated with social status.[36] Another community analysis is represented by the Framingham Study, which, as we have noted, had rather limited data on exercise but recognized it as as a health factor.[37]

Studies based on health insurance plans such as the Health Insurance Plan of New York,[38] which tend to represent data on general populations rather than on special populations, also afford a community view. The failure of some studies of sedentary work groups, such as civil service workers in Los Angeles,[39] to show benefits from exercise may be because leisure-time activities were not considered. Leisure-time exercise habits are relatively important in the energy output pattern of people who do not have jobs that require much physical exertion. In many communities in the United States, programs addressed to community health needs should include attention to leisure-time exercise patterns and facilities. In England a national sports council formed in 1972 has recently launched a "Sports for All, Come Alive!" program to promote leisure-time exercise throughout the country.

One extensive and long-range study of leisure-time exercise patterns and health in the United States is the college alumni study. In this investigation of precursors of chronic disease in nearly 50,000 college alumni (36,500 Harvard University alumni and 13,500 University of Pennsylvania alumni), certain personal characteristics, including exercise habits, were found to correlate with risk of some health problems, heart attack in particular.[40] A study of physical activity as an index of heart attack risk in the Harvard alumni[41] has helped clarify the role of both student and adult exercise patterns, or past and contemporary exercise habits, in coronary heart disease. In this cohort study, which covers the 1962–1972 period, experiences and characteristics of alumni who had entered college as students from 1916 to 1950 were analyzed in relation to their death from heart attacks. Investigators gleaned information from college archives, alumni records and questionnaires, and official death certificates. From student health and athletic records they obtained information about a number of student characteristics: cigarette smoking, systolic and diastolic blood pressure, height and weight (body mass index), body stature, parental death and disease, college varsity athletics, and nonvarsity sports play. In 1962 or 1966, nearly 17,000 alumni replied to a questionnaire concerning their personal characteristics, their exercise habits, and physician-diagnosed disease, including coronary heart disease. To assess their adult exercise habits, alumni were asked how many flights of stairs (using 10 steps as a flight) they climbed each day, how many city blocks or equivalent (using 12 blocks as one mile) they walked each day, and what sports they played in hours per week. Sports or leisure-time activities were classified as "light"— generally considered to require comparatively little energy output, or about 5 Kcal per minute (e.g., bowling, baseball, boating, golf, and yardwork)—and as "vigorous"—requiring more energy, or about 10 Kcal per minute (e.g., running, mountaineering, cross-country skiing, swimming, basketball, and tennis). A physical activity index was devised to provide an estimate of total energy expenditure expressed in kilocalories per week, from stairs climbed, blocks walked, leisure work, and sports played. The physical activity index was divided at 2000 Kcal/week; alumni whose total energy expenditure was on the low side of this index (fewer than 2000 Kcal per week) were classified in the low-energy category, and alumni who expended 2000 or more Kcal per week were placed in the high-energy category. In 1972, a second questionnaire was mailed to each alumnus of classes that entered Harvard from 1916 to 1950 to query men about physician-diagnosed diseases, including coronary heart disease. Weekly updating of death lists by the alumni office provided a way to obtain official death certificates to identify fatal heart attacks. Heart attack deaths were classified as sudden or delayed. Differences in heart attack rates, which were calculated in terms of man-years of observation, were expressed as relative risks, with the rate for men with high levels of activity as base.

Results of the Harvard alumni study of physical activity and heart attack provide a 6- to 10-year follow-up of risk of first heart attack, fatal and nonfatal. A summary of these results follows:

1. Nearly 17,000 Harvard alumni aged 35 to 74 returned questionnaires and reported themselves free of coronary heart disease in 1962 or 1966.
2. By 1972, 572 men had experienced first heart attacks, 357 nonfatal and 215 fatal. Fifty-two of the attacks occurred at ages 35 to 44, 137 at ages 45 to 54, 213 at ages 55 to 64, and 170 at ages 65 to 74.
3. Alumni who reported expending more than 2000 Kcal per week had a 50 percent lower risk of heart attack than did their less energetic classmates.
4. Reduced risk of heart attack with increased physical activity was observed in each age group studied, and patterns were similar in relation to fatal and nonfatal heart attacks.
5. Fifty-six percent of former varsity athletes reported maintaining their active status in vigorous sports or high-energy exercise, and 38 percent of nonvarsity alumni reported activity sufficient to place themselves in the high-energy category (2000 or more Kcal per week).
6. Both groups experienced substantially lower heart attack rates than their currently less active counterparts. Therefore, only a physically active adulthood was associated with lower heart attack rates, regardless of student athletic status.
7. Alumni with any of eight characteristics assessed in 1962 or 1966—cigarette smoking, hypertension, a history of stroke, a history of diabetes, overweight, shorter stature, parental history of heart attack, or parental history of hypertension—were more susceptible to heart attack than men without such characteristics.
8. Even with an adverse characteristic, men with high-energy levels (2000 or more Kcal per week) had an appreciably lower heart attack risk than similarly burdened classmates of the same age who were less energetic. In general, for men with any of these characteristics, rate of heart attack in the less active was half again as high as in the more active.
9. Reduced risk of heart attack was observed with increasing energy output in each category of physical activity, especially in vigorous sports activity, but also in such activities as

climbing stairs and walking blocks. However, at any given level of energy output, risk of heart attack was markedly lower for vigorous sports than for other activities.

10. It was estimated that if all alumni had expended 2000 or more Kcal per week, the number of heart attacks would have been reduced by about 26 percent. If none had smoked cigarettes, heart attacks would have been reduced by about one-quarter. If none had been hypertensive, rates would have been reduced by about 16 percent.

11. If all men had been physically active, nonsmoking normotensives, there would have been only about half the number of heart attacks observed in this population.

Several questions arise in interpreting results of the Harvard alumni study, especially in light of findings from the San Francisco longshoreman study. Again, for those interested in a more detailed presentation of the data, we have included figures and tables on the Harvard alumni at the end of this chapter (see Figures 3.6 to 3.8 and Tables 3.2 and 3.3.) Some parallels and differences between the Harvard alumni and the San Francisco longshoremen studies should be pointed out. First, it is obvious from the physical activity index used in the Harvard study that the reported weekly energy output of the Harvard alumni was considerably lower than the occupational energy expenditure calculated for the longshoremen. In the alumni study, however, no allowances were made for energy expended at times other than when study subjects were walking, climbing stairs, or playing sports. To make the Harvard alumni comparable to the San Francisco longshoremen, an additional 4500 to 5000 Kcal per week should be added to their leisure-time energy expenditure to account for their energy expenditure during a work week. (This figure is based on an estimated metabolic rate of 2 Kcal per minute and a forty-hour work week, an approximate range of 4500 to 5000 Kcal per week.)

As we pointed out earlier, the analyses of each of these study populations are relative: they apply to the groups in the populations under study. Direct comparisons between the Harvard alumni and the San Francisco longshoremen, two extremely different groups, should be made only with caution. One important point, however, should be noted. Although the range of energy output for the college men was a whole stage lower than for the longshoremen, findings ran parallel for heart attack risk—the greater the level of energy expended, the lower the risk of heart attack. Moreover, strenuousness of exercise (i.e., vigorous sports activity) in the Harvard alumni reduced heart attack risk below that associated with simple energy output in kilocalories per week. These results parallel findings for the longshoremen and strengthen the case for a protective effect of exercise against heart attack. Possible selective or hereditary influences in the Harvard alumni are discounted by the finding that varsity athletes had no special advantage over their nonvarsity classmates—unless they continued to be vigorously active in their alumni years. On the other hand, students who had not been varsity athletes or physically active in college but who had adopted vigorous exercise habits in adulthood stood to achieve a lower heart attack risk. The level of physical activity characterizing the lifestyle of Harvard alumni varies over a modest range of energy expenditure at work and at leisure. Since these alumni are engaged in sedentary occupations or are retired, their choice of spare-time activities and activities of everyday living (e.g., stair climbing versus elevator riding) has considerable bearing on their total energy output per week as well as on the vigor of their effort. One difference between the longshoremen and college alumni appeared in their relative risks of sudden death from heart attack. Vigorous activity spared the longshoremen but had no such advantage for the Harvard alumni. This departure may be due to differences in the range of energy output or to differences in data gathering.

EXERCISE IN SECONDARY PREVENTION OF CORONARY HEART DISEASE

Epidemiological evidence on the exercise status and life span of men who have survived a first heart attack is somewhat limited. The longshoremen study suggests that men who returned after heart attack to jobs that required vigorous exercise had a 50 percent lower risk of fatal heart attack than did those placed in less energetic work.[42] Studies in civil service workers indicate that differences greater than twofold may exist between the high risk of death from recurring heart attack in sedentary subjects and the lower risk for those with more energetic lifestyles.[43]

Although many clinical studies have addressed the question of whether regular physical activity is an effective preventive measure against recurrent heart attack, only a few controlled trials have been reported to date. Wilhelmsen and associates randomized 315 patients with myocardial infarction into exercise training and control groups. Over a four-year period, they found 20 percent fewer deaths in the training group than in the controls.[44] Rechnitzer and associates studied a larger group of patients in Canada, using a similar technique of random assignment of patients to an exercise group or a control group.

In a seven-year follow-up, these investigators observed a comparable difference favoring the exercise group.[45] Both studies, however, were limited, were marred by high dropout rates, and lacked adjustment for confounding variables. The most obvious finding from such studies has been that more research is needed.

The ongoing studies of chronic disease among Harvard alumni have included an opportunity to assess on a rather different scale the relationships of exercise and other personal variables to risk of fatal heart attack in survivors of a first attack.[46] (See Tables 3.4 and 3.5 and Figure 3.9.) This study represents an assessment of the natural experience of a free population rather than a set of clinically controlled episodes. Moreover, the pattern of secondary prevention of heart attack in these alumni could be viewed against extensive baseline studies of first heart attack and other chronic diseases in the much larger total population of alumni. The earlier work had developed for the project a long-range acquaintance with the characteristics and activities of all these study subjects.

Among 782 Harvard alumni aged 35 to 74 with history of heart attack (myocardial infarction or angina pectoris) reported by questionnaire in 1962 or 1966, there were 197 heart attack deaths (25 percent) and 82 deaths from other causes (10 percent) in a 12- to 16-year follow-up interval. Relative risks of death from heart attack were related to measures of physical activity, including stair climbing, walking, sports play, and the composite index of these activities expressed in kilocalories of energy expenditure. Men who expended fewer than 2000 Kcal per week were at 42 percent greater risk of fatal heart attack than men who were more active. Relative risks of death from all other causes, however, were unrelated to these same physical activity measures. When the 782 patients were classified as those who had a myocardial infarction with or without angina pectoris (607 patients), or those with angina alone (175 patients), relative risks of death from subsequent heart attack were generally higher for less active men, but there were variations according to the type of activity and the disease category. Parallel differences were found in relative risks for delayed death and sudden death. In general, it would seem that men who suffer an initial heart attack will have a lower risk of death from a recurrent attack, over a period of several years, if they do maintain habits of adequate exercise than if they do not.

Further analysis of exercise and mortality data on the Harvard alumni who had survived a first heart attack indicated a reduced risk of fatal subsequent heart attack in these men as their energy expenditure increased. When a reference level of 100 Kcal per week was used, the data indicated a 25-percent reduction in risk at a 3000-Kcal-per-week expenditure and a 35-percent reduction at a 5000-Kcal-per-week expenditure. Risk reduction from habitual and leisure-time exercise persisted when cigarette smoking, hypertension, obesity, parental heart attack, and student athleticism were taken into account. The salutary influence of exercise was consistent for both angina pectoris patients and myocardial infarction patients at all ages, and in successive periods of follow-up. Men who included vigorous sports play in their weekly activity program experienced a further benefit over those who did not.

Relative and attributable risks of fatal heart attack among Harvard alumni who had a prior heart attack also have been estimated. Potential reductions in fatal heart attack risk were calculated as if specific charactersitics had been eliminated. Among these 782 heart attack patients, the risk of death from subsequent heart attack seemed little influenced during the 12- to 16-year follow-up by the smoking habit,hypertension, or diabetes. A prior stroke, however, led to an eightfold increase in risk of fatal heart attack in patients and may have accounted for 88 percent of heart attack deaths in patients so afflicted. The risk among heart attack patients who expended fewer than 2000 Kcal per week in walking, stair climbing, and sports play was 47 percent higher than the risk in more active patients, and physical inactivity may have accounted for 32 percent of the fatal heart attacks in those less active patients. Although the relationship between physical inactivity and heart attack death is not significant in this small sample of 782 men, if replicated in larger populations of men with coronary heart disease, physical inactivity would represent a formidable risk factor because of its high prevalence.

The findings of this and other studies[47] strongly suggest that men who have suffered an initial heart attack will have lower risk of death from a subsequent heart attack if they maintain habits of adequate exercise than if they do not.

EXERCISE AND CORONARY HEART DISEASE: MECHANISMS OF PROTECTION

The precise mechanisms by which physical activity might reduce the incidence of heart attack are unknown. Various hypotheses have been advanced:

1. An increase in physical activity leads to lower concentrations of triglycerides, very-low-density lipoprotein cholesterol, and low-density lipoprotein cholesterol, while perhaps most importantly increasing concentrations of high-density lipoprotein choles-

terol. Such alterations in blood lipid profiles are strongly related to a lower risk of coronary heart disease.[48]

2. Physical conditioning augments a rise in fibrinolysis induced by venous occlusion[49] and alters platelet stickiness and thrombus formation. Exercise may be implicated favorably in counteracting the pathophysiology of atheriosclerotic processes.

3. Exercise adequate to achieve physical fitness has many salutary effects: it increases maximal oxygen uptake, slows the heart rate, lowers blood pressure, decreases ventricular ectopic activity, increases cardiac output, and increases physical work capacity.[50]

4. Exercise increases insulin sensitivity and may be effective against insulin-resistant states, such as obesity and adult-onset diabetes,[51] both of which are implicated as risk factors in coronary heart disease.

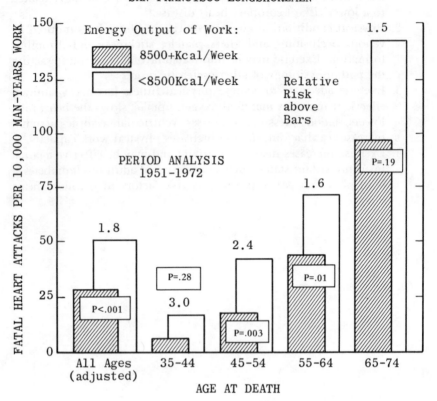

SAN FRANCISCO LONGSHOREMEN

Energy Output of Work:

8500+Kcal/Week

<8500Kcal/Week

Relative Risk above Bars

PERIOD ANALYSIS 1951-1972

FATAL HEART ATTACKS PER 10,000 MAN-YEARS WORK

AGE AT DEATH

Figure 3.1. Period analysis of fatal heart attacks among nearly 4000 San Francisco longshoremen, 1951–1972, per 10,000 man-years of work, by work energy output and age at death.

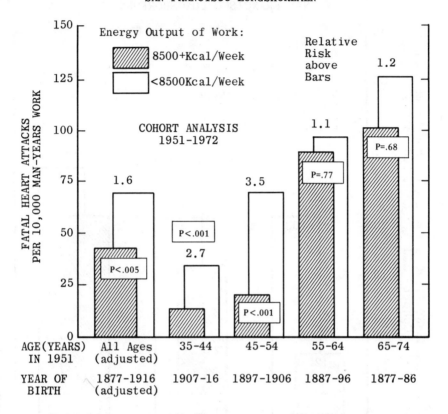

Figure 3.2. Birth-cohort analysis of fatal heart attacks among San Francisco longshoremen, 1951–1972, per 10,000 man-years, by work energy output.

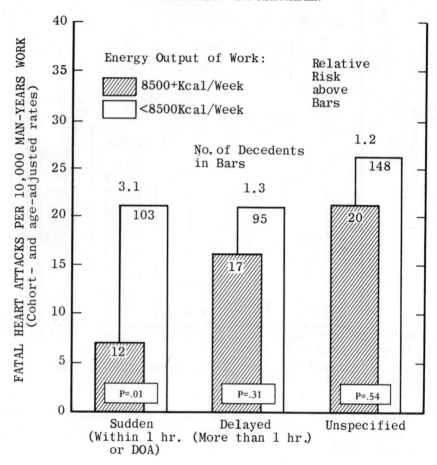

Figure 3.3. Fatal heart attacks among San Francisco longshoremen, 1951–1972, per 10,000 man-years of work, by work energy output and interval from symptom onset to death.

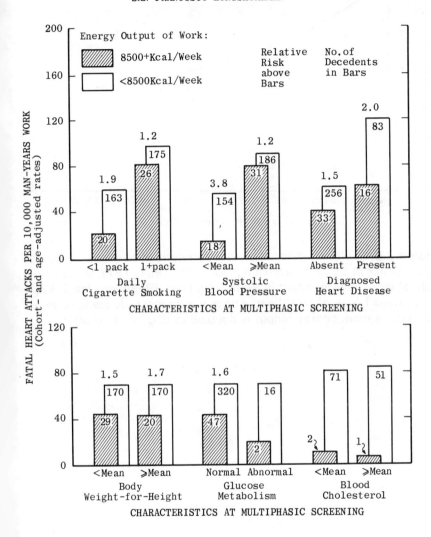

Figure 3.4. Fatal heart attacks among San Francisco longshoremen, 1951–1972, by work energy output and characteristics at multiphasic screening in 1951 (serum cholesterol, 1961).

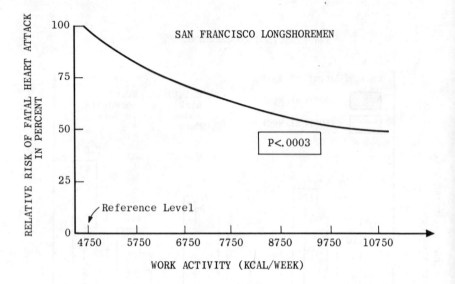

Figure 3.5. Multiple logistic regression analysis of relative risk of fatal heart attack in San Francisco longshoremen, 1951–1972, to delineate role of work energy output in establishing risk. (Reference level, 4750 Kcal/week.) Risk of fatal heart attack is progressively lowered to 50 percent as work energy output is doubled to 9500 Kcal/week.

Table 3.1. Potential Reduction of Fatal Heart Attack (FHA) Rates among San Francisco Longshoremen with Elimination of Specified Characteristics—A Community View of Risk Reduction

Characteristics Eliminated	Prevalence of Characteristic (%)	Man-years Worked with Characteristic	FHA per 10,000 Man-years*	Potential Reduction in FHA Rates (% ± one SE)
1. Low energy output†	68.9	39,247	69.7	48.8± 9.1
2. Heavy cigarette smoking††	37.7	21,457	94.3	27.9± 3.9
3. Higher systolic blood pressure§	40.2	22,916	89.1	28.8± 4.1
1, 2, or both	80.1	45,616	95.7	64.7±10.1
1, 3, or both	81.8	46,598	91.5	73.5± 8.3
2, 3, or both	63.6	36,216	161.6	50.3± 5.3
1, 2, 3, or combinations	88.3	50,303	151.9	88.2± 9.0
None	11.7	6,645	6.7	—

*Age- and cohort-adjusted.
†Fewer than 8500 Kcal expended per week.
††1 or more packs per day.
§Mean level for age.

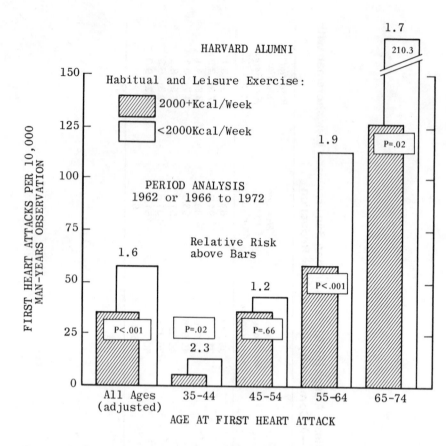

Figure 3.6. Period analysis of first heart attacks among nearly 17,000 Harvard alumni over a 6- to 10-year follow-up (1962 or 1966 to 1972), per 10,000 man-years of observation, by habitual or leisure-time energy output and age at first heart attack.

Table 3.2. Age-Adjusted First Heart Attack Rates per 10,000 Man-Years of Observation among Harvard Alumni in a Six- to Ten-Year Follow-up, by Student and Alumni Activity Patterns

Student Physical Activity Rating	Alumni Physical Activity Index (Kcal/week)		
	< 500	500–1999	2000+
Varsity athlete			
No	70.7	53.3	35.3
Yes	92.7	45.2	35.2
Sports play, hr/week *(excludes varsity athletes)*			
< 5	85.6	54.9	33.3
5+	61.2	49.4	28.4

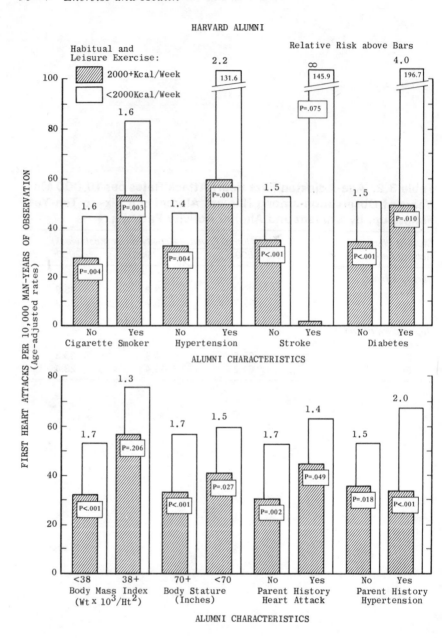

Figure 3.7. First heart attacks among Harvard alumni, over a 6- to 10-year follow-up (1962 or 1966 to 1972), by habitual or leisure-time energy output and personal characteristics assessed in 1962 or 1966.

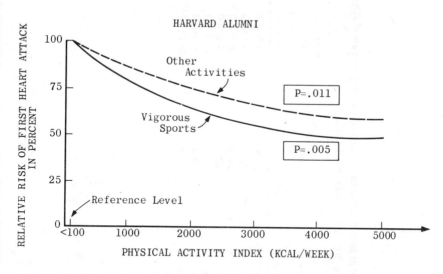

Figure 3.8. Multiple logistic regression analysis of relative risk of first heart attack in Harvard alumni over a 6- to 10-year follow-up (1962 or 1966 to 1972) to delineate roles of vigorous sports as opposed to other activities in establishing risk. (Reference level, 100 Kcal/week.) Reduced risk of heart attack is seen with increasing energy output from each type of activity, but at any given level of output, the risk is far lower for vigorous sports play.

Table 3.3. Potential Reduction in First Heart Attack (HA)—Fatal and Nonfatal—Rates among Harvard Alumni with Elimination of Specified Characteristics—A Community View of Risk Reduction

Characteristics Eliminated	Prevalence of Characteristic (%)	Man-Years Worked with Characteristic	HA per 10,000 Man-years*	Potential Reduction in HA Rates (%±one SE)
1. Sedentary lifestyle†	60.0	49,332	57.9	26.0±5.9
2. Cigarette smoking††	40.0	32,860	70.8	25.1±4.0
3. Hypertension§	8.2	6,784	107.9	16.1±2.5
1, 2, or both	75.6	62,163	57.0	44.6±7.0
1, 3, or both	63.0	51,788	57.7	31.2±6.2
2, 3, or both	44.9	36,912	72.4	36.7±4.4
1, 2, 3, or combinations	77.3	63,596	56.5	48.2±7.3
None	22.7	18,648	26.2	—

*Age-adjusted.
†Fewer than 2000 Kcal expended per week.
††Any amount.
§Doctor-diagnosed.

Table 3.4. Physical Activities and Fatal Heart Attack (FHA) Death Rates among Heart Attack Patients (Harvard Alumni) in a Twelve- to Sixteen-Year Follow-up Interval

Weekly Activity	Patients with Myocardial Infarction (N = 607)		Patients with Angina Pectoris (N = 175)	
	FHA per 10,000 Man-years*	Relative Risk	FHA per 10,000 Man-years*	Relative Risk
Stair climbing				
< 350	319	1.16	128	0.88
350+	275		146	
Block walking				
< 35	300	1.03	157	1.35
35+	291		117	
Sports play				
No	327	1.33	149	1.09
Yes	246		136	
Index in kilocalories				
< 2000	323	1.34	151	3.12
2000+	240		48	

*Age- and interval-adjusted.

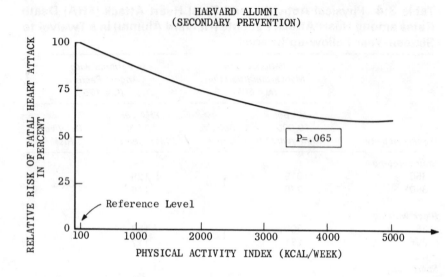

Figure 3.9. Multiple logistic regression analysis of relative risk of fatal heart attack in Harvard alumni who were heart attack patients to delineate role of energy expenditure (habitual or leisure-time) in establishing risk. (Reference level, 100 Kcal/week.) A 25-percent reduction in risk occurs at 2000 Kcal, a 35-percent reduction in risk at 5000 Kcal.

Table 3.5. Potential Reduction in Fatal Heart Attack (FHA) among Heart Attack Patients (Harvard Alumni) with the Elimination of Selected Characteristics—A Clinical View of Risk Reduction

Characteristics	Prevalence of Characteristic (%)	Relative Risk of FHA	P	Potential Reduction in FHA Rates
Cigarette smoking	60.1	1.04	.87	3.7
Hypertension	22.0	1.21	.48	17.0
Diabetes mellitus	5.7	1.20	.69	16.3
Stroke	2.2	8.28	<.01	87.9
Sedentary lifestyle*	71.5	1.47	.14	32.0

*Fewer than 2000 Kcal expended per week.

Exercise and Other Health Problems: Hypertension, Obesity, Diabetes Mellitus, Anxiety, Depression, and Asthma

Exercise has been used for centuries as a way to treat a variety of diseases and to promote health. Indeed, as early as 600 B.C., exercise apparently was used by the Indian physician Sushruta in the management of certain types of diabetes.[1] During World War II, physical-conditioning programs and, later, rehabilitation programs in the U.S. Air Force made extensive use of exercise in the rehabilitation of patients with acute and chronic illness, as well as of those disabled after injury. After World War II, major university-based medical rehabilitation programs were developed, following the pioneering example of Dr. Howard Rusk in establishing the Institute of Rehabilitation Medicine as part of New York University's Medical Center. Rehabilitation of patients with cardiovascular disease, particularly stroke and heart attack, received increasing attention in these centers, as did rehabilitation of patients with other chronic illnesses.

Substantial progress has been made during the past 30 years in the development of therapeutic exercises, including dynamic aerobic exercises, designed to increase physical endurance. Extensive research has been carried out in cardiorespiratory physiology and in the use of exercise in the rehabilitation of patients with cardiovascular disease. Relatively little systematic research, however, has been carried out in other areas. There have been few longitudinal studies of the metabolic and hormonal effects of different types of exercise in normal or obese subjects, or in those with diabetes mellitus.[2] Although evidence related to the role of dynamic aerobic exercise in the prevention and treatment of hypertension, obesity, and diabetes mellitus is limited, the importance of these problems and the burdens that they impose—on individuals, on the health care system, and on society—warrant their consideration. Hypertension ranks second, diabetes mellitus fourth, chronic ischemic heart disease seventh, and obesity tenth among diagnoses of problems that patients bring to general and family practitioners.[3] Among the most common diagnoses by internists are essential hypertension (first), ischemic heart disease (second), diabetes mellitus (third), and obesity (eleventh).[4] These four conditions accounted in 1975 for nearly one-quarter (23.3 percent) of all visits to internists and for 12.7 percent of all visits to general and family practitioners. We also consider the role of exercise in two common emotional problems, anxiety and depression. We consider the evidence related to asthma, primarily because exercise may have an adverse effect on some asthmatics, while it may be of substantial benefit to others.

HYPERTENSION

Hypertension probably affects more than 25 million adults in the United States. Blood pressure measurements were taken for people 6 to 74 years of age as part of the 1971-1974 Health and Nutrition Examination Survey (HANES-1). The prevalence rate of hypertension was 18 percent among those 18 to 74 years of age.* In addition, black adults had higher rates than did white adults.[5] Hypertension accounted for 5.9 percent of the patient visits to general and family practitioners and 9.3 percent of all visits to internists in 1975.[6] Hypertension is important, not only because of its prevalence and the direct burden of the illness imposed on individuals and on the health care system, but also because it is a major risk factor in coronary heart disease, stroke, and chronic renal disease.

Prevention

Since hypertension is a strong predictor of heart attack, the influence of exercise on risk of hypertension was studied in the Harvard alumni population. Figure 4.1 shows the decline in relative risk of hypertension with increasing hours of vigorous sports play per week by Harvard alumni grouped into four weight-for-height levels (body mass indices). In this multiple logistic risk analysis, the reference level is for alumni who did not play vigorous sports, and the data are adjusted for age, follow-up interval, body mass index gain since college, and parental history of hypertension. The results show that obese men, with a body mass index of 36 or higher, were at 50 to 65 percent greater risk of

*An elevated blood pressure was defined as a systolic pressure greater than 160 mm Hg or a diastolic pressure greater than 95 mm Hg.

developing hypertension if they did not engage in vigorous exercise than if they continued this exercise after college years. The gradient relationship to hypertension risk was direct for obesity and inverse for vigorous sports activity. That is, the heavier an individual was for his given height, the greater was his risk of developing hypertension; the more hours a person engaged in vigorous sports, the less was his risk of hypertension.

Exercise was especially significant for obese men, as compared to classmates who weighed less for their height. Risk of hypertension was lower as vigorous sports play increased, but reduced risk was significant only for men 25 percent or more (some 40 pounds or more) overweight for their height. Two hours of vigorous sports play weekly by these overweight men was associated with one-quarter the risk and four hours of vigorous exercise with half the risk of hypertension. A background of collegiate sports did not influence hypertension risk; nor did stair climbing, walking, or light sports play at the time of the study. Obesity, weight gain since college, parental hypertension, and lack of habitual strenuous exertion independently predicted increased risk of hypertension in alumni.

A number of investigators have found that regular dynamic aerobic exercise will lower the systolic and/or diastolic blood pressure of normotensive subjects, but these changes are usually small.[6] In a few controlled studies, those who engaged in heavy work were found to be less likely to develop hypertension than those engaged in sedentary work.[7] In a study of the physical activity of work and coronary heart disease, Morris and Crawford found that the manifestations of hypertension on autopsy were seen less frequently in active than in sedentary people.[8] Morris categorized a large group of English workers into active and sedentary groups based on physical activity required of them on the job and followed them for eight years, performing autopsies on those who died of cardiac and noncardiac diseases. In workers aged 45 to 60 who had a prior medical record of hypertension, he found evidence of the effects of hypertension in the form of focal myocardial fibrosis on autopsy (defined as multiple small scars of the heart) in 4.9 percent of the active workers and 21.5 percent of the sedentary workers. Among older workers aged 60 to 70, the difference was not as striking; 14.4 percent in the active population and 21.6 percent in the less active group had scarring.

Treatment

Exercise may be valuable in the treatment of hypertensive patients, but its value is limited when compared to the benefits of weight reduction, a low-salt diet, and specific antihypertensive drugs. An exercise program should be used as part of the initial therapy of hypertensive patients, however, particularly in those who are also obese, along with a dietary program (i.e., low-salt diet and reduced caloric intake), and a program of stress reduction. Why do we make such a definitive recommendation? What is the evidence that suggests that dynamic aerobic exercise may be an effective means of lowering the blood pressure of hypertensive patients?

The effect of a regular exercise program on the blood pressure of hypertensive patients was reported by Boyer and Kasch in 1970.[9] The study included 23 men aged 35 to 61 with essential hypertension (diastolic blood pressure consistently above 95 mm Hg) and 22 normotensives (systolic pressure lower than 140 mm Hg and diastolic pressure lower than 90 mm Hg). The men participated in a walk-jog interval training program for 30 to 35 minutes twice a week for 24 weeks. The hypertensives had been referred to the investigators by their personal physicians, and all were receiving antihypertensive medication prior to the study and when the pre-exercise program blood pressures were taken. Medications were then held constant throughout the study. Among normotensives, no change occurred in recorded systolic blood pressure after the training program, but diastolic pressures dropped an average of 6 mm Hg. Among hypertensives, systolic and diastolic pressures dropped an average of 13.4 mm Hg and 11.8 mm Hg, respectively. The study results are confounded somewhat by small, although not statistically significant, changes in the subjects' body weight. Normotensives lost an average of 2.04 kg, and hypertensives lost an average of 1.06 kg.

The same variable presents difficulties in the interpretation of data of Strauzenberg and his colleagues on 59 formerly sedentary men, a normotensive group and a hypertensive group.[10] Characteristics of both groups were undefined, except for an average blood pressure of 151/92 mm Hg or above in the hypertensive group. After a brief three-week intensive training program consisting of twice-daily 45-minute sessions of endurance training, these investigators found no significant changes in the blood pressure of the normotensive group, but they did observe an average decrease of 20 mm Hg in systolic blood pressure and of 8 mm Hg in diastolic blood pressure in the hypertensive group. When changes in weight of all of the men were averaged, a small, but again not statistically significant, average weight loss of 2.01 kg was noted.

The effects of exercise on blood pressure were studied by Choquette and Ferguson in 165 middle-aged men, 37 of whom were found to have a systolic pressure greater than 140 mm Hg, a diastolic pressure greater than 90 mm Hg, or both, and 128 of whom were found to be normotensive. All the men as a group then performed endurance exercises weekly for 1½ hours; in addition, 10-15 minutes of calisthenics were carried out daily by individual participants at home. Normotensives experienced drops in their systolic and diastolic pressures of 5 mm Hg and 2 mm Hg, respectively; corresponding pressures in hypertensives dropped by 15 mm Hg and 8 mm Hg, respectively.[11]

Since anxiety may temporarily increase blood pressure, it is possible that the drops in blood pressure observed were due to a lessening of the anxiety surrounding the actual measurement of blood pressure as repeated measurements were taken throughout the training program. This factor is particularly troublesome when interpreting the results obtained by Choquette and Ferguson since the pretraining blood pressure that they used as a baseline was obtained by a single reading rather than an average of readings. In the study of Boyer and Kasch, baseline blood pressure consisted of the average of five readings by laboratory staff on five separate occasions, and these investigators reported that the readings correlated well with readings obtained by the subjects' private physicians.[12] Another important observation about these studies is that, in all the studies, exercise had a more dramatic effect on patients with documented hypertension than on normotensives.

Bonanno and Lies[13] conducted a study of middle-aged male hypertensives in which an experimental group of 12 hypertensives underwent an exercise training program, while a control group of 15 hypertensives remained sedentary. The exercise program consisted of three 30- to 35-minute walk–jog sessions each week for 12 weeks. Weight did not change during the study. When checked after the 12 weeks, mean systolic pressure had dropped 13 mm Hg in the exercising group and 3 mm Hg in the sedentary group, a significant difference. No significant difference was found, however, between the drop in diastolic pressure of 14 mm Hg in the exercising group and 11 mm Hg in the sedentary group. While sample size of this study was smaller than that in studies in which significant decreases in both systolic and diastolic pressures were found, results demonstrate that the evidence relating regular exercise to a lowering of diastolic blood pressure, while suggestive, is not conclusive. On the other hand, systolic blood pressure in men did drop significantly in all these studies. In fact, no studies could be found in which regular aerobic exercise did not result in a moderate, yet significant, decrease in systolic blood pressure.

The implication of these findings for individual treatment of hypertensive patients or for the development of community-based public health programs promoting dynamic aerobic exercise is less clear-cut than for patients with coronary heart disease or for those with multiple cardiovascular risk factors. Williams, Jagger, and Braunwald[14] recommend that all patients with borderline or sustained hypertension, and probably most patients with labile hypertension, should be placed on a nondrug therapeutic regimen that includes regular exercise, relief of stress, modified diet, and control of other coronary heart disease risk factors. They believe that regular exercise, such as jogging or swimming, is indicated based on the evidence that exercise is helpful in controlling weight and that physical conditioning itself may decrease blood pressure. As we indicated at the beginning of this section, we agree. Others, however, are more cautious[15] or do not believe that the available evidence supports the conclusion that exercise is beneficial in the treatment of hypertensive patients.[16]

With regard to policies for community health programs, the findings of the Harvard alumni study suggest that exercise programs to reduce hypertension should be coordinated with those for obesity control. That is, people overweight for their height should be provided with appropriate opportunities to engage in vigorous sports to lower their risk of hypertension. The gradient or dose-response relationships of obesity and exercise toward and against hypertension also should be of interest to planners of community exercise programs, while, of course, these clinical aspects are important to physicians in prescribing individual exercise programs.

Although we recommend exercise both for the individual patients of primary care physicians and for the population at large to reduce the risk of hypertension, particularly in obese individuals, we recognize that most of the evidence to date has been gathered in studies of white, sedentary, middle-aged males. Further study is needed of the effects of exercise in hypertensive and normotensive women, obese and nonobese, as well as the effect of exercise in blacks, Hispanics, and members of other ethnic or minority groups.

OBESITY

Obesity is not easily defined, nor is the prevalence of obesity precisely known. Estimates of the number of obese individuals in the population range from 40 million to 80 million. The Health and Nutrition Examination Survey (HANES) conducted by the National Center for Health Statistics defined as obese "any adult with a triceps skinfold measurement greater than the 85th percentile measurement for people

20-29 years of the same sex."[17] According to this standard, 13 percent of all males, 20 to 74 years of age and almost 23 percent of all females 20 to 74 years were obese.[18] The prevalence of obesity increases with age.

Energy Expenditure and Obesity

Weight is a function of energy input and output. If one increases energy output by exercising more while maintaining constant energy input by not eating more, one will lose weight. Since 1 pound of body fat is equal to 3500 Kcal, and since running or walking 1 mile burns up approximately 100 Kcal[19] (running a mile burns up about 120 Kcal and walking a mile burns up about 80 Kcal[20]), theoretically, one would lose about 1 pound for every 35 miles run or walked over any given period. If, however, food intake increases in proportion' to the increase in energy output, no weight will be lost.

The relationship between energy input and energy output has been studied in adolescents and children. Johnson and her colleagues compared two matched groups of high school girls; 28 obese girls (mean weight 31.6 percent above average for age, height, and sex) and 28 nonobese girls (mean weight 7.8 percent below average).[21] These investigators found that the obese girls actually ate less (an average of 1965 Kcal per day) than the nonobese girls (2706 Kcal per day). Examining the activities of the two groups, they found that nonobese girls participated in an average of 11 hours of "active sports and other strenuous acts" per week, while obese girls participated in only 4 hours per week of such activity. Thomson and her colleagues examined obesity and exercise in a group of 10- to 14-year-old New Zealand schoolboys and girls.[22] They found that the children's skinfold thickness was inversely proportional to the time spent playing games and sports. However, these investigators did find that obese children in this age group consumed a greater average number of calories than did nonobese children.

Exercise Interventions in Obesity

Several studies have examined the effects of an exercise intervention program on acute weight loss in obese individuals. Some interventions combine diet and exercise into a single program, while others attempt to evaluate the effect of exercise alone and subjects are instructed to maintain their regular diets. Balabanski, for example, evaluated the effects of different diets without changing the exercise program that was performed concurrently.[23] Each group of middle-aged men and women who entered a Bulgarian sanitarium over a period of several years participated in the same exercise program (consisting of up to four hours of sports play per day) for a period of approximately nine weeks, while a different diet was tried on each group. (These sanitariums, which are common in Europe, resemble residential health spas.) Balabanski found that all the diets he used—hypocaloric, "normocaloric," hypolipidic, an "Atkins" diet, or a raw food diet—yielded significant weight losses if the diets were combined with the exercise program. The number of calories in the "normocaloric" diet (approximately 2900 Kcal), which was normocaloric in relation to the diet followed by participants prior to entering the sanitarium, was obviously not equal to calories expended by participants while residing at the sanitarium. When the "normocaloric" diet was combined with the exercise program, an average weight loss of 14.6 kg occurred over the nine-week period, a loss of 1.7 kg per week.

Sonka compared the use of diet alone with the use of diet and an exercise program in a group of men and women aged 17 to 45.[24] Again, using up to four hours of daily sports play (but for two rather than for eight weeks), he found a greater weight loss in the exercising and dieting group than in the group that only dieted; the weight losses were 4.0 to 4.5 kg and 2.0 to 3.0 kg, respectively. The average weekly weight loss of approximately 2.1 kg seen in Sonka's group is similar to that achieved by Balabanski's "normocaloric" group (1.7 kg per week). Both investigators, however, asked their subjects to exercise for up to four hours per day. By monitoring nitrogen balance throughout the four-hour-per-day exercise program, Sonka also evaluated the caloric intake necessary to lose body fat but maintain lean body mass in those participating in the program. He found that a caloric intake of 900 to 1000 Kcal per day was required for women and an intake of 1400 Kcal per day for men.

These rather large weekly weight losses (1.7 and 2.1 kg per week) were achieved in rather artificial environments in which the amounts of exercise performed and food eaten could be readily controlled. Exercise performed in a more typical home environment has been found to result in a more gradual weight loss. Lewis and his colleagues, for example, observed a significant but relatively small average weekly loss of 0.23 kg per week during a 17-week semester-long weight control program for obese middle-aged women.[25] Each week the subjects participated in two 20-minute sessions of jogging and walking, two 60-minute sessions of stretching and calisthenics, and one lecture on weight reduction. Questionnaire results revealed that a majority of the women increased their exercise at home as well. After an analysis of total caloric output, it was concluded that the calories expended during exercise accounted for 40 percent of the weight loss; reduced food intake accounted for the remaining 60 percent.

While the study by Lewis and his associates did not include a follow-up analysis to assess whether weight loss was sustained, Stalonas, Johnson, and Christ did a follow-up analysis, although it was for only a one-year period.[26] They compared the use of instruction in behavior modification techniques alone with a program combining instruction and 10 weeks of exercise requiring an energy output increase of approximately 400 Kcal per day. The behavioral modification techniques included eating only at certain times and only in certain places and situations. Weight loss averaged 10.3 kg over the 10-week period in the 13 women in the instruction-only program and 13.1 kg in the 10 women in the combined program. The difference between the two groups was not significant at the end of the 10-week program, but significant differences in weight were found at the 3- and 12-month follow-up examinations. Weight losses of 9.9 kg were seen at 3 months for the instruction-only group; women in the combined instruction-exercise program lost an average of 14.9 kg. After 12 months, the weight losses were 5.2 kg for the instruction-alone group and 16.3 kg for the combined group. (All the programs described above included modification of both diet and exercise patterns.)

Several studies have attempted to measure the effect on obesity of exercise alone. In a study of a group of obese middle-aged men, Strauzenberg and associates utilized only an intensive twice-a-day exercise regimen and observed a weight loss of 4.53 kg over a 23-day period (1.3 kg per week).[27] Oscai and Williams also encouraged their subjects not to concern themselves with their food intake during their 16-week exercise program.[28] In this study, five obese male subjects, aged 35 to 40, walked and jogged 30 to 60 minutes per day, three times a week. A 4.5-kg weight loss was achieved, yielding a weekly loss of 0.28 kg. Gwinup observed a similar rate of weight loss, 0.19 kg per week, over the 52 weeks that he encouraged middle-aged obese women to walk for progressively increasing periods.[29] He imposed no dietary restrictions, but he found that no weight loss occurred until daily walking periods lasted at least 30 minutes. Although he observed a substantial average weight loss over the year (10 kg), his subjects spent a great deal of time walking, up to three hours per day in two cases. Gwinup also observed a substantial dropout rate during his 52-week program, unlike investigators in other studies described, all of which involved exercise programs lasting 24 weeks or less. Of the 34 women who began Gwinup's year-long program, only 11 completed it; weight loss was calculated only for these 11 women. Bjorntorp also has commented on the high dropout rates in an exercise intervention program for weight control.[30] To improve compliance, he suggests that exercise be performed in a group with close supervision and frequent feedback of the results of body measurement changes, including changes in blood lipid levels if possible.

The study of Jette, Barry, and Pearlman is the only one that we have uncovered in which a significant weight loss did not occur in a group of obese subjects after a program consisting either of exercise alone or exercise and diet.[31] In a study attempting to evaluate the psychological changes that occurred during an extracurricular physical activity program for obese adolescents, Jette and his colleagues observed a 2.1-kg increase in weight during the 24-week program, which consisted of twice-weekly 45-minute sessions of lacrosse playing. The control group participants, who did not play lacrosse, also gained weight, an average of 2.5 kg.

Almost all these studies on exercise and obesity reveal a moderate short-term weight loss. None of the studies addresses a more critical problem—long-term weight control. Since the effects of energy expenditure during exercise are cumulative, one might expect that exercise, particularly if continued, would be of substantial assistance in long-term weight control. A longitudinal study of such an exercise intervention program has yet to be conducted. An exercise program is useful, we believe, in both short-term and long-term weight reduction in the obese, especially if ways to improve compliance over the long term are incorporated in the program. Weight loss associated with regular exercise also is important, as we have noted, for obese maturity-onset diabetics, for obese hypertensives, and for those at risk of developing hypertension.

The evidence also suggests that obese patients consulting a primary care physician will do better if they exercise in a group, rather than if they undertake an exercise program alone at home. Certainly a weight-reducing diet also should be followed. For many patients, group or individual counseling also may be necessary. For obese adolescents a program of vigorous physical activity seems particularly useful. Community-based exercise programs should consider the special needs of obese persons, particularly young people and people with maturity-onset diabetes mellitus and hypertension.

DIABETES MELLITUS

Diabetes mellitus is a health problem of major proportions. Of the approximately 10 million diabetics in the United States, about 10 percent—over 1 million—are juvenile-onset diabetics; the remainder are adult- or maturity-onset diabetics.[32] Of the maturity-onset diabetics, at least 75 to 80 percent are overweight.[33] Exercise has long been used in the treatment of patients with diabetes mellitus, particularly in those who are obese and whose disease has manifested itself during adulthood. Factual evidence in support of exercise in the management of diabetes mellitus is, however, limited. Berger and Berchtold have observed:

> Controlled studies on beneficial consequences of different modes of exercise by diabetics or precise recommendations on how to execute useful therapeutic programs of physical exercise are scarce. On the other hand, a multitude of possible therapeutic advantages of muscular exercise has been proposed on the basis of mostly anecdotal reports or clinical experience.[34]

The role of exercise training in the management of diabetes mellitus has recently been reviewed both by Berger and Berchtold[35] and by Vranic and Berger,[36] who have pointed out the need to distinguish between the effects of acute exercise and the effects of exercise training.

Minuk, Vranic, and Zinman documented the fall in blood glucose during acute exercise in 10 obese non-insulin-dependent diabetics, 6 of whom were being treated with diet and an oral hypoglycemic, chlorpropamide, and 4 of whom were being treated with diet alone.[37] From average pre-exercise blood glucose levels of 187 mg per deciliter (dl) in the former group and 226 mg/dl in the latter group, the blood glucose level fell during exercise by an average of 35 mg/dl in each group. In a control group of 7 obese nondiabetics, blood glucose did not fall during exercise. Since hypoglycemia may be a problem for diabetics who exercise, but who do not do so regularly, Zinman suggests that just prior to exercising these patients eat extra carbohydrates of a rapidly assimilated type.[38] He prefers this approach to adjusting insulin dosage on days when one plans on exercising because adjusting dosage restricts the time of day during which exercise can be performed.

Koivisto and Sherwin as well as Vranic and Berger have pointed out that the fall in blood glucose with exercise occurs only in diabetics in whom diabetic control is adequate.[39] That is, if insulin deficiency is mild and/or hyperglycemia is only moderate, glucose levels will fall with exercise. Recent studies by Pedersen, Beck-Neilsen, and Heding indicate that the improvement in glucose tolerance and the diminished insulin requirement in such patients may be due to significantly increased insulin binding in working muscle cells.[40] Acute exercise produces quite a different effect if insulin deficiency is more severe and ketosis is present. In this case, exercise will result in an excessive rise in hepatic glucose production, which exceeds the rate of muscle glucose utilization and causes an increase rather than a decrease in blood glucose. In summary, the metabolic, hormonal, and clinical effects of acute exercise in diabetic patients vary with the degree of metabolic control, the interval between the injection of insulin and the onset of exercise in insulin-deficient diabetics, and the level of exercise.

A key question about regular exercise and physical training is whether these activities will decrease insulin requirements and/or increase tolerance to glucose. Bjorntorp and his associates have shown that in normal, nondiabetic subjects, physical conditioning results in a decrease in basal and glucose-stimulated insulin levels.[41] Since glucose tolerance tests were unchanged in these normal subjects after physical training, one must assume that the body's sensitivity to insulin increased.

Regular exercise plays a role in the treatment of maturity-onset diabetes mellitus as a result of several effects. Exercise often results in weight loss, and the indicator of maturity-onset diabetes mellitus, an abnormal glucose tolerance test, has been shown frequently to normalize after weight loss in maturity-onset diabetics who are obese.[42] Exercise also may be of benefit independent of any weight loss—by increasing insulin sensitivity itself.[43] Thus, as Ruderman and his colleagues point out, exercise may be of most benefit in the large subset of maturity-onset diabetics with hyperinsulinemia and insulin resistance.[44]

Two preliminary studies have begun to test this hypothesis by evaluating the effects of an exercise program on the glucose tolerance of maturity-onset diabetics. Saltin and his colleagues evaluated a group of men aged 47 to 49 characterized as chemical diabetics on the basis of two oral glucose tolerance tests with a plasma glucose concentration above 6.9 millimoles (mM) per liter after 120 minutes.[45] These men then participated in a training program consisting of twice-weekly 60-minute sessions of calisthenics, jogging, and other sports activities. One group of 11 men received solely the physical training for a 3-month period; another group of 25 men was given initial diet instruction and participated in physical training for a one-year period. The diet instruction was given only at the outset of the program and the subjects were encouraged to eat fewer plain sugar products, to eat more fiber and unsaturated fat, and to decrease their total caloric intake. This exercise and diet instruction group lost an average of 4.5 kg by the end of 6 months, while the men in the exercise-only group had not lost weight by the end of their 3-month program. The oral glucose tolerance of subjects in the diet and exercise group was tested at 6 and 12 months and found to have normalized, both in patients who lost weight and in those who did not. The glucose tolerance of the exercise-only group, tested after only 3 months, was significantly improved but had not reached normality at that time.

Ruderman and his colleagues evaluated the effect of physical training on a subset of maturity-onset diabetics characterized by deficient insulin secretion (in contrast to those with hyperinsulinemia and insulin resistance).[46] They studied six middle-aged male maturity-onset diabetics previously treated with diet alone. Glucose tolerance was tested after 3 to 6 months of five weekly 30-minute sessions on a stationary bicycle. These investigators found a signficant improvement in intravenous glucose tolerance tests. No clear-cut changes, however, were found in oral glucose tolerance tests. It is unclear why physical training affected intravenous but not oral glucose tolerance in this study. It is also unclear why training affected oral glucose tolerance in Saltin's but not in Ruderman's studies. Ruderman and his colleagues postulate, however, that, given the results of studies that have demonstrated an increase in insulin sensitivity after a training program, one might expect greater improvement in maturity-onset diabetics characterized by high insulin levels and insulin resistance rather than in those characterized by deficient insulin secretion.[47]

A study on the effects of physical training on juvenile-onset diabetics has been conducted by Engerbretson.[48] During a six-week intensive training program, he found a fall of 10 to 18 units in the required dosage of exogenous insulin in all three of his subjects. Fasting glucose levels also were decreased in all three subjects, indicating an improvement in metabolic control despite the decrease in insulin dosage. Berger and Berchtold point out, however, that while regular exercise can be an efficient therapeutic adjunct in the control of juvenile-onset diabetics, it can be used only with cooperative, well-instructed patients who are accustomed to checking their metabolic state regularly.[49] Insulin-dependent long-distance runners, for example, require careful dosage alterations depending on the length of their run.[50]

Among juvenile-onset diabetics who have angiopathy, McMillan warns against very strenuous exercise.[51] He comments that diabetics fail to achieve as great a cardiac output during exercise as nondiabetics, and that this can result in diminished blood flow to the viscera, including the kidneys, as blood flow is diverted to exercising muscles. Exercise-induced renal cortical ischemia and potential renal insufficiency are, therefore, theoretical considerations in diabetes. McMillan also points out that the rise in blood pressure that occurs during acute exercise could stress the vessels in the eye of a diabetic with retinopathy and cause retinal hemorrhage. Given these considerations, he recommends that activity in diabetics with advanced retinopathy be limited to moderately rapid walking.

Present evidence supports the view that, while moderate exercise can aid in the control of the blood glucose level of juvenile-onset diabetics, it appears that exercise can play a more important role among maturity-onset diabetics. In obese maturity-onset diabetics, exercise can play an important role in a weight-reduction program as well as potentially improving glucose tolerance by increasing insulin sensitivity independent of weight loss.

ANXIETY

Many people who exercise say that exercise decreases the "stress" that they feel. Several studies have been conducted to investigate this effect. According to Folkins, Lynch, and Gardner, exercise does seem to change mood states, especially those of anxiety and tension.[52] Another reviewer, Layman, states that there is some evidence that the acquisition of athletic skills and the development of physical fitness may result in a reduction of anxiety.[53] One of the difficulties in studying this potential effect of exercise, however, is the assessment and definition of anxiety. Different studies use different tests to assess anxiety, and none has been conducted on persons identified as having "high anxiety" states; rather, investigators have focused on people with anxiety levels presumably within the normal range.

Several uncontrolled studies of the effect of regular exercise on anxiety have reported favorable outcomes. More importantly, in a controlled study of the effects of exercise on policeman and firemen, Folkins reported a significant decrease in anxiety in the exercise group.[54] In another study by Folkins, of male and female junior college students, only the women reported decreased anxiety and depression after a 14-week jogging class.[55]

McPherson and his colleagues examined the effects of a twice-a-week, 24-week exercise program on two groups of nine men matched with control groups.[56] The men in one group had recently suffered a myocardial infarction, while the men in the other group were thought to be healthy. A group of nine cardiac patients served as a cardiac control group, meeting once a week to socialize; a group of nine healthy men, who remained sedentary, served as the control group for the exercising healthy men. Using a Manifest Anxiety Scale and Cattell's Sixteen Personality Factors Questionnaire, the investigators found significant reductions in anxiety in the exercising groups, both cardiac patients and healthy individuals. The cardiac control group demonstrated a significant decrease in anxiety as well; the group of normal men who remained sedentary showed an increase in anxiety.

Lion studied the effects of a thrice-weekly, two-month running and walking program on a small group of chronic psychiatric patient subjects in a halfway house.[57] Three subjects exercised while three others were taken to the exercise yard without being instructed to exercise. A decrease in pre- and post-training anxiety, as measured by the State-Trait Anxiety Scale Form, was found in the exercising group; the control group showed an increase in anxiety.

Several possible causes for the apparent effect of exercise on anxiety have been suggested: (1) improved self-image gained from an exercise program; (2) physiological changes in the brain as a result of exercise; (3) the process of confronting and overcoming a challenge, in this case a fitness program; or (4) the process of participating in a group activity.[58] The fourth explanation is particularly critical. Because in all the studies discussed exercise was performed as part of a group activity, the positive effects of exercise could have been a result of peer interaction. In sum, the data indicate that group exercise programs can play a role in anxiety reduction, but further studies are needed before the effect of individual exercise programs on anxiety can be determined.

DEPRESSION

Only a handful of studies have addressed the effect of exercise on depression. In studying depression, we face a problem similar to that in studying anxiety: how should we define it? Among groups with presumably normal levels of depression, male fire and police personnel and junior college women, Folkins found a decrease in the depression scale after an exercise program in the two studies described above.[59]

Naughton and his colleagues examined the effect of an exercise program on a group of post–myocardial infarction patients.[60] When the group was divided into 14 control subjects and 14 subjects who volunteered to participate in the exercise program, the 14 exercisers were found to experience a decrease in the depression score from their pre- to post-training program Minnesota Multiphasic Personality Inventory (MMPI), but the change was not statistically significant. In another study of post–myocardial infarction patients, Kavanagh and his colleagues examined the effects of a 16- to 18-month jogging program on 44 patients with very high depression scores on the MMPI.[61] A significant decrease in depression scores was noted, but the design of the trial did not include a control group and, as the authors point out, the decrease in depression scores over the period of the program also could have been explained by the increased length of time since these patients had suffered their infarctions.

Reports of positive effects of exercise on depressed non-post-myocardial infarction patients have appeared in the popular press;[62] however, little has been reported in the scientific literature. Morgan and his colleagues did report a study conducted with 67 college faculty members, 11 of whom were found to be depressed on the basis of the Self-Rating Depression Scale.[63] Following a three-session-per-week, six-week exercise program, no significant decrease in the depression scale was found in the 56 faculty members who were not initially depressed, but a significant decrease was found in the 11 who were initially depressed. Each of these men had also increased his physical work capacity as a result of the training program. In a study of 167 college students, who had rated themselves as depressed using the Zung Depression Inventory, a variety of exercise activities (e.g., jogging, tennis), with the exception of softball, were found to reduce feelings of depression. Joggers reported the most significant improvement.[64] In a pilot study to determine the effect of regular exercise in patients seeking treatment for neurotic or reactive depression, Greist and associates found that running alone was as effective as time-limited or time-unlimited psychotherapy.[65] The cost of the supervised running program was $115 versus $500 for psychotherapy. The value of running and other types of exercise might be more important in the prevention of recurrent depression than in its treatment.

In sum, the results of the few studies conducted on the effect of exercise on depression in normal and depressed populations are too sparse to draw conclusions for either individual treatment or public health programs.

ASTHMA

It has been known for more than 1800 years that physical activity can provoke wheezing.[66] The phenomenon of exercise-induced bronchoconstriction is a well-recognized clinical entity.[67] Cold-air breathing has been found to magnify exercise-induced bronchoconstriction,[68] while humid air decreases it.[69] The problem of exercise-induced asthma has received increasing attention in recent years, in part because of its frequency and in part because of its value as a diagnostic test for asthma. Godfrey noted a greater than 10-percent drop in peak expiratory flow rate with exercise in 90 percent of asthmatic children tested.[70] Others have found similar responses in 60 to 70 percent of children, using a 15- to 20-percent fall in forced expiratory volume in the first second (FEV$_1$) as their index of response.[71] Exercise-induced asthma can be prevented or substantially reduced by a number of different drugs. Cromolyn sodium, for example, will inhibit exercise-induced asthma if given before exercise, but it is of no value after exercise. This drug appears to inhibit mediator release from mast cells, thus preventing bronchoconstriction. Sympathomimetic, cholinergic, and methylxanthine drugs, by contrast, all elevate baseline lung function.[72]

Although exercise may induce asthma, it is also known that some asthmatics appear to benefit from regular exercise programs. Indeed, some asthmatics have achieved excellence in sports, including victory in the Olympic games.[73] Strick suggests that children with asthma be encouraged to exercise because of their tendency toward a restricted, overprotected, sedentary lifestyle.[74] Swimming has long been the exercise of choice for asthmatics.[75] This assumption was recently examined by Fitch, who compared the bronchoconstrictive effect of four activities—swimming, cycling, kayaking, and running.[76] He measured the decrease in FEV$_1$ that occurred during each of these exercises. Swimming produced the least bronchoconstrictive effect, followed by kayaking, cycling, and running. Fitch then studied the effect of a 24-week daily swimming training program on 46 asthmatic children aged 9 to 16.[77] Diaries were kept by the subjects and their parents for 30 weeks commencing 6 weeks before the training program. Wheeze scores, medications taken, and swimming distances were recorded daily. Drugs prescribed for the subjects remained the responsibility of the subjects' personal physicians, and no request to vary therapy was made by study personnel. Analysis of the diaries revealed a steady fall in both wheezing scores and medication requirements for the first three 6-week periods, with leveling off occurring over the fourth period. The program also seemed to have a salutary effect on resting airway obstruction. Resting FEV$_1$ and forced vital capacity (FVC) were higher at the end of the program than at the beginning. No change, however, could be documented in exercise-induced asthma; asthmatic distress occurred at the same point during the submaximal treadmill running tests performed before and after the swimming training program. Problems in the design of the study also make it difficult to draw conclusions from its results. Lack of a control population tended to invite bias from several sources. First, the decrease in asthmatic symptoms may not have been caused by the exercise, but by a reduction in anxiety resulting from the frequent medical attention that the study necessarily produced. Second, subject bias could have occurred; symptoms experienced and medications taken may have gone underreported by subjects and their parents as a result of the investigators' apparent concern for the children's health and their implicit interest in seeing an improvement in disease manifestations.

Hyde and Swarts and Peterson and McElhenny, who have conducted similar studies, have also reported decreases in self-reported asthmatic symptoms.[78] Hyde and Swarts observed no changes in pre- and post-training pulmonary function tests (including FEV_1 measurements), while Peterson and McElhenny found a beneficial effect in the only pulmonary function test that they conducted, an increase in vital capacity. These studies are subject to the same biases as Fitch's study because they lack a control population. Another problem is that in none of these studies was there an attempt to document the change in aerobic capacity ($\dot{V}O_2$ max), for example, which presumably occurred during the program. If such a change had been documented, one would be on firmer ground when attempting to draw conclusions on the specific effect that dynamic aerobic exercise may have on asthma. Nonetheless, in 1970, the American Academy of Pediatrics Committee on Children with Handicaps and the Joint Committee on Physical Fitness, Recreation, and Sports Medicine approved participation in physical education (under medical management) for the majority of asthmatic children.[79]

For the asthmatic who does exercise, Marley recommends the consistent inclusion of warm-up exercises in order to induce maximum bronchodilation and to improve ventilation/perfusion ratios.[80] The established clinical practice of pretreatment of selected asthmatics with bronchodilators (such as the inhalants, isoproterenol aerosol and cromolyn sodium, or selected oral bronchodilators) also appears to be a substantial benefit. The impact of exercise-induced asthma on psychological development and social adaptation also has been stressed by Oseid and Aas.[81]

In conclusion, exercise does not appear to be contraindicated for the majority of asthmatics. Some studies appear to indicate that regular dynamic aerobic exercise, particularly swimming, may prove to be beneficial. However, more studies, particularly ones that include a control group and that document a change in aerobic capacity, are needed before one can confidently state that regular dynamic aerobic exercise is of physiological benefit for asthmatics.

HARVARD ALUMNI

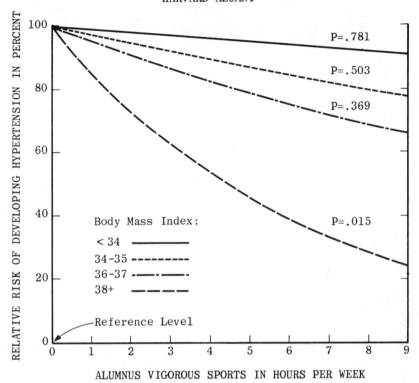

Figure 4.I. Multiple logistic regression analysis of relative risk of hypertension in Harvard alumni, over a 6- to 10-year follow-up (1962 or 1966 to 1972) to delineate the role of vigorous sports play.

Chapter 5

The Prescription for Exercise

Physicians rarely prescribe exercise for patients considered to be healthy. Even patients with cardiovascular disease, including those recovering from myocardial infarction, are only occasionally given specific exercise prescriptions or placed in organized programs of exercise as part of a cardiac rehabilitation program. Although it appears that more and more physicians are prescribing exercise for their patients,[1] in a study conducted in the mid-1970s, 80 percent of those asked could not recall their physician recommending that they exercise.[2] A study in 1978 revealed that, of persons who did not feel that they got enough exercise, 75 percent could not recall their physician ever discussing their getting more exercise.[3] A number of investigators, including Fox, Bruce, Hatch, and Cooper, have recommended that physicians prescribe exercise for their patients.[4] The American Medical Association has done so as well.[5] The American Heart Association developed a handbook in 1972, *Exercise Testing and Training of Apparently Healthy Individuals: A Handbook for Physicians*,[6] and the American College of Sports Medicine has recently issued a position statement on the quality and quantity of exercise for developing and maintaining fitness in healthy adults, as well as guidelines for graded exercise testing and exercise prescription.[7]

Exercise prescription is designed to promote beneficial clinical effects. Like a drug prescription, a prescription for exercise has specific indications, contraindications, and potential adverse effects. Exercise may be prescribed as primary or secondary prevention, as treatment, or as part of a rehabilitation program. This chapter and the next chapter, Chapter 6, provide information on the indications and contraindications for exercise as well as on the possible adverse effects of exercise. Our emphasis is on the prescription of exercise for healthy individuals free of clinically manifest chronic disease. We also consider exercise prescriptions for individuals with cardiovascular risk factors, patients with coronary heart disease, and those with other health problems. For patients with cardiovascular disease, particularly coronary heart disease, the role of exercise in rehabilitation has been accorded increasing attention since the pioneering work of Hellerstein and Ford in the 1950s.[8] Recently, several investigators have reviewed the subject of cardiac rehabilitation. For those interested in detailed information about the role of exercise in the rehabilitation of cardiac patients, excellent resources are available.[9]

The first step in prescribing exercise is to make clear to the patient what is being prescribed. Exercise may mean different things to different people. For example, a patient may consider exercise to include only specific exercises such as calisthenics or jogging, and not sports and games, physical activity associated with work, or physical activities such as sexual intercourse or climbing stairs. Concepts of physical fitness also may vary widely. For some, being fit is being able to carry out the ordinary activities of daily living without distress; for others, it means an optimal level of physical and psychological functioning. Patients will respond to the request for information about exercise, as well as the prescription for exercise, in terms of their own understanding and their own attitudes and beliefs.[10] In addition to making clear to the patient what is meant by the terms "exercise" and "physical fitness," the physician should also clarify the type of physical activity or exercise being recommended, the specifics (i.e., intensity, frequency, duration) of the activity prescribed, and the goals of the exercise program. An exercise program can be designed either for patients who will exercise on their own or for those who will participate in community-based group programs. For patients with coronary heart disease, we strongly recommend a medically supervised exercise program. This may begin in the hospital as the patient is recovering from a myocardial infarction or in a community program when the disease is not as disabling.

EVALUATING HEALTHY PEOPLE UNDER THE AGE OF 35

Most healthy people under the age of 35, including children and adolescents, require no special examinations before an exercise program is initiated. There is little doubt that those under 35 who are exercising regularly can continue to do so without medical clearance. Also, for those under 35 who have been sedentary but who have no known cardiovascular risk factors, no special medical clearance is needed. For a sedentary, overweight, cigarette-smoking male under the age of 35 with a family history of hypertension and coronary artery disease, however, a careful assessment is appropriate.

EVALUATING PEOPLE 35
YEARS OF AGE AND OLDER

Self-Assessment

We agree with Chisholm and his associates that the majority of adults under the age of 65 do not need a major physical examination before they begin a supervised physical activity program.[11] Based on a study of more than 1200 adults in British Columbia, a simple self-administered questionnaire was developed by these investigators for adults to determine whether they should consult a physician prior to initiating an exercise program. An intensive validation of the questions was conducted, including physician review of all questionnaires with an affirmative response, an age-specific physical examination, a 12-lead resting electrocardiogram, and a bicycle ergometer exercise test with electrocardiographic monitoring and physician supervision. The original questionnaire triggered 52.4 percent of all subjects to contact a physician, far higher than the estimated 11.2 percent in which unsupervised exercise was deemed medically contraindicated.[12] After further refinement, a questionnaire was developed that was better able to detect those who should not exercise without a physician's clearance and those who did not need such clearance to exercise on their own.

This self-administered Physical Activity Questionnaire (PAR-Q), which includes only seven questions, is in widespread use at the present time as part of the Canadian Fit-Kit,[13] and the questionnaire also is undergoing further evaluation and verification.[14] The PAR-Q questions are simple and straightforward:

1. Has your doctor ever said you had heart trouble?
2. Do you frequently have pains in your heart and chest?
3. Do you often feel faint or have spells of severe dizziness?
4. Has a doctor ever said your blood pressure was too high?
5. Has your doctor ever told you that you have a bone or joint problem such as arthritis that has been aggravated by exercise, or might be made worse by exercise?
6. Is there a good physical reason not mentioned here why you should not follow an activity program even if you wanted to?
7. Are you over age 65 and not accustomed to vigorous exercise?[15]

Those who respond "yes" to one or more questions are advised to consult their personal physician, and, after medical evaluation, to seek advice about physical activity (unrestricted or restricted/supervised).

Those who answer "no" to all the questions are given "reasonable assurance" that they are suited for a graduated exercise program and a home fitness test.

A home fitness test developed in Canada is also part of the Fit-Kit, and this test has been found simple and safe to use.[16] A person is instructed to step to music at a speed adjusted for his or her age and sex for three minutes and to count the radial pulse for 10 seconds. If the pulse rate does not exceed a given rate, the person proceeds to a second three-minute step test, after which the pulse rate is again taken for 10 seconds. This test determines whether a person has an undesirable, minimal, or recommended level of fitness.[17] Based on the fitness level and the person's age, sex, height, and weight, a simple walk–jog exercise program has been designed to stress the person to 60 percent of $\dot{V}O_2$ max.[18]

Medical Assessment

There is by no means universal agreement about the need for a medical examination, including monitored performance testing, for adults before they begin any kind of fitness or exercise program. Although there is no medical consensus about the need for medical assessment, many physicians and professional organizations, including the American Heart Association, recommend it. Certainly it is indicated when the physician considers the patient to be at increased risk for coronary heart disease or other cardiovascular diseases that might modify an exercise prescription. The purpose of this medical assessment is twofold: to detect diseases that contraindicate exercise or require special precautions, and to provide information for the prescription of an exercise program suitable for a patient's age, sex, weight, height, level of fitness, health status, and personal interest.

The physician's evaluation begins with a careful history, including information about present and past levels of physical activity, as well as information about cardiovascular disease (e.g., myocardial infarction, cardiac arrest) or symptoms suggesting cardiovascular disease, arthritis, infection, or other disorders that might contraindicate exercise. (See Tables 5.1, 5.2, and 5.3.)

The physical examination is equally important, with particular attention being paid to resting heart rate, blood pressure, weight, and any sign of cardiovascular disease (e.g., murmur of aortic stenosis, absent pedal pulses).

Laboratory studies should be based primarily on the history and physical examination. We recommend as routine measurements a complete blood count, urinalysis, fasting blood sugar, serum cholesterol, and resting electrocardiogram.

The physician's first obligation is to determine the presence or absence of diseases that would contraindicate exercise or require special precautions.

Contraindications to Exercise

Conditions that are an absolute contraindication to initiating an exercise program are congestive heart failure, acute myocardial infarction, rapidly increasing angina pectoris with effort, and a variety of other conditions (Table 5.1). In addition to these absolute contraindications, there are a number of relative contraindications (Table 5.2) and conditions requiring special consideration and/or precautions (Table 5.3). The relative contraindications may be time limited (e.g., toxemia or pregnancy), may respond fully to treatment (e.g., thyrotoxicosis), or may persist or grow worse (e.g., cardiac enlargement). Conditions requiring special consideration and/or precautions include conduction disturbances, severe hypertension, severe anemia, marked obesity, severe rheumatoid arthritis, as well as severe neurological disorders and psychoses.

Exercise Tests

Exercise tests are often considered an essential component of pre-exercise program evaluation. The most common exercise test methods are the treadmill, bicycle, and step-test protocols. These tests are useful, particularly with patients with cardiovascular disease, to provide a basis for an objective evaluation of physical work capacity and for provoking symptoms that may provide clues to mechanisms limiting physical work capacity. The tests are not, however, a satisfactory means of screening for coronary artery disease. Exercise (stress) tests have been found to produce many false-positive and false-negative results.[19] Given the likelihood of a false-positive test, the physician is faced first with the problem of what to recommend for a person whose pre-exercise program stress test is positive. If such a test is definitively positive, an exercise tolerance test with Thalium-201 may be indicated to decrease the likelihood of a false-positive result. A positive stress test presents the physician with an additional problem. By finding a person whose stress test is positive, the physician has identified just the individual being screened for—the individual at greater risk of developing a myocardial infarction or arrhythmia with exercise (although this identification may still be inaccurate because of the large number of false positives even with the addition of the Thalium scan). Should this individual then be discouraged from entering an exercise program? When one considers the studies discussed in Chapter 3, which show exercise to be somewhat protective against death from coronary heart disease in persons who have the disease, this individual is probably an excellent candidate for an exercise program because of the positive stress test. Clear-cut recommendations concerning exercise prescriptions also are lacking for individuals with negative pre-exercise program stress tests. While the number of false-negative test results is probably fewer than the number of false-positive results, some individuals with coronary heart disease will have a negative stress test with or without the added benefit of a Thalium scan.[20] In a study of 13 cardiac deaths that occurred during or shortly after jogging, Thompson and his colleagues found that, of the four who had undergone stress tests within two years of death, three had had negative stress tests and one had had a test with an equivocal result.[21] Based on the evidence to date, Jones feels that "we can no longer expect this non-invasive test to provide a cost-effective, reliable measure for screening the asymptomatic population in search for persons with coronary disease."[22] Many other physicians apparently share Jones's sentiment; when a large number of middle-aged physicians who were joggers themselves was surveyed, few had undergone stress testing prior to beginning their own exercise program.[23] There are others, however, who recommend an exercise (stress) ECG for men above 40 years of age prior to their engaging in any exercise program.[24] We agree with Jones that stress testing is not necessary as a routine procedure to screen people over age 35 or 40 who wish to begin an exercise program.

The principles of exercise testing, the methods used, and the criteria for evaluation have been thoroughly reviewed.[25] Stress testing, while not a necessity as a pre-exercise screen, can be helpful in determining an appropriate exercise prescription. The purposes of this evaluation have been succinctly defined by Hellerstein and his associates:

> The evaluation must be multi-level, steady state (also ideally non-steady state), on a calibrated ergometer (bicycle, treadmill, steps). The magnitude and duration should be sufficient to tax the individual's capacity, safely, to his highest safe level, or to elicit evidence of strain if at a lower level, as assessed by continuous measurements of cardiovascular functions (heart rate, blood pressure, electrocardiogram) and clinical signs and symptoms.[26]

Stress testing, as noted, may be performed using treadmill, bicycle, or step-test protocols, all of which are capable of providing comparable measures of maximum oxygen intake ($\dot{V}O_2$ max). Differences among the results obtained by these three methods are unimportant from a clinical point of view.[27] It is necessary to obtain data about the intensity and duration of the work performed during the stress test, as well as to record the heart rate, arterial blood pressure (indirect), electrocardiogram, and respiratory rate at rest and during the last minute of exercise at each workload.

Maximum oxygen intake is the goal of a dynamic exercise test, but the test should be terminated before that level is reached if certain symptoms, signs, or electrocardiographic abnormalities occur before that point. Endpoints during clinical exercise testing include the following:

maximum level of oxygen uptake ($\dot{V}O_2$ max);
chest pain, unless minor and clearly extracardiac;
symptoms and signs of cerebral ischemia;
undue or unusual dyspnea, weakness, fatigue, pallor or cyanosis;
fall in blood pressure or heart rate with increasing work load, or blood pressure exceeding 260/130;
leg pains suggesting claudication; and
significant electrocardiographic abnormalities, if not present at rest.[28]

Test results, particularly $\dot{V}O_2$ max or the appearance of other endpoints, determine the initial exercise prescription for cardiac patients. The heart rate, blood pressure, and their product can be used as an indirect measure of $\dot{V}O_2$ max. Each measure—physical work capacity, heart rate, arterial blood pressure, heart rate–systolic blood pressure product, and elecrocardiographic response to exercise—provides valuable information for the physician writing the exercise prescription for the cardiac patient.[29] Any primary care physician wishing to initiate or to supervise exercise stress testing for cardiac patients should be thoroughly familiar with the principles and practice of performance testing.

BASIC FEATURES OF THE EXERCISE PRESCRIPTION

The basic elements of an exercise prescription are the same for healthy participants as for those with cardiovascular or other diseases. Four factors need to be considered when determining the content of an exercise prescription: (1) the type of activity; (2) the intensity of the activity; (3) the duration of the activity; and (4) the frequency with which the activity is performed.

Type of Activity

Many different dynamic aerobic activities and sports can be prescribed for a patient, including walking, running, swimming, and tennis (see Table 5.4). In determining which activity is most appropriate for an individual patient, a primary factor is the patient's interest in a specific activity. The patient's health and estimated physical capability also are important. Limiting factors may include the patient's work and time commitments, the facilities available, and the cost of alternative exercise programs.

Intensity of Activity

The most important element in any dynamic aerobic exercise program is the intensity of the exercise relative to the individual's initial aerobic capacity. For most people, the intensity of exercise can be monitored most simply by the heart rate. To achieve the desired result—a training effect—the heart must be beating at 70 percent of its maximum rate. (The maximum rate can be estimated by subtracting an individual's age from 220.) Hellerstein and his associates have observed: "The heart rate expressed as percent of maximal heart rate bears significant relationships with coronary blood flow, myocardial oxygen intake, oxygen consumption as percent of maximal oxygen consumption, respiratory exchange ratio, lactate production, and catecholamine excretion."[30]

There are limits, however, to the use of the heart rate as a fraction of the maximal rate, particularly in patients with coronary heart disease or other heart diseases that may result in a target heart rate lower than 70 percent of the maximum heart rate. It may also be true of patients taking drugs, in particular propranolol. Signs or symptoms that preclude exercise at a higher work level include exertional hypertension, angina pectoris, hypotension, ventricular ectopic activity in salvos or paroxysms, sinoatrial or high degrees of atrioventricular block, 3 or 4 mm ST-T displacement, or other severe symptoms. In such patients, Hellerstein designates the heart rate at which the above symptoms or signs develop as the Maximum Safe Heart Rate and uses an average of 70 percent of this heart rate and a peak of 85 percent of this heart rate (rather than the maximum heart rate) as a guideline in training prescriptions.[31]

For the healthy adult, the target for the average exercising heart rate should be 70 percent of maximum heart rate (220 minus the patient's age) with periodic peaks to 85 percent of the maximum rate. Although 70 to 85 percent of the maximum heart rate is the target range, the initial goal should be an exercising heart rate that is 60 percent of maximum. While the physician may be able to judge the exercise intensity that would bring a particular patient's heart rate into the target range, the patient should be taught to check his or her pulse to verify the physician's judgment of the intensity required. The carotid artery is recommended for checking the pulse rate because it is often easier to feel than the radial artery at rapid heart rates. Both pulses are difficult to feel while actually in the process of exercising, and the patient should be instructed to stop exercising briefly at periodic intervals to check his or her pulse. If the pulse is not in the target range, the pace of exercise can be increased or decreased to bring the rate into the proper range. During the first few weeks of an exercise program, the participants will need to stop and check their pulse rates several times during each workout to ensure the proper exercise intensity, but with experience most will soon be able to judge the intensity required with only occasional pulse checks. A very rough guide to attaining the necessary exercise intensity is the "perspiration test." When one is exercising hard enough to perspire in a cool environment, one's pulse is generally above 70 percent of maximum. Exercise at this intensity need not be exhausting; the participant should finish the workout feeling pleasantly fatigued rather than at the point of collapse. A workout of appropriate intensity and duration should leave a person feeling rested, fully recovered, and not fatigued within an hour after exercise. For persons whose exercise program features jogging as the chief aerobic activity, a particularly useful guide to ensure that the intensity of the workout is not above the target heart range is the "talk test."[32] If a runner is going too fast to talk while running, the pace should be slowed down to the point at which the runner can carry on an intelligible conversation with a fellow runner. Most people find exercise at the "talk test" level of intensity to be more pleasant than exercise performed at greater intensity. The added benefit is that the runner can interact with others on the road. Therefore, for a person in a jogging program, the target heart rate generally can be achieved at a pace fast enough to pass the "perspiration test" but not so fast that a person cannot pass the "talk test."

Individuals over the age of 35 who have not been given stress tests and who have not recently participated in a regular exercise program should be started on an exercise program of lower intensity than individuals who have undergone stress testing and have been judged with some confidence to be free of aysmptomatic coronary heart disease. The intensity of the exercise programs for the former group should be designed initially to reach a target heart rate of 60 percent of the maximum rate. If cardiac symptoms do not develop during the first several weeks of this lower-intensity program, exercise intensity can be increased gradually to the point at which the pulse rate is in the target range of 70 to 85 percent of the maximum predicted heart rate. Most of these patients are best begun on exercise programs with walking as the chief activity. The patient may start by walking one mile, stopping occasionally to do a pulse check, and then adjusting his or her pace accordingly. As time passes and the training effect begins to occur, the pace necessary to maintain the pulse at the prescribed rate will increase. As this occurs in patients over age 35 who have not been stress tested, the prescribed heart rate can be increased gradually into the 70- to 85-percent target range. Once the exerciser can cover a mile in 15 minutes and still be in the target range, a jogging or jogging/walking program can be begun. The walk–jog program consists of alternate segments of walking and jogging, with each segment performed for either a set period or a set distance.[33] For example, the participant might jog for one minute and then walk for one minute, then jog for one minute and walk for one minute, and repeat this sequence for the duration of the exercise period. As the exerciser's condition improves, the jogging periods can be increased and walking decreased, and the exerciser moves gradually to the point at which jogging consumes the entire exercise period. Once the exerciser reaches this point, he or she may elect to continue jogging or move on to another activity, a racquet sport, for example. A combination of activities also is perfectly acceptable and is often the most practical way to increase the chance of exercising with the frequency needed to maintain or to improve fitness.

Individuals who have been stress tested and found to have negative results can be placed in a program with the initial target range of 70 to 85 percent of maximum heart rate. Often, however, their musculo-skeletal system requires conditioning that can be obtained during a lower-intensity program (60 percent of maximum heart rate) prior to their participation in the 70- to 85-percent target range program.

Any newly exercising adult should be warned of symptoms that might occur during exercise that could indicate the presence of coronary heart disease: (1) chest, arm, neck, or jaw pain; (2) significant increase in shortness of breath with exercise; (3) lightheadedness or fainting; (4) irregular heart beat; (5) nausea or vomiting during or after exercise; (6) prolonged fatigue after exercise; (7) weakness or uncoordinated movements; (8) unexplained weight changes; or (9) unexplained changes in exercise tolerance. It is a good idea to list these symptoms on the written exercise prescription. Patients should be instructed to discontinue exercise immediately if symptoms develop and to consult their physician. If cardiac symptoms develop during an exercise program, a stress test with Thalium may prove useful. The importance of warning newly exercising patients of cardiac symptoms was demonstrated in the previously mentioned study by Thompson and his colleagues.[34] They found that of 13 persons who experienced cardiac death during or shortly after jogging, 6 had noticed either new onset or worsening of cardiac symptoms in the weeks prior to their death. Only 2 of the 6 notified their physicians of their change in symptoms.

As an alternative to exercise prescription by percentage of maximum heart rate, the MET unit system can be used. One MET unit is the amount of energy expended at rest multiplied by a factor of 1.1. This approach has been used by Fletcher and Cantwell.[35] Exercises range from a low of 3 to 4 METs (walking three miles per hour) to 12 or more METs (running eight miles per hour). (See Table 5.5.) Measuring the patient's exercise tolerance with a stress test (step, bicycle, or treadmill) will determine the maximum tolerance for work. If this tolerance is 10 MET units, the exercise prescription should fall within the target range (7.0 to 8.5 MET units).

Frequency and Duration of Activity

For the training effect to occur, the exercise must be performed for 20 to 30 minutes three to four days per week.[36] Greater levels of fitness can be achieved with activity performed more frequently and for longer periods, but satisfactory levels can be attained with even 20 minutes of activity performed three days per week; once a desired level of fitness is attained, 30 minutes of activity on two nonconsecutive days may be enough to maintain fitness.[37] In addition to the 20 minutes or more of dynamic aerobic activity, time must be spent warming up and cooling down. Warmup, which should last approximately 5 to 10 minutes, should consist of an activity of an intensity intermediate between the activity that the individual was doing before beginning the workout and the dynamic aerobic activity that will constitute the bulk of the workout. Stretching, calisthenics, walking, and jogging are excellent warmup exercises. For the individual whose aerobic activity is walking or jogging, warmup can be incorporated into the workout by simply starting off at a slow pace and gradually increasing the pace over the first 5 to 10 minutes. Ideally, cool-down consists of 3 to 5 minutes of gradually decreasing activity. This is often impractical, however, such as after a game of tennis. When a period of gradually decreasing activity is not practical, this period can be replaced by a few minutes of relaxation. The relaxation will help avoid acute changes in body temperature, as might occur when a person goes directly from vigorous activity to a shower or a sauna. This should be avoided, as should very hot or very cold showers. During cool-down when gradually decreasing activity is not possible, some people will find it helpful to rest with their feet and legs elevated to avoid syncope.

GETTING THE PATIENT STARTED

The simple recommendation to exercise may be adequate to motivate self-starters among a physician's patient population, but most patients will need more direction. Some patients who need more direction may require only a brief discussion of benefits and principles of exercise and the recommendation of a good how-to-exercise book that they might be interested in. Examples of good resources for patients include *Jim Fixx's Second Book of Running, Run to Health, Women's Running, The Aerobic Way, The Wonderful World of Walking, Get Fit With Bicycling, Aerobic Dancing, Tennis Everyone, The Science of Swimming, Swim for Fitness, Total Swimming,* and *Racquetball.*[38]

Some patients may respond to a question on exercise asked during a routine history and physical examination. If patients are asked how much exercise they get and whether they think that they exercise enough, they may well turn the question around and ask the physician for his or her opinion on the question. This is often a good time to initiate discussion about the value of exercise, the nature of an exercise prescription, and alternatives available for carrying out a program of dynamic aerobic exercise. After discussing with a patient how exercise might be of value, a referral to an appropriate community resource might be in order if the doctor feels that the patient's participation is more likely to be sustained in a group. Exercise programs often are available in YMCAs and YWCAs, YMHAs and YWHAs, community centers, city parks and recreation departments, hospitals, high schools, colleges, universities, medical groups, and for-profit exercise centers. (See Chapter 8.) One of the chief benefits of these programs is that exercise is usually performed with others in a group; peer support can be a valuable adjunct to a physician's advice and encouragement.

Patients in whom pre-exercise evaluation reveals one of the conditions requiring special consideration and/or precautions (Table 5.3) are more appropriately placed in a medically supervised exercise treatment program than in a program supervised only periodically during visits to the prescribing physician.[39] These programs, which are available in most U.S. metropolitan centers, may be organized by a community hospital, a medical group, or a community organization. Persons who should be placed in medically supervised exercise treatment programs fall into two categories: those with known cardiovascular disease for whom such supervision is essential, and those at high risk of developing cardiovascular disease. The first category includes (1) patients with past myocardial infarction (who may be admitted to a treatment program as early as three weeks after infarction); (2) patients with stable angina pectoris; and (3) patients with coronary artery bypass (who may be admitted four to eight weeks after surgery).[40] The second category, those at high risk of developing cardiovascular disease, includes (1) patients particularly vulnerable to coronary heart disease based on presence of several risk factors; (2) aymptomatic patients with a positive stress test; (3) patients with or without other clinical evidence of coronary heart disease with arrhythmias induced or aggravated by activity; and (4) patients with significant hypertension and a low functional capacity.[41] (Hypertensive patients with normal functional capacity do not require a supervised program.) Primary care physicians experienced in prescribing exercise may want to prescribe home exercise programs for some of these patients.

Patients with coronary heart disease are, of course, at increased risk of such cardiac events as myocardial infarction and cardiac arrest, and they also are at risk of musculoskeletal injuries that may occur with exercise (see Chapter 6). To provide these at-risk patients with a safe environment for exercise, it is necessary that physicians, nurses, and others involved in exercise testing and training be knowledgeable and skilled not only in relation to coronary heart disease, but in safety practices and procedures as well. Emergency equipment should be immediately available, including defibrillator, cardiovascular monitoring equipment, oxygen, respiratory assist equipment, and appropriate drugs and intravenous fluids. Emergency procedures should be posted and clearly visible.

Patients' decisions to enter an exercise program will be as varied as physicians' reasons for prescribing dynamic aerobic exercise. For the healthy 35-year-old woman who wants to "get in shape" or "feel better," the motivation may be strong. For a sedentary, overweight, middle-aged man who has hypertension and other cardiovascular disease risk factors, the story may be quite different. Motivation is a critical factor in the patient's decision to enter an exercise program. The healthy individual may be motivated to begin an exercise program for his or her own reasons; in response to pressure from family, friends, or peers; or as a direct result of an exercise prescription from the physician. Patients with coronary heart disease, particularly those in cardiac rehabilitation programs, may be motivated by fear of another attack, while healthy individuals may be more likely to be motivated by a general belief in long-term benefits of exercise. One explanation for the high dropout rates in exercise programs observed in patients who have recovered from a myocardial infarction may be that, as time passes and their fear subsides, so does the urgency to maintain an exercise program, especially if exercise has not been previously a part of a person's lifestyle. In contrast, people who are motivated by a general belief in the benefits of exercise are better able to continue a program after the immediate urgency and fear disappear.

Among a randomly selected group of nonparticipants in a program of regular physical exercise made available by the National Aeronautics and Space Administration, job-related factors, such as heavy workload, travel schedule, and lack of time, were cited most frequently as reasons for nonparticipation.[42] Social or environmental factors, such as low income, also have been found to affect participation in regular exercise.[43] In a study of beneficial health behaviors among Canadians, Mackie found that respondents with a high school education or fewer years of education were less likely to exercise than were those with some university training.[44] Regular exercise was less likely also when spouses did not exercise and when respondents were obese. Exercise was judged least enjoyable by working-class respondents and most enjoyable by lower-middle-class and upper-middle-class respondents. If religion, work, and good health were important to the respondent, exercise was judged more enjoyable and the respondents were more likely to engage in regular exercise. Future-oriented people were more likely to exercise and to see exercise as enjoyable than were people who lived day to day. Age, too, was an important factor; those over 60 believed that exercise was less necessary than did younger respondents.

CONTINUED PARTICIPATION IN EXERCISE PROGRAMS, DROPOUTS, AND REASONS FOR NONCOMPLIANCE

Continued participation by healthy individuals and by those with cardiovascular disease in regular exercise programs is extremely variable. In studies of healthy individuals, including sedentary middle-aged males, and of patients with coronary heart disease, compliance rates range from 18 to 86 percent, with overall compliance for a mean of 12 months of approximately 55 percent.[45] In studies of compliance of post–myocardial infarction patients to exercise programs, patients have been found to drop out for a variety of reasons: psychosocial reasons (lack of interest or motivation, lack of family support), medical reasons (cardiac and noncardiac), and unavoidable reasons (change of jobs, change of residence).[46] In one particularly interesting study, Oldridge found that "95 of 100 subjects who are smokers, blue collar workers, who do not participate in leisure-time physical activity involving more than a walk three times a week, and who have low energy demand in their job are likely to become dropouts within 23 months of entry."[47] Smoking was the single most discriminating variable in this study—59 percent of those who smoked on entry dropped out. Earlier, Taylor, Buskirk, and Remington found that, in recruiting volunteers for controlled trials of exercise, cigarette smokers tended to volunteer less often than nonsmokers, and men whose off-the-job level of activity was high tended to volunteer more often.[48] In examining the features of healthy males who were dropouts, Massie and Shephard found that excess weight was a striking feature of this group.[49] They characterized the likely dropout as overweight, stronger than average, extroverted, and a smoker.

Noncompliance with prescribed regimens is complex and may be related to a number of factors. First of all, it is very difficult to change already established lifestyle patterns, particularly cigarette smoking, diet, and physical activity. Rosenstock has identified a number of other factors:[50]

health motivation;
perceived susceptibility to a particular illness;
perceived severity of illness;
perceived benefits of professional intervention;
perceived barriers to taking action; and
knowledge of the medical condition and the prescribed regimen.

Haynes, after a thorough review of literature related to noncompliance with therapeutic regimens, found five factors of major importance: (1) the disease (particularly a psychiatric diagnosis); (2) the regimen (complexity, degree of behavior change, duration); (3) the therapeutic source (inefficient and inconvenient clinics); (4) patient–therapist interactions (inadequate supervision, patient dissatisfaction); and (5) the patient (inappropriate health belief, previous or present noncompliance with other regimens, family instability).[51]

In analyzing the social and psychological factors that influence continued participation in exercise programs, Heinzelman found that individuals in higher social classes were more likely to recognize and accept the need to exercise than those in lower classes.[52] There are a variety of reasons for this circumstance, not the least of which is a more flexible work schedule and more time to exercise. These findings related to the importance of social and environmental factors in compliance are consistent with those of other investigators. Such factors as financial constraints (particularly low income), transportation problems, time constraints, and competing demands can affect compliance.[53] Similar problems were identified in a study of participation of federal employees in exercise programs.[54] Factors most often cited as having a negative influence on continued participation were directly related to the individual's job (e.g., workload, travel schedule). Physical problems (e.g., orthopedic problems involving muscles, joints, or tendons) were cited by 13 percent of participants.

Physicians prescribing exercise should attempt to take these factors into account. A convenient location, group participation, and adequate supervision are likely to enhance exercise participation. The first step, however, is to provide the patient with the information needed to facilitate the patient's decision to participate in an exercise program. Information is needed about individual health status, the value of exercise, why the physician is recommending exercise, and exactly what is involved in carrying out the exercise program. Information and patient education, however, are not enough. Some studies that have measured patients' knowledge of their disease and therapies show a positive relationship between knowledge and compliance, but many studies show no association. Indeed, it has been observed that ". . . there appears to be no relationship between patients' knowledge of their disease and its therapy and their compliance with the associated treatment regimen."[55]

One problem is that the educational effort is generally part of a multifaceted intervention. As a result, it becomes difficult to isolate the independent effects of patient education. Usually, education is accompanied by periodic monitoring and support from a physician or another health professional. Once this interpersonal contact is terminated, compliance tends to decline to its original level. Obviously, more than information transfer seems to be at work. If only transmission of information were involved, one would think that it would have a stable effect over time. The patient would become informed and knowledgeable, and would have no need for supervision and periodic interpersonal contact with a health professional.

A basic assumption since the work of Rosenstock, Hochbaum, Leventhal, and Kegeles, as well as that of Kasl and Cobb, has been that the patient's motivation, beliefs, attitudes, and perceptions play a pivotal role in determining compliance.[56] The basic points of this "health beliefs model" are, first, that patients are more apt to be compliant if they perceive themselves as being subject to some threat, that is, if they see themselves as susceptible to a disease or a problem and if they view that disease as severe. Second, patients will be more likely to engage in a given health behavior (in this case, compliance with an exercise program) if they perceive the exercise as valuable, that is, if the benefits are seen as outweighing the costs. Third, a patient may perceive himself or herself to be under threat, and perceive the therapy as valuable, but still need some cue or trigger to action, some suggestion that it is appropriate to engage in a given activity.[57]

The "health beliefs model" was first used to predict acceptance of preventive health recommendations related to annual checkups, screening tests, and immunizations. Empirical research based on hypotheses derived from this model demonstrates that the approach has real promise in enhancing patients' compliance with therapeutic regimens.[58] However, a major problem with this model is its emphasis on attitudes and perceptions to the exclusion of knowledge. The "health beliefs model" focuses so much on patients' motivation and attitudes that it neglects the fact that some patients may not be exercising regularly because they have misconceptions about exercise or are lacking in knowledge about how to do the exercises properly.

The problem of noncompliance also can be viewed as a problem in physician–patient communication and interaction. For patient compliance with a prescribed regimen to occur, the physician must be able to function as an effective motivator, teacher, and persuader. To motivate the patient, the physician must use strategies designed to attract the patient's attention so that he or she is ready to listen to what the physician is going to say about the exercise program. As a teacher, the physician has to use communication skills to ensure that the patient understands and remembers what is conveyed. Finally, even if the patient is motivated to listen to the physician's message, and even if he or she understands and remembers the message, it will not be acted upon unless the patient accepts it. Thus, the physician must also function as a change agent or persuader. Studies have shown that physicians' use of these multiple communications skills is associated with increased patient understanding of and compliance with medical advice.[59] However, no studies have been done to assess whether physicians who receive training in these skills can master them and increase compliance among their patients.

Teaching, motivating, and persuading patients is a dynamic process involving flexibility in physicians' communication styles, willingness to listen to patients' points of view, and adaptability in altering regimens to meet the patients' needs. Specifically, the communication process includes the following elements:

1. trying to anticipate the patient's needs for information;
2. designing and delivering a "message" based on principles of learning;

3. eliciting feedback from patients in an effort to identify communications barriers;
4. redesigning ("tailoring") messages to meet individual needs, seeking a different regimen if necessary, and/or providing other assistance;
5. periodically monitoring the patient's knowledge, motivation, and ability to identify the patient's changing needs and problems.

Periodic visits to the physician can help motivate the patient, and they can provide the opportunity for needed alteration of the exercise prescription and the treatment of musculoskeletal or other complications that may develop. To continue to have a beneficial effect, exercise must be a lifelong activity and thus something that the patient likes to do and something that fits into his or her lifestyle. Therefore, if the patient grows weary of the activity prescribed, the physician should suggest new activities until the patient finds one that he or she enjoys and looks forward to. Many people enjoy exercising with others and, if the patient expresses such an interest, he or she should be encouraged to seek out friends or family with whom to exercise. As mentioned previously, exercise groups in the community also can provide fellowship. Another technique to improve compliance is to have the patient keep an activity diary. Recording the day's exercise in a diary can provide a patient with a feeling of accomplishment, stimulating him or her to get out and exercise on the next prescribed exercise day. The tangible benefit of being able to record the workout in the diary is often enough to get a person to exercise on a day on which motivation is particularly low. Periodic physician visits also provide the opportunity to discuss other risk factors, smoking, for example.

For patients with orthopedic and other limitations, dynamic aerobic exercise may not be the most appropriate exercise prescription; the physician may want to prescribe another type of exercise. For patients with obesity, osteoporosis, peripheral vascular disease, anxiety, or depression, low-intensity exercise (e.g., stretching, calisthenics) may prove helpful. Exercise performed for relaxation (e.g., leisurely walks or whatever type of exercise relaxes the patient) may be useful in the treatment of depression and anxiety, and, to a lesser degree, in weight management.

Once the physician has prescribed exercise, he or she must be prepared to handle many of the minor complications that may arise. Because dynamic aerobic exercise involves the continuous, repetitive use of large muscle groups, it may result in injury to these muscle groups and to joints as well. A previously sedentary adult is particularly susceptible to developing these musculoskeletal injuries. The experienced athlete stressing his or her body to the limit, however, also may experience similar problems via the same overstress mechanism. The jogger, for example, may develop knee problems, achilles tendonitis, or a host of other orthopedic problems. Most of these problems respond promptly to reduced pace or to temporary discontinuation of jogging. By beginning at an easy pace and by increasing the pace gradually over a period of months, the new jogger can avoid many of these problems. These complications as well as other risks of exercise are discussed in detail in the next chapter.

Certain other precautions are necessary to minimize potential cardiovascular or musculoskeletal complications.[60] This is particularly true for patients with cardiovascular disease. The patient should:

begin slowly, with one to four weeks of gradual buildup at subtraining intensity;

avoid exercise during illness;

allow adequate time for warmup and cool-down;

stop exercise immediately if chest discomfort develops;

avoid eating a large meal fewer than two hours before or one hour after exercise;

avoid cigarette smoking at all times, but particularly after exercise;

avoid cold or very hot showers, tub baths, or saunas before or immediately after exercise;

avoid going outdoors in cold weather if still perspiring after exercise or undergoing other extreme temperature changes;

avoid "all-out" efforts that increase the risk of cardiovascular complications; and

avoid exercising alone when there might be special risks (e.g., jogging alone in a public park).

In summary, the prescription for exercise, like the prescription for a drug or a diet, must be based on sound knowledge of the benefits and risks of exercise as well as on knowledge of the patient for whom the exercise is to be prescribed. When this is the case, the benefits of exercise can be great.

Table 5.1. Absolute Contraindications to Exercise

1. Manifest circulatory insufficiency ("congestive heart failure")
2. Acute myocardial infarction
3. Active myocarditis
4. Rapidly increasing angina pectoris with effort
5. Recent embolism, either systemic or pulmonary
6. Dissecting aneurysm
7. Acute infectious disease
8. Thrombophlebitis
9. Ventricular tachycardia and other dangerous arrhythmias (e.g., second and third degree atrioventricular block [multifocal ventricular activity])
10. Severe aortic stenosis

Source: Adapted from American College of Sports Medicine, *Guidelines for Graded Exercise Testing and Exercise Prescription* (Philadelphia: Lea & Febiger, 1975).

Table 5.2. Relative Contraindications to Exercise

1. Uncontrolled or high-rate supraventricular dysrhythmia
2. Repetitive or frequent ventricular ectopic activity
3. Untreated severe systemic or pulmonary hypertension
4. Ventricular aneurysm
5. Moderate aortic stenosis
6. Uncontrolled metabolic disease (diabetes, thyrotoxicosis, myxedema)
7. Severe myocardial obstructive syndromes (subaortic stenosis)
8. Marked cardiac enlargement
9. Toxemia of pregnancy

Source: Adapted from American College of Sports Medicine, *Guidelines for Graded Exercise Testing and Exercise Prescription* (Philadelphia: Lea & Febiger, 1975).

Table 5.3. Conditions Requiring Special Consideration and/or Precautions

1. Conduction disturbance
   a. Complete atrioventricular block
   b. Left bundle branch block
   c. Wolff-Parkinson-White syndrome
2. Fixed rate pacemaker
3. Controlled dysrhythmia
4. Electrolyte disturbance
5. Certain medications
   a. Digitalis
   b. Beta-blocking drugs and drugs of related action
6. Clinically severe hypertension (diastolic over 110, grade III retinopathy)
7. Angina pectoris and other manifestations of coronary insufficiency
8. Cyanotic heart disease
9. Intermittent or fixed right-to-left shunt
10. Severe anemia
11. Marked obesity
12. Renal, hepatic, and other metabolic insufficiency
13. Deforming arthritis
14. Central nervous system disease
15. Psychoses

Source: Adapted from American College of Sports Medicine, *Guidelines for Graded Exercise Testing and Exercise Prescription* (Philadelphia: Lea & Febiger, 1975).

Table 5.4. Dynamic Aerobic Sports and Activities

Requiring only one participant
Bicycling (briskly)
Cross-country skiing
Dancing (briskly)
Ice skating (briskly)
Jogging/Running
Rollerskating (briskly)
Swimming
Walking (briskly)

Requiring at least two participants
Badminton
Basketball
Fencing
Football
Handball
Platform tennis
Racquetball
Soccer
Squash
Tennis
Volleyball

Requiring two participants or more
Basketball
Football
Soccer
Volleyball

Table 5.5. Classification of Exercise by MET Units

3–4 METs
walking (3 mph)
cycling (6 mph)
softball
dancing (moderate)
volleyball
3 METs = treadmill (2 mph, 3.5% grade)
4 METs = step-up (24 steps/min., 12 cm ht.)

4–5 METs
tennis (doubles)
walking (3½ mph)
cycling (8 mph)
Ping-Pong
raking leaves
dancing (vigorous)
4 METs = treadmill (2 mph, 7% grade)
5 METs = step-up (24 steps/min., 18 cm ht.)

5–6 METs
walking (4 mph)
cycling (10 mph)
ice skating
swimming (1 mph)
5 METs = treadmill (2 mph, 10.5% grade)
6 METs = step-up (24 steps/min., 25 cm ht.)

6–7 METs
walking (5 mph)
cycling (11 mph)
lawnmowing (hand mower)
skiing (easy downhill)
square dancing
tennis (singles)
swimming (1.6 mph)
7 METs = step-up (24 steps/min., 32 cm ht.)

7–8 METs
jogging (5 mpg)
cycling (12 mph)
sidestroke (1 mph)
mountain hiking
8 METs = step-up (24 steps/min., 35 cm ht.)

8–9 METs
jogging (5½ mph)
cycling (13 mph)
basketball (vigorous)
paddleball
9 METs = step-up (30 steps/min., 28 cm ht.)

10–11 METs
running (6 mph)
handball (vigorous)
swimming backstroke (1.6 mph)
10 METs = treadmill (3.4 mph, 14% grade)
11 METs = step-up (30 steps/min., 36 cm ht.)

12 METs
running (8 mph)
rowing
12 METs = step-up (30 steps/min., 40 cm ht.)
12 METs = treadmill (3.4 mph, 18% grade)

Source: S.M. Fox, *et al.,* "Physical Activity and Prevention of Coronary Heart Disease," *Annals of Clinical Research* 3:404–432 (1971).

Chapter 6

Risks of Exercise

with Kenneth G. Campbell, M.D.

Exercise is accompanied by certain risks and complications. The adverse effects of exercise testing and dynamic aerobic exercise may be classified as cardiac and noncardiac complications. The cardiac complications of exercise, particularly ventricular arrhythmia and myocardial infarction, are rare; however, they are very serious and may cause death.[1] The noncardiac complications range from heat stroke and hyperthermia in marathon runners to shin splints, tennis elbow, and blisters in other exercisers. The most common adverse effects of dynamic aerobic exercise are musculoskeletal problems, which we will discuss in detail.

CARDIAC COMPLICATIONS

In an analysis of deaths associated with 170,000 exercise (stress) tests performed in 73 medical centers, the mortality rate was one death per 10,000 exercise tests, while the combined mortality/morbidity rate was four incidents per 10,000 tests.[2] Certain cardiac arrhythmias, particularly multifocal ventricular premature complexes, frequent ventricular premature beats (more than 10 per minute), and ventricular tachycardia are more likely to occur with vigorous exercise in the presence of coronary heart disease and should alert the physician to proceed cautiously with an exercise prescription until the nature of the patient's underlying disease is determined. After carefully studying the problem of cardiac arrhythmias in both normal subjects and those with coronary heart disease, Morris and McHenry observed:

. . . Among patients with known coronary artery disease, the incidence of multiple-vessel disease and/or abnormalities of left ventricular wall motion

---

Dr. Campbell is an orthopedist practicing at the Palo Alto Medical Clinic, Palo Alto, California.

is higher in those with exercise induced ventricular arrhythmias than in those without. Finally, preliminary data from our laboratory indicate a significantly greater incidence of sudden death in coronary disease patients who manifest complex ventricular arrhythmias at exercise heart rates below 70 percent of their predicted maximal heart rate.[3]

Exercise training or vigorous exercise at levels of 70 to 85 percent of the maximal heart rate may be associated with cardiac arrhythmias, myocardial infarction, and sudden death. However, in patients who have recovered from an acute myocardial infarction and who have participated in cardiac rehabilitation programs, including exercise training, the rate of reinfarction is lower than in those with similar characteristics who do not participate.[4] The Harvard alumni study, discussed in Chapter 3, also provided evidence of a lower rate of heart attack in normal subjects and in regularly exercising post–heart attack patients than in subjects who did not exercise. Ventricular arrhythmias and myocardial infarction may occur both with exercise testing and with dynamic aerobic exercise. The presence of coronary heart disease increases this risk, yet with proper precautions patients who are asymptomatic or who have minimal limitations will be less likely to suffer these adverse effects than will comparable patients who do not exercise.

Among patients who have recovered from myocardial infarction, the risk of sudden death due to ventricular arrhythmia can be reduced if physical training takes place in a medically supervised environment with proper equipment (see Chapter 5). Thirty medically supervised, outpatient cardiac rehabilitation programs reported 1,480,000 man-hours of participation with the occurrence of 33 nonfatal cardiac arrests, 8 fatal cardiac arrests, 4 nonfatal myocardial infarctions, 2 fatal myocardial infarctions, 2 fatal pulmonary emboli, 1 fatal pulmonary edema, and 1 fatal cardiogenic shock. For every 29,020 man-hours of participation, there was a fatal or nonfatal cardiac event; of the 41 cardiac arrests, resuscitation was successful in 33 (80 percent).[5] To detect patients at special risk of ventricular arrhythmias, Morris and McHenry suggest frequent "spot-check" electrocardiographic monitoring during or immediately after exercise training sessions.[6]

A likely mechanism for cardiac arrhythmias during or immediately after vigorous exercise, particularly long-distance running, has been suggested by Pickering, who notes:

. . . during long distance running, plasma levels of norepinephrine, potassium and lactic acid may all be very high, and ventricular premature beats are very frequent. The stage is thus set for malignant arrhythmias to occur, particularly in the immediate post-exercise period, when blood pressure and presumably coronary perfusion, suddenly decrease.[7]

The appearance of signs or symptoms such as dyspnea, tachycardia, hypertension, or angina pectoris should, of course, serve as a warning for both the patient and the physician.[8]

The athlete's heart syndrome has recently attracted renewed attention.[9] In the past, studies had been limited to clinical examination, electrocardiograms, and chest radiographs. In recent years, additional radiographic, electrocardiographic, and echocardiographic studies have been carried out in trained athletes, including swimmers, runners, and weight lifters. Bradycardia is a universal finding in runners, swimmers, and other athletes who have participated regularly in dynamic aerobic exercises. Sinus arrhythmia is also quite common, and occasionally first-degree or second-degree atrioventricular block is found. Although echocardiographic studies of runners and swimmers reveal an increased left ventricular end diastolic volume, conflicting results have been found with respect to left ventricular thickness.[10] It is important to be aware that some abnormalities found in athletes are not necessarily evidence of cardiovascular disease.

NONCARDIAC COMPLICATIONS

Climate and Exercise

Heat stroke and hyperthermia are among the most serious complications associated with long-distance runs, particularly marathons. Heat stroke results from a failure in temperature regulation, with a cessation of sweating and a marked rise in core temperature.[11] When environmental temperatures are cool and marathon runners have adequate amounts of water to drink at regular intervals during a race, they will generally be able to sweat enough to remain in thermal balance with high rates of aerobic heat production. Cases of heat stroke in runners and cyclists have been reported as a result of prolonged intense physical activity in hot humid weather. Prevention is clearly better than treatment; Wyndham has recommended cancelling a running or cycling marathon if wet bulb globe temperature exceeds 28 degrees centigrade.[12] Treatment depends on prompt recognition of the problem and rapid cooling of the patient. Exercise at high altitudes or in particularly cold climates also can be harmful both to healthy adults and to those with coronary heart disease.[13]

Genitourinary Problems

Another problem observed in marathon runners is exercise-related hematuria. In a study of 50 marathon runners, exercise-related hematuria was observed in 9 (18 percent). No formed elements other than red blood cells were seen, and all abnormalities cleared within 48 hours.[14] The primary cause of this hematuria is probably repeated impaction of the flaccid posterior wall of the bladder against the bladder base during running.[15] Hematuria may be associated with kidney damage, particularly if hyperthermia, hypotension, dehydration, and hypokalemia occur. Hematuria also may be associated with rhabdomyolysis, myoglobinuria, and hyperuricemia.[16] If exercise-related hematuria does not clear within 48 hours or if it recurs more than once or twice, the physician should investigate for more serious underlying abnormalities of the kidneys or lower urinary tract.

Asthma

The problem of exercise-induced asthma, which we discussed in Chapter 4, is particularly important in children and adolescents, but it may occur at any age and may be the first clinical manifestation of asthma.

Accidents

A potential hazard for any runner who uses public roads is death or injury caused by an automobile or other vehicle. The exact number of joggers killed or injured in such accidents is not known, but, like other pedestrians, they are at some risk. It is easy to exaggerate the risk, as Burch has done.[17] Milvy points out that in 1977 there were an estimated 100,000 pedestrian injuries and 8700 pedestrian deaths in the population under 1 year of age to over 65 years of age.[18] How many of these injuries or deaths have involved joggers or long-distance runners is not known.

Musculoskeletal Overload and Other Orthopedic Problems Associated with Exercise

The rapid and widespread increase in the number of people exercising has meant that more people are applying stress to variably resistant body systems. The body is composed of a number of biological and mechanical systems, which can become overloaded or injured when overused or stressed. Musculoskeletal overload can result from either a single high loading force or a lesser force applied over a longer period. Obviously, the strength of the system loaded is important in determining how much stress can be tolerated. Stress means many things to many people. To some, it is the body's response to external stressors; to others, it is the environmental factor causing the bodily response. In examining the impact of stress on the musculoskeletal system, it is necessary to agree on a definition of the term. We define stress in this context as an applied force or a system of forces that tends to strain or deform a body. Strain is the deformation produced by stress.

A sudden, violent force or stress applied to the musculoskeletal system will produce an acute overload or injury. Repetitive stress applied through frequent and prolonged use will produce a chronic overload syndrome. Examples of acute overload include skin laceration, acute bone fracture, ligament rupture, and muscle strain. Obviously, the stress applied has "deformed" one or more parts.

A repetitive force or stress, such as in running or in tennis, can result in strain or deformity via chronic overload. Here the problem is the application of force without adequate rest—the body's maintenance system cannot keep up. The result may be a stress fracture of bone, tendonitis, or synovitis. "Repetitive microtrauma" is a term used to de- cribe this mechanism of overuse. Chronic overload is complex because of the many factors involved. These factors include age and the basic strength of the musculoskeletal system; hereditary factors in part determine the continuing strength of the bones, joints, and supporting tissues. Conditioning can improve strength and hence the capacity of the musculoskeletal system to do work. Degenerative changes reduce the resistance to stress, as do illness, vitamin or other nutritional deficiencies, hormone imbalance, and osteoporosis. Other more subtle factors, such as the basic pliability of connective tissue (called the "fibroelastic diathesis"), and the sensitivity of connective tissue ("connective tissue sensitivity syndrome") can alter the endpoint for soft tissue failure. For some individuals, such as ballet dancers and acrobats, the connective tissues are remarkably pliable and resilient. For other individuals, however, connective tissues seem to be their weak point. They suffer from nagging recurrent bursitis, tendonitis, synovitis or fasciitis, low-back pain, or other musculoskeletal disabilities. The baseball pitcher can overload the shoulder system and through microtrauma can develop a tendonitis. The long-distance runner can pound on an asphalt surface and develop a stress fracture. The stress fracture will predictably heal, but the tendonitis may be chronic or recurrent. Once soft tissue is overloaded and a chronic pain pattern develops, it is more the product of inflammation than of injury. The result is an unpredictable amount of discomfort or disability, an indefinite period of recovery, and a variable response to a variety of treatment modalities. Ice, heat, ultrasound, rest, aspirin and other oral anti-inflammatory drugs, cortisone injections, and many other treatment methods may be employed. A basic problem is that we do not understand why connective tissue becomes inflamed other than to say it is a direct result of overuse. Even more frustrating is our inability to plot a consistent course toward recovery. All this makes advising an individual about the possible consequences of a course of exercise more difficult.

Age and Musculoskeletal Overload

Childhood and Adolescence. The young have tissue systems that are growing, have a faster healing and remodeling rate, and generally are more elastic than those of middle-aged or older adults. These tissue systems usually are resistant to both acute and chronic overload conditions. Children have as their major problem the sequelae associated with rapid growth and the various osteochondritis syndromes, problems that account for many of the "growing pains" of childhood and adolescence. For example, pain and swelling at either end of the patellar tendon or in the elbow usually represent the inflammation of osteochondritis. Many of the complaints of backache in the adolescent represent juvenile epiphysitis and can be confirmed by vertebral changes seen on x ray. Whereas the usual overload patterns in children respond quickly to rest, the symptoms of osteochondritis may last for one or more years. The nature and cause of osteochondritis are as yet unknown. Rest in varying amounts for varying periods is the basic treatment. The growing child develops tight connective tissue in association with longitudinal bone growth. The hamstrings are a good example of a system that becomes tight and should be stretched on a regular basis during growth. Aching in the thigh after exercise is a good indication that the hamstrings are too tight.

Acute fractures in children generally heal rapidly, and because of remodeling a certain amount of displacement is usually tolerated. The exception are fractures that involve the epiphyseal areas. The potential for deformity in these fractures in the growing area of bone is great and in degree of harm compares to the intra-articular hip fracture in the adult. Accurate assessment and early treatment are vital.

Low back pain is an increasingly common problem, as more and more adolescents engage in active sports throughout the school year. Overuse injuries, such as stress fractures, must be considered in differential diagnosis, as must neoplasms, infection, and other inflammatory processes. The most common causes of low back pain in adolescents are: (1) osteochondrosis of vertebral epiphyses (Scheuermann's disease or juvenile epiphysitis); (2) disc disease; (3) low-back anomalies (such as spondylosis and spondylolisthesis); and (4) mechanical back pain due to acute or chronic musculotendinous or ligamentous injuries of the spine.[19]

The particular susceptibility of adolescents to repetitive microtrauma is due, in part, to imbalances resulting from the adolescent growth spurt in which the soft tissues, ligaments, and musculotendon units do not keep pace with bone growth. Improper pretraining and conditioning are a frequent cause of low back pain due to musculoskeletal overload in growing athletes. In all sports, stretching and muscle-strengthening exercises are important, as is gradual progress rather than instant achievement.

Parents, coaches, recreation directors, and physicians, as well as children and adolescents, should try to find individual and team activities that will provide the opportunity to develop endurance, strength, and skill and at the same time minimize the risk of injury. Some activities are far more dangerous than others. In a study of 800 children aged 6 to 17 participating in six supervised sports (football, soccer, basketball, baseball, swimming, and gymnastics), football was found to be by far the most hazardous sport. Using an injury index factor to estimate the degree of risk in the 800 children, Chambers found that the risk of a participant sustaining an injury in football was twice as high as it was in basketball and gymnastics.[20] Soccer and baseball were low-risk sports; swimming had a risk factor of zero. It should be noted that in the group Chambers studied, supervised athletics accounted for only one-third of clinically severe orthopedic injuries (fractures and joint dislocations). Unsupervised recreational activities (tree climbing, running, and especially skateboarding) contributed twice as many extremity injuries. In Chambers's view, soccer is an excellent team sport and swimming an excellent individual sport for children and adolescents because of the benefits in terms of fitness, low cost, and low risk.

Skateboarding and rollerskating are popular sports among children and adolescents. The rapid increase in the number of skateboarding children has been accompanied by a rapid rise in the number of children injured in skateboarding accidents.[21] Although most skateboard injuries are trivial, there is the danger of more serious injury, including fractures, rupture of the spleen, hemorrhage, and serious renal damage. Similarly, most rollerskating injuries are trivial, although fractures and more serious injuries may occur. Unfortunately, awareness of these problems has not led to effective strategies for prevention. Skateboard riders and rollerskaters should be advised to avoid city streets, particularly at dusk or after dark. Injuries might well be reduced by the use of protective equipment, but there is little evidence on this point at present.

Advising parents and adolescents about contact sports, particularly football, also can pose a difficult dilemma. Although fatal or even serious injuries are rare, and although relatively minor injuries—sprains, strains, contusions, and abrasions—account for more than 70 percent of all football injuries,[22] the apparent increasing frequency of cervical spine injuries merits the special attention of the personal physician. In an analysis of data on football fatalities and injuries from 1971 to 1975, Torg and his associates found that of 1,275,000 players, 77 died, 99 became permanent quadriplegics, and 259 received injuries to the cervical spine involving fracture-dislocations.[23] Of the quadriplegics, 77 were high school players, 18 college players, and 4 played at other levels. Although both the number of deaths and the death rate have declined as equipment has improved, the present design of the football helmet has led many players, with their coaches' encouragement, to use the helmet as a "battering ram" in tackles, blocks, and running. Physicians should advise their football-playing patients about the dangers of "spearing" and take an active role in the community to stop such tactics if they are taught.

The myth that all children are active and do not need to be reminded to exercise regularly is still prevalent. The notion that children need to participate in competitive sports is equally erroneous. In addition, the concept that all children are limber and do not need regular stretching exercises is categorically wrong. As children grow, bones lengthen and connective tissue becomes tight. Therefore, children should develop a habit of stretching early in childhood and continue it on a lifelong basis. Regular exercise also should begin in childhood. The physician as teacher and counselor should encourage these habits.

Children who participate in organized sports—such as baseball, soccer, and swimming—may be subject to emotional stress that is reflected in a variety of physical symptoms. These symptoms usually are not caused by the vigorous nature of the sport or by the youngster's involvement in a team effort. Too often they are instead related to parental pressure or to an over-zealous coach who puts too much emphasis on winning and not enough on participation. Some parents drive their athletically gifted children in ways that other parents drive their academically gifted youngsters. As a result, a youngster may become easily fatigued or may develop vague physical symptoms that point more to a problem of psychological origin than to one of physical origin. A careful history and physical examination often are the first steps toward resolving this problem.

In childhood and adolescence, the personal physician's role in advising about exercise is threefold: (1) to encourage the habit of regular exercise; (2) to help the child, the adolescent, and the parent make decisions about appropriate sports based on differences in constitutional makeup and the existence of physical disability; and (3) to recognize physical problems or injuries, to prescribe adequate treatment, and to give good counsel regarding return to athletic participation. Examples of these roles would be encouraging the obese, less than well-coordinated child to embark on a regular exercise program; guiding the small, thin, delicate-boned adolescent away from football toward a noncontact sport; diagnosing osteochondritis early, prescribing adequate treatment, and counseling parent and child regarding acceptable sports.

Middle Years (21 to 55). With normal growth and maturation, the body develops strong bones and muscles as well as pliable connective tissue and no longer has the potential for epiphyseal fractures. The middle years are the athletic years: the body is resistant to injury and should be in good physical condition. Acute overload problems do occur, however, because of the vigorous nature of many sports. Some chronic overload also is seen because of the intense nature of athletic training. For example, the 16,000-yard-per-day swimmer may impinge the rotator cuff mechanism of the shoulder and develop tendonitis; the distance runner may overwhelm the metatarsals and develop a stress fracture. By and large, the young, mature body accepts the punishment of training and competition, and, if an overload occurs, healing is relatively rapid. Genetic expression of early degenerative changes (e.g., osteoarthritis of the hip), and connective tissue sensitivity syndrome, and other problems, however, may become apparent during middle life. These problems usually are manifested by chronic overload problems such as tendonitis or synovitis. Individuals endowed with strong muscles, flexible tissue, good coordination, and no tissue or architectural defects will be more resistant to overload. Given any genetic predisposing factors, individuals who maintain their musculoskeletal system in good condition are less likely to develop overload problems.

An intelligent conditioning program is vital at this stage in life. Habits formed at this time will pay dividends throughout one's lifetime. The individual should establish a regular pattern of exercise and accord it a priority in relation to other activities. The major conditioning needs of the middle years and beyond are cardiovascular fitness and stretching. Muscular strengthening and sport-specific conditioning are of secondary importance, but they still should be given priority. Coaching and appropriate lessons will enable weekend athletes to compete successfully at their level by using the best biomechanics and by avoiding faulty use of the musculoskeletal system.

The onset of overload can be prevented or delayed. Proper rest is vital to tissue recovery. Overindulgence in the offending exercise may be disastrous, a situation seen all too often in tennis players and runners. Both sports seem to be addictive and are overdone for a variety of psychological reasons. The tennis player who is having a good day and whose game is "on" keeps playing until there is no one else around. The runner who goes three miles per day wants to increase to five, then to seven, then to a mini-marathon, and finally goes on to a marathon without proper conditioning. Both are destined for failure, particularly connective tissue overload failure. The tennis player will develop tendonitis of the shoulder or elbow; the runner will develop back pain, achilles tendonitis, a stress fracture, or other injuries. Adequate rest means allowing exercised tissue to recover. Recreational swimming can be done every day, but overzealous tennis playing or running cannot. We see many returnees from a week at tennis camp who started having knee pain after four days of continuous play—and who kept playing. It may take weeks or months to recover from this kind of overindulgence in physical activity.

A physician's analysis of such problems, whether degenerative or structural, is vital, so that remedial exercise, supportive equipment, coaching, or a change in sport can be prescribed. Obviously, old injuries with sequelae will affect how much a system can be used. Fractures with deformity, severe sprains, strains, dislocations, and other injuries will dictate what sports and how much activity can be advised. Anatomic inadequacies such as spondylolisthesis, severe bow legs, or rigid, highly arched feet, may keep a person from participating in certain sports such as jogging but will allow cycling or swimming. There is usually some sport or exercise for everyone. However, proper initial treatment and rehabilitation are a must to minimize long-term disability.

As a rule, patients who have orthopedic back or weight-bearing joint problems will be better advised to exercise in water and should consider swimming as a sport in place of running. On a decreasing trauma scale, contact sports (football and rugby) would be at the top, then the vigorous racquet sports (racquetball and squash), serious running and tennis, mild jogging and relaxed doubles tennis, cycling, swimming, and, finally, walking.

In advising adult patients, particularly those over 30 or 35 years of age, the physician also needs to be familiar with the problems posed by the more popular physical activities in which patients are likely to engage. These range from relatively low-risk activities, such as walking, jogging, and swimming, to those that may pose a range of hazards, such as scuba diving and horseback riding.

Swimming, although it is a low-risk sport for most participants, may cause "swimmer's shoulder" in competitive swimmers who swim free style, backstroke, or butterfly. This complication, frequently called an impingement syndrome,[24] is the result of chronic irritation of the humeral head and rotator cuff on the coracoacromial arch during abduction of the shoulders.[25] Knee problems may occur in swimmers who use the whipkick with the breast stroke.[26] Rest and proper swimming technique are the best means of treatment—and prevention.

Runners and joggers, particularly those who run 20 to 30 miles per week, are subject to a host of problems, from blisters to stress fractures. Orthopedic problems include shin splints, compartment syndromes, patellar tendonitis, plantar fasciitis, and achilles tendonitis. To avoid many of these common orthopedic problems, the jogger or runner should have good shoes and orthotics if needed. Conditioning should start slowly and build up gradually. For many people, it is better to begin exercising on alternate days to give the body a chance to rest. It will probably take about six weeks to reach a steady-state level of 30 minutes of running or jogging three or four times per week. Stretching exercises are essential before jogging or running. An excellent approach to exercise warmup and cool-down, as well as to a gradual buildup (over 12 weeks) to a full exercise program, has been described by Wood.[27]

Tennis, another very popular sport, may cause eye, neck, shoulder, arm, elbow, hand, low-back, leg, heel, and toe injuries.[28] The keys to prevention are good techniques—tennis lessons help—and a regular program of stretching and muscle strengthening. Playing tennis when it hurts is possible, but it requires that both the physican and the patient be sensitive to the patient's specific problems.[29]

Skiing also has become a popular sport. In recent years, the rate of injury has decreased, particulary the rate of lower extremity equipment-related injuries.[30] Proper training is again an important factor in reducing injuries; less skilled skiers have higher injury rates than do more highly skilled skiers. Because skiing is an endurance sport, adequate conditioning is essential to prevent fatigue-related injuries. Many preseason conditioning programs are available.

The physician advising middle-aged patients should (1) encourage the discipline of exercise; (2) explain the lasting values of cardiovascular fitness, maintenance of normal body weight, and a well-conditioned musculoskeletal system; and (3) understand the concepts of wellness and risk factors so that a tailored preventive maintenance program can be prescribed for each patient. Knowledge of behavior modification and other patient education techniques is also valuable (see Chapter 5). Other well-trained health professionals are available to help the primary physician educate patients in health and exercise principles. If the physician does not have the time or knowledge to prescribe exercise, he or she can refer the patient who has no underlying problems to community exercise programs or centers that provide guided physical activity programs. A referral to a consultant is particularly important when a patient has physical problems or limitations. If he or she has low-back pain, an adequate assessment and diagnosis is needed so that an intelligent exercise program can be designed. For most people with physical or medical problems, exercise may be good for general well-being and for the specific condition. Examples of these conditions include rheumatoid arthritis and degenerative lumbar disc disease.

The Later Years (Age 55 and Beyond). With advancing age, all the orthopedic problems encountered in middle life continue to affect the musculoskeletal system. Old injuries lead to degenerative changes; once-pliable connective tissues become tighter and less resilient. Genetic factors may predispose to demineralization of bone or to degenerative changes in the hips, spine, and knees. Illness, damage, or degenerative changes in other systems produce alterations in the musculoskeletal system through inactivity or nutritional deficiency. Hormone imbalances, such as estrogen or androgen deficiencies, thyroid imbalance, or diabetes mellitus may affect the entire body. There are, however, marked differences among individuals. Some who have maintained a normal weight, exercised regularly, and avoided cigarette smoking may be remarkably fit and vigorous. Others may be overweight or hypertensive, and may have multiple coronary heart disease risk factors, osteoarthritis, and degenerative disc disease as well. The advice given to these two types of pateints will be quite different. A patient with almost any of these conditions can pursue some level of physical activity on a regular basis to achieve a goal, whether it be cardiovascular, neuromuscular, or psychological.

The great variation among older patients, as well as their greater susceptibility to musculoskeletal overload with exercise, should not preclude exercise. Almost everyone aged 55 years or over should exercise regularly. Because of clinically manifest or subclinical conditions in this age group, however, an adequate health inventory is necessary before an exercise program is initiated. The degenerative joint that is allowing a reasonable amount of walking may not allow jogging, but it may permit swimming without difficulty. Chronic shoulder tendonitis will not allow a regular tennis serve, but it may respond to a professional's advice about altered body mechanics. A patient with chronic obstructive pulmonary disease will need a specialist's advice about conditioning or exercise, but this patient usually can participate in a walking program.

No matter what the age of the patient, but particularly for those age 55 and over, the physician can provide sound advice about avoiding musculoskeletal overload. The first step is to correct, minimize, or ameliorate whatever chronic problems are present. If this cannot be done, cognizance must be taken of the problem in designing an exercise program. In some cases it may be necessary to avoid specific activities (e.g., jogging for a middle-aged or elderly woman with osteoarthritis of the hip, carrying a heavy briefcase for an elderly man with chronic shoulder pain). In others, a routine of stretching, strengthening, and warming up can work wonders in prevention. In still others, specific remedial exercises may be needed to correct such problems as chronic low-back pain.[31]

Even if the primary care physician cannot be a sports medicine specialist, he or she can serve as the patient's ombudsman in relation to exercise.

A PREVENTIVE PROGRAM FOR EXERCISERS OF ALL AGES

Stretching

People vary in flexibility, that is, in the pliability of their connective tissue. Everyone is more limber during the second half of the day and tightens up at night. With age, connective tissue becomes more brittle and relatively more "stiff." Certain connective tissue disorders and genetic factors may increase this tightness. Therefore, it is important to work on a stretching program daily. The major areas of tightness include the neck, shoulders, lumbar spine, hip area (adductors and hamstrings), and the achilles tendons. Because low-back pain (often associated with degenerative disc disease) is a common problem, it is important to give very careful consideration to basic stretching exercises. Not all these areas need to be stretched regularly, but one or more probably need regular attention. Stretching exercises depicted in popular books[32] or on television programs that stress both stretching and aerobic exercise can be used as guides. The most important point about stretching exercises is that they must be initiated gradually but done regularly. Unlike dynamic aerobic exercise, which can be done for 20 minutes or more three times per week, stretching exercises are best done daily. When doing the stretch, a person should not "bounce." It is vital to hold the stretched position as instructed. Stretching helps prevent chronic overload and often acute strains by allowing more motion before tissue deformation occurs. Increased motion also results in a better force transfer through improved biomechanics. For the healthy adult, yoga can supplement stretching exercises.

Strengthening

More muscle means more power and greater endurance. This translates into running more quickly and for a longer time or hitting a tennis ball with more authority. Increasing muscle quality and quantity is helpful at any age, but it becomes more important with advancing age. Aging joints are better protected by good-quality muscle surrounding them. Without daily use, muscles lose their tone just as connective tissue tightens. To counteract this problem, muscle can be protected or developed by three different modes of exercise: (1) isometric; (2) isotonic; and (3) isokinetic.

In isometric exercises, muscles are contracted against a resistance, but no motion is involved. Opposing muscle groups can be used as the resistance; for example, rather than exercising one arm by pushing it against a wall or other stationary object, one can push it against the other arm. Isometric exercise is not an efficient way to build muscle, but it is an effective way to prevent some muscle atrophy. No equipment is needed, and the exercises can be performed at a desk, in bed, in a cast, on a plane, or even in outer space.

Isotonic exercises are the most frequently used exercises to strengthen muscles. To do them, one contracts one's muscles against a resistance with motion. Push-ups and pull-ups are common examples; so is weight lifting. Weight rooms, health spas, and training quarters have a variety of equipment, ranging from simple to sophisticated, to help people develop necessary muscle. In general, muscle is built for power or endurance. It is important for everyone to have well-conditioned muscles, particularly in the trunk and around the shoulders and thighs. In addition, sports require certain muscle groups to have more power or more endurance. Such sports-specific training is best undertaken with the guidance of a coach, a professional in the sport, or a trainer.

In isokinetic exercises, a part of the body is moved against a constant resistance through a range of motion at a fixed speed setting. Hydraulic equipment such as the Fitron® or the Orthotron® can increase the power and endurance of many muscle groups.

The physician, in advising a patient who wishes to begin or expand an exercise program, may wish to ask for advice from a sports medicine specialist, a coach, a professional in a particular sport, or an exercise specialist in a YMCA, YWCA, or health spa in planning a specific exercise program.

Warming up

Warming-up exercises are designed to ready an individual mentally and physically for a specific sport. These exercises help to stretch tight connective tissue and to ready the body physiologically to meet the task at hand. This means (1) metabolic readiness for increased oxygen consumption; (2) neuromuscular readiness and shortened reflex time; and (3) psychic readiness as demonstrated by concentration and confidence. Warming-up exercises prior to running or tennis might include stretching, arm rotation, side bends, knee hugging, and head circling,[33] as well as sports-specific repetition of those motions or actions that will be performed during the sport. Warming-up exercises should always precede active exercise such as running, tennis, or vigorous swimming.

Protective Equipment

Specific sports require protective equipment; good examples are football and ice hockey. Recreational sports sometimes also require protection—

for example, raquetball players wear eye protectors, and bicycle riders and horseback riders wear helmets. When areas of the body show weakness, degenerative changes, or symptoms of overload, those areas should be protected. For example, the elbow with symptoms of tendonitis can be partially protected by a counterforce brace called a "tennis elbow" band, which helps reduce the amount of force transmitted up the arm to the elbow. A jogger with excessive pronation and soreness in the foot or knee may be helped by an orthotic.

Having the right sports equipment and apparel is also important. For example, a tennis raquet must not be too heavy and the grip size must be right. Adequate clothing must be used on cold days. A proper, precisely fitting athletic shoe is essential for runners, joggers, and tennis players.[34]

The Responsibility of the Individual

The individual's responsibility is to stay within the tolerance of his or her musculoskeletal system. To know those limits may require a physician's advice, but it also requires individual judgment. This means that a tennis player should not play that extra set, and that a runner should not attempt that extra three miles. It also means that a tennis player should not string the raquet too tight and that a runner should obtain the best running shoe for the conditions that he or she will encounter. It means, too, that the physician should provide the interested patient with as much information as possible about exercise—its potential benefits, its risks, the most appropriate way to carry out an individually tailored exercise program, and the importance of "listening to your body."

The individual who wishes to exercise more actively and more regularly should be confident that if an injury or other problem develops there is usually a solution. If the problem is not solved, there is almost always some other sport to provide exercise and fun. The runner can change to cycling, the tennis player can swim. The best advice to the patient is usually: "Don't quit."

Chapter 7

Exercise and Public Policy

Exercise has a place in federal, state, and local strategies to improve the health of Americans. To understand how exercise fits into broader strategies to improve health, it is useful to examine the context in which public policies on health are emerging, the evolution of new health promotion and disease prevention strategies in the United States, and the role of specific federal, state, and local government agencies in promoting exercise.

HEALTH PRIORITIES AND HEALTH POLICIES IN THE 1970s AND 1980s: THE CONTEXT FOR CHANGE

During the past decade, several developments have contributed to a growing interest at all levels of government in such concepts as "prevention," "health promotion," "health maintenance," "wellness," and "fitness" and to an increasing awareness of behavior or lifestyle as a major determinant of health and illness. First, during the 1970s and continuing into the 1980s, public policymakers, particularly at the federal level of government, have been confronted with a series of recurring "health care crises." These crises have centered on the cost, effectiveness, and quality of health care, as well as on the problem of access to care. The issues commanding the most attention have been the rapidly rising cost of care, especially hospital care, and questions about the effectiveness of health care—or more precisely, the role and perhaps the limits of medicine—in further improving the health status of the American people. In the mid-1970s people both inside and outside government began to press for a reassessment of health priorities and health policies in the United States. With costs climbing and with well over 90 percent of the nation's health expenditures devoted to financing health care or to supporting in some way the health care system, sharp questions began to be raised about the return on this investment, in terms not only of meeting the needs of the sick but also of improving the health and well-being of the American population as a whole.

Public policymakers in the United States were not alone in raising these questions. In Great Britain, Canada, Australia, and other industrialized countries, government leaders were concerned about similar issues. Under the leadership of Minister of National Health and Welfare Marc Lalonde, the Canadian government undertook a thorough reexamination of its health policies and issued in 1974 a report entitled *A New Perspective on the Health of Canadians*.[1] This report, which presented a detailed picture of the health problems of the Canadian people and the major factors affecting their health, laid out a new set of strategies for improving their health status. The most controversial idea in the report was that health care is not the major determinant of health, and that providing access to and improving the quality of health care are not the only steps that might be taken to improve a population's health. This reexamination of Canadian health policies was undertaken after the establishment of a publicly funded and administered program of national health insurance, which provided access to necessary physician and hospital services for all Canadians. After examining the major factors affecting health, the Canadians grouped these factors into four broad categories—human biology, environment, lifestyle, and health care organization—and proposed five intervention strategies:

1. a health promotion strategy, stressing health education and the acceptance of greater responsibility for health by individuals and organizations;
2. a regulatory strategy, aimed at hazards to both physical and mental health;
3. a research strategy, stressing diseases of high incidence or mortality, such as mental illness and cardiovascular disease;
4. a health care efficiency strategy, aimed at achieving a better balance between cost, accessibility, and effectiveness; and
5. a goal-setting strategy, setting goals for mental and physical health as well as goals for improving the efficiency of the health care system.[2]

The promotion of exercise and physical fitness was an important element in the Canadian government's health promotion strategy. As part of that strategy, a home fitness test—the Fit-Kit—was developed and marketed, an extensive mass media campaign on exercise and fitness was launched, and the active participation of medical, scientific, sports, and lay groups was encouraged.[3]

The ideas set forth in *A New Perspective on the Health of Canadians*, which was probably one of the most widely read of government policy documents on health, did not meet with the universal acceptance of American policymakers or health professionals. There were widely diverging views among policymakers both before and after the Canadian report was issued in 1974 about the major thrust of a plan that would improve health, provide access to needed health care, and control costs. In dozens of books, different writers approached these problems from different perspectives—economic, social, political, ethical, historical, epidemiological, and clinical. The titles of these books hint at the nature of health policy debates: *Who Shall Live? Health, Economics, and Social Choice; Medical Nemesis: The Expropriation of Health; The End of Medicine; The Role of Medicine: Dream, Mirage, or Nemesis?; Doing Better and Feeling Worse: Health in the United States; Life and Death and Medicine; Humanizing Health Care: Alternative Futures for Medicine; Promoting Health: Consumer Education and National Policy; Expanding Health Care Horizons; The Healer's Art: A New Approach to the Doctor-Patient Relationship; Lives of a Cell: Notes of a Biology Watcher; Effectiveness and Efficiency: Random Reflections on Health Service.*[4] These books were published in the space of only five years, from 1972 through 1977.

Debates about the direction of health policy also took place at a number of national conferences. Two of these conferences were sponsored by the Health Policy Program of the University of California, San Francisco, the Blue Cross Association, and the Rockefeller Foundation. The first conference, "Future Directions in Health Care: The Dimensions of Medicine," was conceived because representatives of the sponsoring institutions were convinced that "a new perspective of health is essential if we are to achieve substantial improvement in the health status of the population."[5] The follow-up conference, "Future Directions in Health Care: A New Public Policy," also sponsored by the Institute of Medicine of the National Academy of Sciences, focused on the policy implications of a broader view of the influences on health—a view that encompasses biological, behaviorial, sociocultural, and environmental determinants of health.[6] Still another important conference was "The National Conference on Preventive Medicine," sponsored by the John E. Fogarty International Center for Advanced Study in the Health Sciences of the National Institutes of Health and the American College of Preventive Medicine.[7]

Several points of view on health policy emerged from these and other books and conferences, as well as from the myriad articles about health published during the past decade. Three ideas, which are still central to health policy debates in the United States in the 1980s, are particularly important to the evolution of health-promotion and disease-prevention policies. Each of these points of view has different implications for a plan of action to improve the health of Americans. These three viewpoints can be summarized as follows:

1. The problem with health in the United States is the health care system.

2. The problem with health in the United States is the behavior of the American people.
3. The problem with health in the United States is that health is everybody's business but no one's responsibility.

The problem with health in the United States is the health care system. The health care system is essentially a "treatment" system or a "sickness" system geared toward the care of acute episodes of illness in physicians' offices or in short-stay hospitals. This system does not mesh with the population's health problems. The major health problems of Americans today are chronic and degenerative diseases—coronary heart disease, stroke, arthritis and rheumatism, diabetes mellitus, chronic obstructive pulmonary disease—malignant neoplasms, accidents and violence, mental and emotional disorders, and the abuse of alcohol, tobacco, and drugs. With an increasing number of elderly people, whose chief health problems are chronic and degenerative diseases, there is a need for continuing care in managing illness and for other types of assistance directed toward helping the elderly maintain an independent level of functioning in their daily activities. There is little emphasis within the health care system on providing continuing care and support for those with chronic illness. There is also little room in the system for heatlh promotion and disease prevention for people of any age. Few preventive health services are routinely available in physicians' offices or in hospital outpatient clinics; in addition, few are routinely reimbursable through public or private health insurance. The major way to improve health and to control costs, according to proponents of this view, is to make the heatlh care system more efficient and more responsive to the population's health needs—to improve the way health care is delivered and financed.

The problem with health in the United States is the behavior of the American people. Many of America's major health problems have been labeled "behavioral" or "lifestyle" problems or problems whose root causes lie in "self-imposed" risks. These "bad habits" are directly related, some say, both to rising health care costs and to medicine's limited capacity to improve the health of the population. Curtailing costs directly depends on curbing or eliminating these habits, and a preventive strategy focused on altering individual behavior should be a major tool in any long-term cost-containment strategy. This point of view was expressed by the late John Knowles in an essay entitled "The Responsibility of the Individual":

> Prevention of disease means forsaking the bad habits which many people enjoy—overeating, too much drinking, taking pills, staying up at night,

engaging in promiscuous sex, driving too fast, and smoking cigarettes. . . . The cost of sloth, gluttony, alcoholic intemperance, reckless driving, sexual frenzy, and smoking is now a national, and not an individual, responsibility. This is justified as individual freedom—but one man's freedom in health is another man's shackle in taxes and insurance premiums. I believe the idea of a "right" to health should be replaced by the idea of an individual moral obligation to preserve one's own health—a public duty if you will.[8]

As evidence of the potent influence of behavior on health, proponents of this view point to the results of studies by Breslow and Belloc.[9] After conducting studies of a sample of nearly 7000 persons in Alameda County, California, during a 5½-year period from 1965 through 1970, these investigators found that "good" individual health practices—not smoking, drinking alcoholic beverages in moderation, eating breakfast, not eating between meals, maintaining normal body weight, sleeping for 7 to 8 hours daily, and engaging in regular physical activity—were related to increased life expectancy, especially for men. Based on the age-specific death rates of men during the study period according to the number of health practices that they had reported following, a 45-year-old white man who followed all the health practices could be expected to live on an average 11 years longer than a man who had reported following fewer than four of the practices. The difference between the two health practice groups for women was less, a little over 7 years. A 9½-year follow-up study of this population conducted in 1974 showed that mortality rates continued to be much higher among those with poor health habits and to be much lower for both men and women who followed good health practices. In this study, reported by Breslow and Enstrom, men following six to seven health practices had a standardized mortality ratio only 37 percent that of men following zero to three health practices; women following six to seven health practices had a mortality ratio only 50 percent that of women who followed zero to three health practices.[10] In another recent study of health practices in the Alameda County population by Wiley and Camacho, the practices were analyzed to see if they could be used to predict future health status. These investigators found that certain components of lifestyle, individually and in combination, do appear to predict future health, in particular a person's resistance to illness and disability. In this 9-year follow-up study, five behavioral factors—cigarette smoking, alcohol consumption, leisure-time physical activity, hours of sleep, and body weight—appeared to be the most potent predictors of a person's future health status.[11]

To define the problem with health in the United States as the behavior of the American people, however, is to oversimplify a complex problem. For example, other studies of the same population have shown the vital link between social and community ties and health. In a nine-year follow-up study of the Alameda County population, Berkman and Syme found that people who lacked social and community ties—for example, marital ties, contacts with friends and relatives, church membership, and informal and formal group associations—had higher mortality rates than did people who reported having such ties. The higher death rates in the group without ties, or with only minimal ties, could not be explained by self-reported physical health status at the time that the group was studied initially in 1965; by socioeconomic status; by health practices such as smoking, alcoholic beverage consumption, obesity, and physical activity; or by the utilization or nonutilization of preventive health services.[12]

All the major health problems confronting us today have multiple causes: biological, behavioral, sociocultural, and environmental. Multiple causes mean multiple opportunities for intervention. However, multiple causes also decrease the probability that any one intervention aimed toward any one factor or group of factors, behavioral or otherwise, will have a significant impact on any major health problem. The current fashion of labeling many of our major health problems as "lifestyle" problems, "behavioral" problems, "individual" problems, or "self-imposed" risks will lead inevitably to less than satisfactory policy solutions. "Blaming the victim" for his or her health problems has several causes and consequences. As Crawford points out:

> [There is an] emergence of an ideology which blames the individual for her or his illness and proposes that, instead of relying on costly and inefficient medical services, the individual should take more responsibility for her or his health. At-risk behavior is seen as the problem and changing lifestyle, through education and/or economic sanctions, as the solution. . . . The ideology of individual responsibility promotes the concept of wise living which views the individual as essentially independent of his or her surroundings, unconstrained by social events and processes. When such pressures are recognized, it is still the individual who is called upon to resist them. . . . [This ideology] poses an alternate social control formulation. It replaces reliance on therapeutic intervention with a behavioral model which requires only good living. . . . [T]he new ideology argues that individuals, if they take appropriate actions, if they, in other words, adopt lifestyles which avoid unhealthy behavior, may prevent most diseases. "Living a long life is essentially a do-it-yourself proposition," as it was put by one pundit. Policy, it is argued, must be redirected away from the extension of social programs which characterized the 1960s toward a health promotion strategy which calls upon the individual to become more responsible for his or her own health . . . The emergence of the ideology is explained by the contradictions arising from the threat of high medical costs, popular expectations of medicine along with

political pressures for protection or extension of entitlements, and the politicization of environment and occupational health issues. These ideological initiatives, on the one hand, serve to reorder expectations and to justify the retrenchments from rights and entitlements to medical services, and, on the other hand, attempt to divert attention from the social [and environmental and occupational] causation of disease.[13]

The problem with health in the United States is that health is everybody's business but no one's responsibility. At the federal level of government alone, a conservative count of agencies with responsibilities or functions related to health shows 12 departments, 17 independent agencies, 3 quasi-official agencies, several permanent or temporary offices within the Executive Office of the President, and 4 agencies within the legislative branch.[14] (This count does not include congressional committees and subcommittees with jurisdiction in health-related areas.) In fact, many health activities at the federal level lie essentially outside the Department of Health and Human Services, especially those that involve regulation in the areas of nutrition, environmental protection, and consumer product safety. Food and nutrition programs are administered by the Department of Agriculture; occupational health and safety programs are administered by the Department of Labor; environmental control programs are administered by the Environmental Protection Agency and other agencies; consumer product safety programs are administered by the Consumer Product Safety Commission; and recreational safety programs, the regulation of home safety codes and standards, and fire prevention programs are administered by independent agencies or departments whose primary emphasis is not health related. This problem is compounded by still other problems: (1) there are few intraagency mechanisms for sharing information about health policy development; (2) there are few interagency mechanisms to encourage cooperation in health policy development; (3) health policy responsibility in the Congress is even more fragmented than in the executive branch; and (4) the federal–state–local infrastructure to plan for health, which is only now beginning to emerge, is outside the long-established federal–state–local public health network.

The pursuit of health in the United States, however, is the exclusive enterprise neither of government nor of medicine. It is a mutual enterprise including government, business and industry, health professionals, voluntary and health professional organizations, civic and community groups, and families and individuals. While public policymakers have been preoccupied with the "health care crises" of the 1970s, a consumer health movement—including "holistic" health and wellness groups, self-care, self-help, and mutual aid groups, women's health groups, and exercise and fitness advocates—has helped set the stage for new initiatives in health promotion and disease prevention in the United States.

HEALTH PROMOTION AND DISEASE PREVENTION: A NATIONAL STRATEGY FOR THE 1980s

Policymakers in the United States have yet to reach consensus on a broad-based approach to improving the health of the population. However, several events during the past six years have led to the development of a national strategy for health promotion and disease prevention.

One of the potentially most significant of these events was the passage of the National Health Planning and Resources Development Act (Public Law 93-641) in 1974, the year that Canada's Department of National Health and Welfare issued its report, *A New Perspective on the Health of Canadians.* In the U.S. House of Representatives Committee Report on this legislation, one statement reflected an intended effect of the act:

> If health planning is actually to improve people's health, it must not be limited just to planning for medical care. In recent years it has become increasingly clear that our health, both individually and collectively, is determined by the environment we live in (physical, work and home), our culture and our individual lifestyles as much as by the availability of medical care.[15]

Two of the 10 national health priorities set forth in the act deal specifically with disease prevention and consumer health education:

8. The promotion of activities for the prevention of disease including studies of nutritional and environmental factors affecting health and the provision of preventive health care services.
10. The development of effective methods of educating the general public concerning proper personal (including preventive) health care and methods for effective use of available health services.[16]

Initial guidelines issued to State Health Planning and Development Agencies (SHPDAs) and local Health Systems Agencies (HSAs) to aid them in complying with the provisions of Public Law 93-641 introduced general goals and objectives as well as a new taxonomy to be used in planning for health. According to these guidelines, both State Health

Plans and Health Systems Plans must include plans for health promotion, health protection, disease detection and prevention services, and treatment and rehabilitation services. The National Health Planning and Development Act was enacted when decentralization of government authority and "New Federalism" were still primary strategies for achieving national objectives and when the role of special interests, such as organized medicine, was expanding. SHPDAs and HSAs, created by the law, resisted efforts to impose what they considered to be too much federal direction and regulation. With few exceptions, HSAs were not part of local government, but rather nonprofit private agencies strongly influenced by health care providers (e.g., physicians and hospitals) represented on their boards of directors. With their broad and ambiguous mandates, with pressure to do something about the rapidly rising cost of health care, and with their inexperienced staffs and limited resources, it would not be surprising if HSAs did not attach a high priority to planning for health promotion and disease prevention. Also, the development of complete national health guidelines and of State and Health Systems Plans has been painfully slow, and, at this point, probably represents only a small step forward in terms of delineating and planning a full range of interventions with an impact on health.

Nevertheless, a survey of 65 HSAs conducted in 1979 by the Bureau of Health Planning in the Health Resources Administration of the Department of Health, Education, and Welfare revealed that 62 of these agencies selected health promotion and education as prime concerns and established goals for them in their "first-year" Health Systems Plans.[17] Seven of the 62 plans had exercise- or fitness-related goals. An earlier survey undertaken in 1978 by Higgins, Philips, and Bruhn assessed the involvement of 203 HSAs in health promotion.[18] Responses were received from 72 percent of these agencies; more than 90 percent of the responding agencies reported planning activities for health promotion, and more than one-half of those agencies were actively working to develop health-promotion programs in their areas. A computer search of 110 first-year Health Systems Plans in July 1980 showed that 33 plans had exercise and fitness goals.[19]

The second major event influencing policy development in health promotion and disease prevention was the passage of the National Consumer Health Information and Health Promotion Act of 1976 (Public Law 94-317). This legislation, in turn, was influenced by earlier efforts of task forces created by the John H. Fogarty International Center for Advanced Study in the Health Sciences within the National Institutes of Health and the American College of Preventive Medicine.[20] Public Law 94-317 added a new title to the Public Health Service Act—Title XVII,

Health Information and Health Promotion—that gave the Secretary of Health, Education, and Welfare broad authority to:

> formulate national goals and a strategy to achieve such goals with respect to health information and health promotion, preventive health services, and education in the appropriate use of health care;
> analyze resources for implementing these goals and this strategy, recommend educational, quality assurance, and manpower resources needed; and
> undertake and support research and demonstrations respecting
> health information and health promotion, preventive health services, and education in the appropriate use of health care.

Section 1706 of Title XVII also directed the secretary to establish an Office of Health Information and Health Promotion within the Office of the Assistant Secretary for Health as a focal point for coordinating departmental and private-sector activities relating to health information and health promotion, preventive health services, and education in the appropriate use of health care.

Since 1977, several other developments have led to the further definition of policy directions in health promotion and prevention. In December 1977 a task force composed of representatives of all agencies within the Department of Health, Education, and Welfare was convened to review and analyze departmental activities in disease prevention and health promotion as well as activities in other federal agencies. This internal effort was aided by the efforts of many others outside of government—the Institute of Medicine of the National Academy of Sciences and the Health Policy Program of the University of California, San Francisco, among them.[21] In November 1978 the Health Services and Centers Amendments of 1978 (Public Law 95-626) were passed.

Title II, the health services extension, provided for the following:

> Health incentive grants for comprehensive public health services. The intent of these grants was to supplement existing categorical programs of federal assistance to the states by a national program of stable generic support for such public health activities as the prevention and control of environmental health hazards, prevention and control of disease, prevention and control of health problems of particularly vulnerable population groups, and regulation of health care facilities and health service delivery systems.
> Project grants for preventive services. These grants include grants for hypertension control (programs for screening, detection, diagnosis, prevention, treatment referral, follow-up on compliance with treatment); immunization of children (e.g., against measles,

rubella, poliomyelitis, diphtheria, pertussis, tetanus, and mumps); and rodent control.

Formula grants to states for preventive health service programs. These grants are to assist states in planning, developing, and providing preventive health service programs designed to reduce, through primary or secondary prevention of risk factors or causative conditions, the mortality rate for one or more of the five leading causes of death in a state or the burden of illness associated with one or more of the five leading causes of morbidity in the state. States are required to develop detailed program plans in prevention to qualify for these grants; each program is required to have a separate health communications component that describes how the communications media, including the electronic media, will be used to further the purposes of the program.

Projects and programs for the prevention and control of venereal disease.

Lead-based paint poisoning prevention programs.

A select panel for the promotion of child health.

Title IV, resources for disease prevention and health promotion, provided for:

Five intensive and comprehensive community-based demonstration projects in both rural and urban areas. These projects are to demonstrate and evaluate optimal methods of organizing and delivering comprehensive health services to defined populations.

A comprehensive program to deter smoking and the use of alcoholic beverages among children and adolescents. This program includes support of biomedical and behavioral research to understand biological and behavioral determinants of smoking and the use of alcoholic beverages among children and adolescents (emphasis on children under 12), as well as grants to states for community- and school-based demonstration projects in the areas of smoking and alcohol.

Title V directed the Secretary of Health, Education, and Welfare to establish a new office—the Office of Health Information, Health Promotion, and Physical Fitness and Sports Medicine—within the Office of the Assistant Secretary for Health to supplant the Office of Health Information and Health Promotion.

As a fitting climax to these activities, in July 1979, the Department of Health, Education, and Welfare published *Healthy People: The Surgeon General's Report on Health Promotion and Disease Prevention.*[22] A companion document, *Healthy People: The Surgeon General's Report on Health Promotion and Disease Prevention: Background Papers,* is a more detailed publication prepared by the Institute of Medicine; it contains state-of-the-art background papers on several discrete areas of prevention.[23] The importance of both the Surgeon General's Report and the final report of the Departmental Task Force on Prevention, *Disease Prevention and Health Promotion: Federal Programs and Prospects,*[24] is that these documents establish a conceptual framework for prevention, develop criteria for setting prevention priorities, and set several priorities for action. The task force made recommendations for departmental action in 15 areas, ranging from hypertension to environmental toxicology.

The Surgeon General's Report sets health goals and subgoals for infants, children, adolescents and young adults, adults, and older adults. Both the Surgeon General's Report and the Task Force Report identify "actions for health" as health promotion, health protection, and preventive health services. Target areas in health promotion include smoking cessation, reducing alcohol and drug abuse, stress control, improved nutrition, and exercise and fitness. Priorities in health protection include toxic agent control, occupational safety and health, accidental injury control, fluoridation of community water supplies, and infectious agent control. Major emphasis under preventive health services is given to family planning, pregnancy and infant care, immunizations, sexually transmissible disease services, and control of high blood pressure.

The Health Policy Program has developed a framework similar to that used in both the Surgeon General's Report and in the Canadian policy document, *A New Perspective on the Health of Canadians.*[24] This framework also defines actions for health as health promotion, health protection, and preventive health services.

Health promotion activities, which are designed for broad population groups, are aimed at sociocultural and behavioral factors that affect health. These activities are directed toward families, special vulnerable groups—for example, mothers, infants, children, adolescents, and the elderly—communities, and the general population. The setting for such activities can be schools, places of work, churches, civic groups, and clubs. The aim is to augment people's knowledge, skills, and/or resources so that they can make positive decisions about health. Program areas include

mass health education and information programs relating to smoking, diet and nutrition, alcohol and drugs, driving, exercise and physical fitness, human sexuality and contraceptive use, family development, and mental health;

food and nutritional programs; and
family and group support

Health protection activities, which are also designed for population groups, are aimed at specific or identified hazards to health and safety in the biological, chemical, and physical environment. Program areas include efforts aimed at controlling hazards, essentially through regulatory strategies, in:

the general environment (air pollution, water pollution, noise pollution, radiation, pesticides and other toxic substances);
special environments (workplace, home, hospital, transportation, recreation); and
consumer products (food, drugs, medical devices, diagnostic products, alcohol, tobacco, firearms, tools, toys, apparel, household products and appliances, and motor vehicles).

Preventive health services, which are tailored to individuals, are aimed at behavioral and human biological factors that influence health. These services include:

personal health education and information programs relating to smoking, diet and nutrition, exercise and physical fitness, alcohol and drugs, and other factors noted above;
pre- and postnatal care, including nutrition counseling;
family planning services;
genetic counseling services;
immunization; and
screening services aimed at the early detection of hypertension, diabetes, cancer, cardiovascular disease, sexually transmitted diseases, vision and hearing problems, lead poisoning, and congenital diseases.

In August 1979 the Department of Health, Education, and Welfare took still another step in defining health objectives for the nation when it published *Preventing Disease/Promoting Health: Objectives for the Nation*, a document containing drafts of working papers developed in 15 areas by participants in a public, department-sponsored conference held in Atlanta in June 1979.[26] This document was widely circulated for public review and comments. Whether these prevention objectives will become departmental objectives or will be recommended as objectives in guidelines for state and local programs is as yet unclear. Objectives have been developed in the following 15 areas:

1. hypertension
2. family planning
3. pregnancy and infant health

4. immunization
5. sexually transmitted diseases
6. toxic agent control
7. occupational safety and health
8. accident prevention and injury control
9. fluoridation
10. surveillance and control of infectious diseases
11. smoking and health
12. alcohol and drug abuse
13. nutrition
14. physical fitness and exercise
15. stress

The best available evidence indicates that exercise has an important place in broader strategies to improve the health of the American population. As mentioned previously in this book, epidemiological and clinical studies conducted during the past 25 years have clarified the role of exercise in the primary and secondary prevention of coronary heart disease and in the rehabilitation of cardiac patients; studies also have suggested an important role for exercise in the control of hypertension, diabetes mellitus, and obesity, as well as a potential role for exercise in the prevention or alleviation of anxiety and depression. Regular physical activity also can increase stamina and physical work capacity and can enhance the quality of life, often encouraging a change in health habits.

A major campaign to promote exercise is an attractive policy option for all levels of government for the following reasons:

Substantial evidence points to the health benefits of regular exercise.

Public interest in exercise and physical fitness is strong and growing.

A campaign to promote exercise, unlike campaigns to change smoking, drinking, and dietary habits, would not be met by a strong lobby or a coalition of special interest groups—or health professional groups—united against it.

Business and industry and organized medicine have thus far been supportive, if not enthusiastic in some cases, about promoting exercise—either in their own self-interest for public relations reasons, or in the case of the former group, in the interest of employee relations.

A campaign to promote exercise lends itself to a continuum of support at the federal, state, and local levels.

Costs would appear to be low at the federal, state, and local levels.

Mechanisms to administer various programs are already in place at all levels of government and at the federal level within the jurisdiction of the Department of Health and Human Services as well as of other departments and agencies.

The campaign need not be aimed at a particular segment of the population; all Americans could potentially benefit from such a program, and it is a "positive" program, unlike an antismoking initiative.

Although this campaign can best be carried out by a coordinated public and private effort, the role of specific federal, state, and local government agencies is highlighted in the following section. (A description of the mobilization of key resources to promote exercise at the community level is included in Chapter 8.)

EXERCISE AND THE FEDERAL GOVERNMENT

The involvement of federal agencies in the development of policies and programs related to exercise and physical fitness has been growing during the past 25 years. To assess the present direction of federal policy on exercise, we recently analyzed the policies of federal agencies in three departments: the Department of Health and Human Services, the Department of Education, and the Department of the Interior.[27] This analysis was based on a review of the legislative mandates of each agency and on interviews with agency staff on the policy direction of exercise-related activities, as well as on the agency's level of involvement in these activities in terms of budgetary and staff commitments.

Department of Health and Human Services

The Office of Health Information, Health Promotion, and Physical Fitness and Sports Medicine has broad mandates deriving from two separate pieces of legislation—the National Consumer Health Information and Health Promotion Act of 1976 (Public Law 94-317) and the Health Services and Centers Amendments of 1978 (Public Law 95-626). The purpose of the office is to coordinate all activities within the Department of Health and Human Services that relate to health information and health promotion, preventive health services, and education in the appropriate use of health care and to coordinate these activities with similar activities in the private sector. In Title V of Public Law 95-626, the Congress recognized physical fitness and sports medicine as integral components of a broader health-promotion and disease-prevention strategy at the federal level of government, and several specific functions were outlined for the office with respect to physical fitness and health and sports medicine. The office is to:

1. assist and foster research, investigations, and model projects on the

nature of physical fitness, the development of physical fitness, and the relation of physical fitness and health;

2. assist and foster research and investigations into the utilization of sports medicine, the development of sports medicine techniques, and the application of sports medicine throughout organized systems of athletic competition and in personal physical fitness development activities at every age and competition level;

3. foster and assist research into the proper role of nutrition in physical fitness programs;

4. promote the coordination of research and model programs conducted by the office with similar programs conducted by other agencies of the federal government and other public and private organizations;

5. communicate the results of studies in the widest possible manner to the American people and to special groups with particular interests and special needs in the development of physical fitness, such as young children, the handicapped, senior citizens, and workers in occupations that present special risks of physical disability.

Title V of Public Law 95-626 contains four other significant provisions with regard to exercise. The title provides for project grants to State Councils on Physical Fitness; project grants for physical fitness improvement and research projects; a National Program on Sports Medicine Research; and a conference on education in lifetime sports.

Project grants to State Councils on Physical Fitness may be made by the Office of Health Information, Health Promotion, and Physical Fitness and Sports Medicine to each state, providing that the state matches federal funds. State Councils must consist of at least 15 members, chosen by the governor to serve terms of four years, and appointed from among people who have distinguished records in the areas of physical fitness, sports medicine, public health, athletic competition, education, labor, business management, and nutrition. The functions of State Councils include the following:

1. To promote the development of physical fitness with the assistance of local health and educational agencies; business; labor unions; health action and advocacy groups; religious, fraternal, and social organizations; community-based multiservice recreational agencies; and health maintenance organizations.

2. To assess the physical fitness and nutrition status of residents of the state.

3. To plan and administer a program of grants-in-aid to support physical fitness projects, research projects, and public information efforts.

4. To evaluate and improve the availability and quality of sports medicine and athletic trainer programs in the state.

Although the legislative language is unclear, it appears that each state could receive up to $60,000 in matching grants. Thus far, the Congress has not made any of this money available.

Project grants for physical fitness improvement and research projects may be made to public or private groups to conduct research and establish model projects with regard to the improvement of physical fitness. Projects encompassed under this provision may include the following: (1) entire small communities, both urban and rural; (2) educational settings for a variety of age groups; (3) occupational settings; (4) groups of handi-capped individuals; and (5) groups of senior citizens. No moneys have yet been appropriated for these grants.

The National Program on Sports Medicine Research includes a program of project grants to conduct research into the problem of athletic injuries, the development of training and conditioning techniques, and the development of athletic protective equipment as well as a Clearing-house on Sports Medicine Research to disseminate the results of that research to practitioners in relevant fields of health care and physical fitness. This clearinghouse would be a cooperative venture with the President's Council on Physical Fitness and Sports. To fund the National Program on Sports Medicine Research and the Clearinghouse, the Congress authorized $1.5 million for each fiscal year ending September 30, 1980 and 1981. Again, these funding authorities have not been met with appropriations.

The Office of Health Information, Health Promotion, and Physical Fitness and Sports Medicine has recently developed national goals and objectives related to exercise and physical fitness as part of a national health-promotion and disease-prevention strategy.[28] Plans for implement-ing this proposed national exercise policy, which targets specific populations, are unclear; to meet these goals and objectives related to health, the office would have to rely on other federal departments and agencies as well as on state and local government agencies and private-sector organizations to develop programs, to provide services, to undertake research, and to provide technical support. The office is handicapped by the minimal budget—$800,000 for fiscal year 1980—and the small amount of staff time available to support exercise-related initiatives. The Office of Health Information, Health Promotion, and Physical Fitness and Sports Medicine operates as a program office under the Deputy Assistant Secretary for Disease Prevention and Health Promotion, Office of the Assistant Secretary of Health.

The President's Council on Physical Fitness and Sports has the longest history of involvement in exercise-related activities of any federal agency.

Created by Executive Order by President Eisenhower in 1956 and reestablished and restructured by succeeding Executive Orders of presidents throughout the years, the council's purpose is to enlist the active support and assistance of individual citizens, civic groups, professional associations, amateur and professional sports groups, private enterprise, voluntary organizations, and others in efforts to promote and improve the health of all Americans through regular participation in physical fitness and sports activities. The council is an established name in physical fitness and sports, and it has worked very successfully to stimulate private-sector support for educational and informational materials, programs and events, and conferences related to sports and physical fitness, and to cosponsor such activities. Although it is an official Advisory Body to the Office of Health Information, Health Promotion, and Physical Fitness and Sports Medicine on all matters relating to physical fitness, the council has devoted little attention to health-related fitness activities or to coordinating its activities with those of other federal agencies. It has concentrated instead on working with private industry, insurance companies, and schools. It is governed by Public Law 92-463, which sets standards for the formation and use of advisory committees, and is located within the Office of the Assistant Secretary for Health, but the council chairman reports to the Executive Office of the President, rather than to the Deputy Assistant Secretary for Disease Prevention and Health Promotion, as does the Director of the Office of Health Information, Health Promotion, and Physical Fitness and Sports Medicine.

The council consists of 15 members, including the chairman, who are not officers or employees of the federal government. These members, who are appointed by the president, are selected from among the fields of medicine, business and industry, physical education, amateur sports, and research. The council is supported by a professional staff of five, and in 1980 its budget was $800,000. The staff and budget have increased only modestly since 1962.

The National Institutes of Health have no defined policies or programs relating specifically to research on exercise and health. However, in six of the institutes, there are approximately 80 projects related to exercise, ranging from subcellular responses of the heart to exercise to the relationship of exercise to coronary heart disease risk, obesity, and hypertension. The National Heart, Lung, and Blood Institute supports the majority of work on exercise and health. The National Heart, Blood Vessel, Lung, and Blood Act of 1972 (Public Law 92-423) as well as the 1975 and 1977 amendments to the act expanded the institute's general responsibilities. The 1972 legislation established the position of Assistant Director for Health Information to disseminate information on cardiovascular and pulmonary diseases, with emphasis on the effects of such factors as exercise, diet, and stress. Also included in this legislation was a provision to establish prevention and control programs, a maximum of 30 national research and demonstration centers, and an interagency technical committee. The National Heart, Lung, and Blood Institute will soon publish a pamphlet on exercise, *Exercise and Your Heart*, which clarifies the institute's position on the benefits—and risks—of exercise.[29] Although there is substantial evidence of the health benefits of exercise, much remains to be known about the type, amount, frequency, duration, and intensity of exercise required to achieve these benefits in specific individuals or in specific populations. The National Institutes of Health could play a vital role in establishing a broader scientific data base on the relationship of exercise to health and its role in the prevention, treatment, and rehabilitation of specific health problems. The narrowly defined research objectives of individual institutes, however, are often an impediment to those proposing to study exercise.

The National Institute of Mental Health has untapped potential for examining the role of exercise in the prevention and treatment of emotional and mental problems, including stress or anxiety and depression. New research priorities within the institute focus on the prevention of mental health problems, particularly stress and violent behavior. The institute has just begun to support research on exercise, however.

Department of Education

The Department of Education and its predecessor, the Office of Education, have played a very limited role in school health education, including physical education. The Division of Comprehensive School Health was established in 1979 to promote school programs with a comprehensive health education component and to build linkages with those programs and health-related agencies. The division is encouraging comprehensive, sequentially planned K–12 school health education programs. In the past, categorical curricula have been developed in such areas as smoking, nutrition, alcohol, and drugs. Rather than promoting the development of categorical programs in exercise and physical fitness, therefore, the division recommends that exercise components be integrated into comprehensive school health curricula.

Department of the Interior

Public Law 89-29, signed May 23, 1963, established "adequate outdoor recreation" for the American people as a national priority. This legislation mandated the Department of the Interior to regularly inventory, classify, and evaluate outdoor recreation needs and resources; to prepare a nationwide outdoor recreation plan every five years; to provide technical assistance on outdoor recreation to states and localities and private interests; to encourage interstate and regional cooperation in planning, purchase, and use of outdoor recreation resources; to conduct research and set up educational programs to increase public use of outdoor recreaton; and to coordinate plans and activities related to outdoor recreation with those of other federal agencies. The National Urban Recreation Study (1978) and the Third Nationwide Outdoor Recreation Plan (1979) described the recreational needs of the country and established priorities for the Department of the Interior. Physical health, mental health, and economic activity were defined as the three primary social benefits of recreation.

Within the department, the Heritage Conservation and Recreation Service has programs directed specifically toward promoting these social benefits. The Urban Park and Recreation Recovery Program was established in 1978 by Title X of the National Parks and Recreation Act of 1978 (Public Law 95-625). The purpose of the Urban Park Act was to provide federal funds to distressed urban communities for the rehabilitation of existing facilities for recreational, health, social, and community activities and for the development of innovative projects with a nationwide demonstration potential. At this point, activities are focused primarily on urban, community-based programs, but a rural assessment study is currently in the process. The Community and Human Resource Division, also a part of the Heritage Conservation and Recreation Service, was created specifically to coordinate Department of Interior recreational activities with related activities of other federal agencies. Some of its staff members have the sole responsibility of federal agency coordination. The division has developed a variety of formal interagency agreements, including a memorandum of understanding with the Public Health Service, Department of Health and Human Services, to promote health and physical fitness objectives in park and recreation settings through cooperation of health and recreation officials at the local level. In addition, the Community and Human Resources Division has assisted the Public Health Service in a literature search on the role of recreation in improving physical and mental health; the division also has assisted the Public Health Service in disseminating information on risk-reduction programs targeted to local communities. The Administration on Aging, Department of Health and Human Services, has a memorandum of understanding with the Heritage Conservation and Recreation Service to provide assistance in policy planning and project implementation for strategies to provide recreation services to the elderly.

Coordinating Federal Efforts to Promote Exercise

The major findings of our analysis of policies on exercise in federal agencies can be summarized as follows:

1. The federal government has no clear or consistent policy on exercise.
2. Among the federal agencies surveyed, there are five existing or emerging policy strategies related to exercise: a health-promotion/disease-prevention strategy; a sports and physical fitness strategy; a health research strategy; a physical education strategy or a school health education strategy; and a recreation strategy.
3. All these policy strategies are interrelated and complementary. However, the six federal agencies work relatively autonomously to develop individual strategies, some agencies to fulfill specific legislative mandates, and others to meet general agency goals and objectives.
4. No lead agency has been identified to develop an overall federal policy on exercise, including national goals and objectives related to exercise, or to coordinate existing or emerging policies and programs in the range of federal agencies.
5. One agency—the Office of Health Information, Health Promotion, and Physical Fitness and Sports Medicine—has several legislative mandates supporting its identification as lead agency to develop a federal exercise policy based on evidence of the health benefits of exercise and to coordinate its exercise-related activities with those of other federal agencies as well as other public and private organizations.
6. This agency has already defined national goals and objectives to promote exercise and physical fitness as part of national goals and objectives to promote health and to prevent disease.
7. This agency is presently handicapped in assuming a lead agency role in federal exercise-related activities, however, because funds authorized by the Congress to support the majority of agency exercise-related activities have not yet been appropriated, and only a minimal amount of staff time is devoted to these activities.
8. A health-promotion/disease-prevention strategy related to exercise is not in conflict with other existing and emerging policy strategies.
9. Current evidence on exercise suggests that different types of exercise may have different health benefits—and risks—for different populations, and that there may be other benefits of exercise that are not strictly health related.
10. A clear, consistent, and coordinated federal effort to promote exercise is necessary for several reasons: (a) to clarify and to maximize the health and nonhealth benefits of exercise for different target populations; (b) to integrate existing and emerging exercise-related policies and programs within the Department of Health and Human Services, the Department of Education, the Department of

the Interior, and other federal departments and agencies; (c) to create a federal focal point of support for state and local government efforts to promote exercise; and (d) to capitalize on the strong and growing public interest in exercise and physical fitness and on the current trend toward exercise promotion in the private sector (e.g., business and industry, professional and voluntary health associations).

We believe that the priority of exercise and physical fitness activities should be raised throughout the federal government. The potential benefits of exercise have yet to be realized by a majority of Americans—only about one-third to one-half of all Americans report exercising regularly. Children and adolescents, women, the elderly, the poor, nonwhites, the handicapped, and innercity and rural residents are underrepresented in the exercising population. We also believe that national goals and objectives related to exercise and physical fitness should reflect the health benefits— and risks—of different types of exercise for different populations as well as the nonhealth benefits of exercise and the need to integrate existing and emerging policy strategies related to exercise in various departments and agencies. Each of the policy strategies now being developed by federal agencies can serve to promote health and nonhealth benefits of exercise and physical fitness. To integrate these strategies, each federal department or agency with an existing or emerging policy strategy related to exercise— a health-promotion/disease-prevention strategy, a physical fitness and sports strategy, a health research strategy, a physical education or school health education strategy, a recreation strategy—should be represented on a federal Interagency Working Committee on Exercise. This committee should review and refine the national goals and objectives on exercise and physical fitness developed by the Office of Health Information, Health Promotion, and Physical Fitness and Sports Medicine, and it should delineate individual and mutual agency goals and objectives related to exercise. All federal agencies involved should agree on national goals and objectives, and interagency memoranda of agreement should be used to implement these goals and objectives.

Clearly, the Congress has acknowledged the importance of exercise by outlining specific provisions in the wording of Public Law 95-626. However, funds authorized to be appropriated for the support of exercise activities—including funds for the operation of the Office of Health Information, Health Promotion, and Physical Fitness and Sports Medicine itself—are either very modest or nonexistent and pose a major stumbling block to the office in carrying out its new mandates. If funds authorized are not appropriated, the mandates of the office will be further undercut. This office has potentially the major role to play in developing a coherent federal effort with regard to exercise. That potential, however, is yet to be realized.

Lack of appropriations is not the only problem hampering the Office of Health Information, Health Promotion, and Physical Fitness and Sports Medicine. There are a number of serious flaws in the legislation that created the office and then broadened its mandates—the National Consumer Health Information and Health Promotion Act of 1976 (Public Law 94-317) and Title V of the Health Services and Centers Amendments of 1978 (Public Law 95-626). Coordination of "all activities within the Department and the private sector that relate to health information and health promotion," one of the principal functions of the tiny office, is a difficult job at best. When few resources are provided, it is impossible. The coordination strategy requires the office to obtain the voluntary cooperation of totally independent organizational units, including private businesses and industries and voluntary health organizations, in the absence of political or economic incentives. A similar problem plagues other federal programs, including health planning agencies and agencies created by the Older American Act.[30] This problem has been described clearly and crisply by Pressman and Wildavsky:

> Telling another person to coordinate . . . does not tell him what to do. . . . Everyone wants to coordinate—on his own terms. Invocation of coordination does not necessarily provide either a statement of, or a solution to, the problem, but it may be a way of avoiding both when accurate prescription would be too painful. . . . Coordination means getting what you do not have.[31]

Coordination as a policy strategy creates a variety of implementation problems, each related to the definition of coordination. Six different problems, each calling for a different implementation strategy, have been described by Marmor and Kutza: (1) fragmentation; (2) duplication of services; (3) gaps in services; (4) inaccessibility of services; (5) discontinuity of serial and sequential services; and (6) incoherency among simultaneous services.[32] Although there is no agreement on what coordination means, and certainly no evidence that the Congress had any specific definition in mind in enacting Public Laws 94-317 and 95-626, one common element is that the problem requiring "coordination" is nearly always considered from the standpoint of service providers rather than of service beneficiaries or consumers.[33] Conceptual fuzziness creates serious problems in evaluation and accountability. Particularly difficult will be measures of outcome, as opposed to input or process measures. Estes has described these difficulties and others in assessing problems in the Older Americans Act:

Implementation problems are likely to occur in broad multiple-aim programs that require extremely complex, highly uncertain, and often contradictory implementation processes for accomplishment. For coordination policies in particular, the requirement of joint action extends the number of relevant actors and decision points, increasing the unpredictability of action and decreasing the probability of program success. Perhaps most important, policy failures are easily attributed to implementation failures and weaknesses in the agencies and actors responsible for implementation rather than the mismatches between ends and means in the policy design.[34]

In spite of formidable obstacles, the Office of Health Information, Health Promotion, and Physical Fitness and Sports Medicine has performed yeoman service. It has been a rallying point for those interested in health promotion and disease prevention. It has spearheaded the Surgeon General's efforts in policy development in this area, and it has managed to keep issues in health promotion and disease prevention before policymakers in the Department of Health and Human Services and in the Congress. Our concern is not with the quality or intensity of effort, but with the flawed legislative mandate and lack of appropriations.

A Health-Based Federal Strategy to Promote Exercise

A strong federal effort to promote exercise can be launched as an integral part of broader strategies in health promotion and disease prevention, health care, and health research.

Health Promotion and Disease Prevention. Activities focused on exercise and physical fitness at the federal level of government might focus on two basic goals: getting people interested in exercise, especially dynamic aerobic exercise, and providing opportunities for them to exercise. Both the Stanford Three Community Study in California and the North Karelia, Finland, study have demonstrated that a mass media campaign can be an effective tool in decreasing major cardiovascular risk factors in target populations.[35] Lalonde called for a mass media campaign by the Canadian government to promote exercise, and this campaign has been well accepted by the Canadian people. [36]

In the United States, the President's Council on Physical Fitness and Sports has begun a small-scale media campaign, which could be substantially improved in terms of its coordination, size, and direction. Funds to finance this media campaign come almost exclusively from sources outside government—businesses, industries, and other private sources with some incentive for promoting exercise and physical fitness.

Recently the Blue Cross Association, the American Medical Association, and a host of companies marketing sports and exercise apparel and equipment have begun media campaigns. These campaigns in part may be responsible for stimulating the increased public interest and participation in exercise.

It seems reasonable that the Congress could capitalize on the current private-sector enthusiasm for promoting exercise by appropriating adequate funds for the Office of Health Information, Health Promotion, and Physical Fitness and Sports Medicine to conduct a major mass media program. Since other groups are promoting exercise or fitness in general in their campaigns, perhaps the best role for the office to play is to develop and air more specialized fitness messages. Television, radio, magazine, and newspaper messages might instruct people on the need for regular, not just weekend, physical activity, as well as on the differences between dynamic aerobic and low-intensity exercise and the importance of cardiovascular conditioning. Messages could be targeted to low-income populations, the elderly, minorities, and women, who are underrepresented in the exercising population. Special messages could be developed for children and adolescents as well as for handicapped persons. The office also could assume greater responsibility for providing information on the prescription of exercise to physicians by working with county medical societies and medical schools conducting courses in continuing education. Efforts to provide physicians with this kind of information and to encourage them to write individualized exercise programs for patients on prescription pads are still small and unfocused.

The second major role for the federal government with regard to exercise in a health promotion context is in providing opportunities, either directly or indirectly, for people to exercise. Both the provision of exercise programs and the provision of exercise facilities are ways to enhance opportunities for exercise. Perhaps a logical place for the federal government to begin is to provide more of these opportunities for its own workers.[37] The President's Council on Physical Fitness and Sports has had some success in the past in convincing federal agencies to provide exercise facilities for their own employees. The National Science Foundation, National Aeronautics and Space Administration, Environmental Protection Agency, Smithsonian Institute, the Federal Reserve Board, and the Departments of Justice, Defense, State, and Agriculture have offered exercise programs to some or occasionally all of their employees. Only about 40,000 federal employees, however, are now offered exercise programs, in which 15 percent actually participate either formally or informally. This represents a tiny fraction of the federal civilian work force of nearly 3 million.

Several years ago, a study in Region IX of the Department of Health,

Education, and Welfare indicated employee interest in a physical fitness program; it also pointed out potential barriers to the development of such a program for federal employees.[38] Among the barriers to the development of such a program were cost, lack of space, and apparent lack of management support for an organized program of health maintenance. The Region IX study is a prototype of the kind of study that might be undertaken by employee and employer groups within the federal government to define precisely the objectives, the resources, and the likely costs of such a program.

The Office of Health Information, Health Promotion, and Physical Fitness and Sports Medicine has recently developed a proposal for a health promotion program for employees of the Department of Health and Human Services.[39] The program, which would initially be made available to employees in the Washington, D.C., headquarters of the department, would emphasize risk assessment and lifestyle change. The purpose of the demonstration project is to determine the feasibility, acceptability, and effectiveness of establishing a health-promotion program at department worksites. The major intent is to document changes in risks and to assess both behavior change and changes in morbidity and mortality, particularly those associated with cardiovascular disease. Program components include exercise (jogging, aerobic dance, conditioning exercises), smoking cessation, and nutrition/weight control. For those individuals deemed to be at high risk of cardiovascular disease or at some medical risk, a stress test or some equivalent will be recommended, and these individuals will be referred to a Public Health Service health unit for counseling and for subsequent referral to a private physician before being permitted to enter the exercise program. It is interesting that this exercise demonstration project was proposed 12 years after a similar project was initiated jointly by the National Aeronautics and Space Administration (NASA) and the U.S. Public Health Service (PHS). The joing NASA/PHS project, which was evaluated in 1972, clearly demonstrated the feasibility and benefits of both supervised (stress laboratory exercise and jogging) and unsupervised exercise programs for federal employees.[40]

Health Care. The Health Care Financing Administration within the Department of Health and Human Services is responsible for the administration of the Medicaid and Medicare programs. One possible area for consideration might be Medicaid and Medicare reimbursement for cardiac exercise rehabilitation programs. Careful analysis of these exercise rehabilitation programs as well as their costs is imperative, however, before such a change is undertaken on a large scale. It also would be appropriate to examine carefully the question of reimbursement for preventive health examinations, including those that might be carried out prior to the initiation of an aerobic exercise program. Perhaps the newly established National Center for Health Care Technology in the Office of the Assistant Secretary for Health could undertake such a study.

Health Research. Pivotal studies on the role of exercise in the prevention of coronary heart disease and in the treatment or control of hypertension, diabetes mellitus, and obesity have been described in Chapters 3 and 4. Although these studies provide substantial evidence of the health benefits of exercise, there are still many unanswered questions about the relationship between exercise and health as well as about the relationship between exercise and specific health problems. The Department of Health, Education, and Welfare Task Force on Prevention identified a number of health research needs, ranging from studies of the relationship between physical activity and aging to the role of physical fitness in the reduction of mental health disorders.[41] A major prospective research effort in the field of physical activity has been called for by Fox, Naughton, and Haskell, by Morris, and by Mann.[42] A well-controlled, large-scale, prospective intervention program might do much to provide additional information about the effect of physical activity on coronary heart disease and on other problems for men and women of different racial and socioeconomic backgrounds. Since the cost of such a study would be large, however, the feasibility of actually carrying it out has been questioned. The need for such epidemiological studies also has been questioned. Havas, for example, believes that we do not need more epidemiological studies, but rather a synthesis of the findings of studies that already have been conducted.[43] We believe, however, that there is a serious lack of data on the effect of different types of exercise on the health and health problems of women, minority populations, the elderly, and low-income populations. Other unanswered research questions about the role of exercise in specific health problems and in other specific areas are summarized briefly below.

Cardiac Diseases. Because we do not know why dynamic aerobic exercise seems to exert a protective effect against coronary heart disease, expanded funding for research projects investigating this question is warranted. A better understanding of this question might lead to clarification of the type, intensity, duration, and frequency of physical activity needed to achieve a protective effect. Therapeutic actions, other than exercise, that might produce similar effects also should be investigated. Expanded research funding for the study of the relationship between exercise and lipids, particularly high-density lipoproteins, might provide the most immediate rewards.

The use of exercise as a tool in the long-term rehabilitation of myocardial infarction patients and of patients who have undergone coronary artery bypass surgery is a relatively recent innovation. Thus, few studies have examined the effectiveness of exercise as a secondary or tertiary preventive measure. With perhaps 20 percent of the nation's deaths due to second heart attacks in post–myocardial infarction patients, expanded research funding for an examination of this topic, too, is indicated.

Noncardiac Diseases. Studies have shown that dynamic aerobic exercise may also play a useful role in the treatment of many noncardiac diseases, including diabetes mellitus, hypertension, and obesity. Perhaps half of the adult population of the United States has one of these health problems. More research is needed to determine the role of exercise in both the prevention and the treatment of these problems.

The public seems to be more convinced than health professionals of the psychological benefits of exercise. Research into the potential usefulness of exercise as a treatment for depression, anxiety, and psychic stress, which are common medical problems, deserves increased emphasis by mental health funding sources.

Injuries resulting from exercise have unfortunately kept pace with the recent exercise boom. Much work needs to be done in this field, particularly in the development of more effective preventive measures and improved treatment methods.

Compliance with Exercise Prescriptions. With the increasing prescription of exercise by physicians, compliance in beginning and continuing exercise programs will undoubtedly become a larger problem. Too little is known about the motivation to exercise; much more could be learned about compliance in healthy children, adolescents, and adults as well as in the obese and in persons with hypertension, coronary heart disease, or diabetes mellitus. Examination of the motivation and past background of adults who have continued to exercise since childhood might prove useful. Large-scale studies of the effects of various promotional messages and methods, such as the Stanford Three Community Study, also are needed. Not only do the specifics of mass media messages need to be carefully evaluated in relation to reducing cardiovascular disease risk factors, but smaller scale studies are also needed to evaluate the effects on attitude and exercise behavior of specific information provided to patients by physicians. The National Institutes of Health—in particular, the National Heart, Lung, and Blood Institute, the National Institute on Aging, the National Institute of Child Health and Human Development, the National Institute on Arthritis and Metabolic Diseases, and the National Institute of Mental Health, as well as the Office of Health Information, Health Promotion, and Physical Fitness and

Sports Medicine, and the National Center for Health Services Research—could provide funding for exercise research.

Other Federal Strategies to Promote Exercise

Other federal strategies to promote regular exercise include an education strategy and a recreation strategy. The newly organized Department of Education could take the lead in developing a national program of physical fitness and sports in all the nation's public schools—elementary schools, secondary schools, community colleges, and four-year colleges and universities. These institutions provide a network of facilities and staff that is accessible not only to those attending school but also to all people who are not homebound or institutionalized. Federal matching grants to states could be made available for the development of a curriculum related to the teaching of lifetime sports and the health benefits of regular exercise, as well as the development of dynamic aerobic exercise programs for children, adolescents, and adults who want to participate. Funds also could be made available to create the necessary school exercise facilities (e.g., swimming pools) where these are lacking. The advantages of this strategy are that existing schools and school systems already provide facilities and exercise programs, including competitive sports programs, and that schools have the capacity to reach the general population easily if they are provided with the resources to do so. The secretary of the new Department of Education promised at the First National Conference on Physical Fitness and Sports for All in Washington, D.C., in March 1980 to review departmental programs that "affect physical fitness teaching and training." She also has indicated that she is "pleased by recent increases in sports participation among women and girls, and hoped that there would be similar improvements in opportunities for the elderly and the middle-aged."[44]

A recreation strategy is already being planned and implemented by the Department of the Interior. The department already has provided funds for the development of exercise and recreation facilities. The National Parks and Recreation Act of 1978 (Public Law 95-625) as well as other legislation has laid the groundwork for this involvement. Title X of the act provides for "rehabilitation grants," "innovation grants," and "recovery action program grants" to local communities to augment indoor or outdoor parks, buildings, sites, or facilities. A recreation strategy, implemented through state and local government park and recreation departments, would build on an already existing network with a variety of recreational facilities and services that are meeting the recreational exercise needs of millions of people.

Other federal departments and agencies also have a potential role to play in the promotion of exercise.

The Department of Transportation could make highway trust funds available for fitness trails and bicycle paths, if the Congress were to give it clear authority to do so.

The Department of the Treasury could assess the cost and incentive value of tax credits to industry for qualified fitness/lifestyle programs in the private sector. Such credits might permit a significant expansion of existing programs.

The Department of Labor could fund exercise programs as part of occupational health demonstration projects. Industries with large numbers of sedentary workers would be prime targets for such programs.

The Department of Defense has the potential capability for promoting exercise in a major way. Two million Americans in the armed services could receive not only instructions in dynamic aerobic exercise, but also the stimulus to continue exercise after they leave the service.

The range of possible actions to promote exercise is broad. It encompasses exercise education and information; exercise services, programs, and events; exercise and recreation facility development; legislative and regulatory initiatives; and economic measures. Now is the time for the federal government to set priorities and to assess which of these actions, or which combination of actions, should be part of a national strategy to promote exercise, particularly dynamic aerobic exercise, in the American population, and which agencies can work cooperatively to advance a coherent federal effort in exercise promotion.

EXERCISE AND STATE GOVERNMENT

How can state governments increase the number of people participating in exercise, particularly dynamic aerobic exercise? A variety of actions can be taken, but the effort might begin with the establishment of a Governor's Council on Physical Fitness and Lifetime Sports. If federal funds become available under provisions of Title V of Public Law 95-626, Governor's Councils may become a reality in more states. While their numbers are increasing, only about 30 states now have Governor's Councils on Physical Fitness. Few states have active programs for the promotion of exercise for state employees or for the population as a whole. Some critics have questioned the usefulness of Governor's Councils as a vehicle to promote exercise at the state level. Perhaps the chief value of such councils is to raise the visibility of exercise and physical fitness as a policy issue within states.

Three departments of state government are most likely to be involved in efforts to promote exercise: the Department of Parks and Recreation, the Department of Health (Health Services or Public Health), and the Department of Education.

The authority exists for many State Departments of Parks and Recreation to provide facilities and natural areas for exercise and recreation and to promote the use of these facilities and areas. Unfortunately, funds are often lacking even to maintain existing park and recreational facilities. Oregon has emphasized the development of recreational facilities, using a portion of its highway funds for the construction of more than 300 miles of bikeways and footpaths.[45]

Many State Departments of Health (Health Services or Public Health) have taken the lead in promoting exercise. Existing federal legislation—the National Health Planning and Resource Development Act of 1974, the National Consumer Health Information and Health Promotion Act of 1976, and the Health Services and Centers Amendments of 1978—gives states ample authority to request initial financial support from the federal government to initiate health-promotion and disease-prevention programs stressing regular exercise. Again, policy priorities and the shortage of federal and state appropriations for these programs have severely limited their development within the state health department structure. The Commonwealth of Massachusetts, through its Department of Public Health, has used the mass media to inform the public of the availability of health promotion resources, including exercise facilities in each community.[46] Other states—including Kansas, Rhode Island, Georgia, Wisconsin, and Connecticut—have launched innovative health-promotion and disease-prevention campaigns with exercise components. State health or public health departments have been the focal points for the planning and initiation of these campaigns, some of which are described as case studies in exercise promotion in Chapter 8.

State Departments of Education are in a unique position to influence the policies and programs of local school districts. In many states, these departments could stimulate and support the development of a physical education curriculum geared toward the teaching of lifetime dynamic aerobic exercise habits. At the present time, elementary and secondary school physical education instruction is inadequate to prepare children to participate in regular exercise when they become adults. The teaching of team sports—such as football, basketball, baseball, and softball—is emphasized in schools rather than the teaching of individual or two-person sports, which are better suited for integration into an adult lifestyle. Tennis, racquetball, running, jogging, aerobic dancing, and cross-country skiing are examples of such lifetime sports. Several of these sports (e.g., skiing) are beyond the financial means of low- and middle-income students, but almost everyone can run or jog.

Schools offer little or no instruction about the fundamentals and health benefits of dynamic aerobic exercise. For example, children are not taught that to improve cardiovascular fitness exercise must be moderately strenuous and must be carried out for at least 20 to 30 minutes three times per week. Since schools have a great potential to promote regular exericise, we have explored several alternatives for statewide initiatives. (See Chapter 8.) We are in full agreement with the American Academy of Pediatrics and the American Medical Association in urging schools to provide regular participation in cardiovascular endurance activities for all children from kindergarten through the twelfth grade. The academy notes that "it is ironic that public school physical education programs are being decreased at the very time there is increased awareness of their long-term value."[47]

EXERCISE AND LOCAL GOVERNMENT

Actions to promote exercise also can be initiated by local governments. These actions are described in detail in the following chapter, which suggests how community resources might be mobilized to promote exercise.

EXERCISE AND PUBLIC POLICY: A CONCLUDING NOTE

The health prospects of Americans during the last two decades of the twentieth century will depend on the quality of decisions made by federal, state, and local government, by business and industry, by community organizations, by voluntary and professional health associations, by health professionals themselves, and by families and individuals acting on their own behalf. In short, if the health of Americans is to improve, both individual and collective actions will be necessary. These actions will be guided to some extent by perceptions of health and disease, particularly by perceptions of the potential benefits of measures to enhance health and the quality of life and to reduce the risk of disease. Interest in exercise as a way to promote health and to prevent disease has grown rapidly, both among policymakers and the American public, during the past decade. This interest has paralleled the growing interest in diet and nutrition and in other risk factors in chronic disease, particularly cardiovascular disease. Dr. Henry Blackburn of the University of Minnesota, one of the nation's leading investigators of the role of cardiovascular risk factors and their reduction, notes, "Talk about prevention is being replaced by policy and programs and by research and practice."[48] He goes on to say:

> One of the important impediments to an effective preventive practice is the idea that "habits don't change." . . . Significant changes *are* accomplished in personal behavior and in risk factor levels, but success or failure to change [is] still incompletely explained . . . . [Risk] factors *are* changed and change is maintained. . . . Much remains uncertain, however, about the best ways of reducing risks, about which strategies are more propitious than others, and about the long-term impact of these changes on health and rates of premature illness.[49]

Despite uncertainties about risk factors and their reduction, particularly in cancer and cardiovascular disease, some dramatic changes in health behavior and risk factors have taken place during the past 20 years. American men by the millions have abandoned smoking since the first Surgeon General's report on smoking and health was issued in 1964. This dramatic change is related, in part at least, to the risks of lung cancer and coronary heart disease in cigarette smokers. Serum cholesterol levels have decreased by approximately 5 percent during the last 10 to 15 years, as millions of Americans have reduced the animal fat and cholesterol content of their diets. Americans have been modifying their eating patterns prob-ably as a result of a combination of factors—increased public knowledge and awareness about nutrition and the relationship between diet and heart disease, the rising cost of beef and dairy products, and new food labeling and "truth in advertising" policies. The percentage of American adults who report that they participate in some form of exercise also has changed dramatically in the past 20 years.

Improvements in the health of the American people during the past 20 years have not been due exclusively to individual changes in lifestyle. The enactment of Medicare and Medicaid in 1965 opened the door to more adequate health care for millions of the aged and the poor. A number of special health programs, such as neighborhood health centers and maternal and infant care projects, were targeted to high-risk populations, particularly poor women and children. Neonatal intensive care units, established in hospitals throughout the country, have played an important role in reducing infant mortality. Intensive care untis for coronary heart disease patients also have been established in hospitals throughout the nation. Also, the federal government, in cooperation with state and local governments, professional organizations, and community groups, has launched a massive effort to reach and provide appropriate care for the 25 million or more people with hypertension in the United States.

Mortality rates for coronary heart disease, cerebrovascular disease, and hypertensive disease have been declining, particularly during the past decade, as changes in lifestyle, health care, and public policy have affected the lives of millions of people. It seems clear that changes in lifestyle, including changes in patterns of physical activity, are making contributions to the decline in mortality rates.

There are some real risks, however, related to policy initiatives in health promotion and disease prevention themselves, especially those centered on behavior change. The first risk is that both government policymakers and individual Americans will become impatient because results from these changes are not occurring rapidly enough. Mortality rates may not dip sharply enough to satisfy policymakers authorizing increasing public investments in prevention. Personal lives may not be transformed overnight by personal successes in achieving weight loss, an unflagging daily jogging routine, or a victory over a lifelong smoking habit. "The time frame of Americans must be lengthened," reads a recent report from the Rhode Island Department of Health. "Americans tend to place overwhelming importance on the present and the short-term."[50]

The second risk of health-promotion and disease-prevention initiatives is that impressive strides will be made in conquering some widespread disease or some personal health problem, and that the reason for this victory will be oversimplified or tied to successful action in one area, such as hypertension control with drug therapy, when the actual reason may be diet change or, more likely, simultaneous success in altering several risk factors.

The third risk is that federal policymakers will retreat from national health insurance because they feel that they have "done something" to improve health by investing a minimal amount in health-promotion and disease prevention programs. In the absence of national health insurance—particularly when 40 million people have little or no health insurance—it will be difficult to implement health-promotion and disease-prevention programs on a large scale. These programs will simply be viewed as "a cheap way out" for the federal government.

The fourth risk is that lifestyle change will be isolated from the economic, political, social, and environmental contexts in which it occurs, and that health-promotion and disease-prevention efforts will focus exclusively on changing individual behavior and not on reducing or eliminating structural barriers, such as unemployment and poor housing, to lifestyle change. There are powerful incentives for individuals within themselves and within society to pursue and to persist in certain behaviors. These forces begin with the society and its values. To attempt to change an individual's behavior and leave his or her world unchanged is very likely futile.

The fifth risk is that the responsibility for changing behavior will be seen either as the sole responsibility of the government or of the individual—or of the health professional—rather than as a shared responsibility of others in the community at large: business and industry, unions, voluntary organizations, community and service organizations, mutual-aid and self-help groups, women's support groups, senior citizen groups, families, and individuals.

The importance of all these caveats has been expressed by A.B. Morrison, Deputy Minister, Health Protection Branch, Canadian Department of National Health and Welfare. Describing the problems and progress of Canada's ambitious initiative in prevention nearly five years after the publication of the Canadian health policy document, *A New Perspective on the Health of Canadians*, he reports:

> I cannot tell you of great victories already won, nor can I say that all parts of the immensely complex system involved in prevention always mesh together just as they should. . . . However, [there] is a deep sense of commitment to prevention, and creative beginnings aimed at translating the philosophies of a new perspective on health into policies and programs. . . . We have recognized that effective prevention demands the active support of people at the federal, provincial, municipal, and community agency level. It needs the private sector, too—companies and their industry organizations, the professions, health and fitness organizations, trade unions, key figures in the media; and it needs acceptance and understanding among the general public. We have recognized that a modified physical and social environment can be built up incrementally by small advances, such as access to exercise facilities, the introduction of exercise breaks, and the building of confidence to say "no thanks" to various temptations such as "one for the road." . . . When we speak of modifying lifestyles, we are speaking ultimately of influencing values, indeed our whole culture. When we speak of influencing numerous systems other than the health care system—the workplace, the urban environment, the food system, education, and transport—over which the health system has no control—we are speaking of affecting our entire social organization. . . . We are aware of the difficulties in persuading private enterprise and public agencies to include the health variable in their decisions, especially when protection of health may not be in the interest of economics.[51]

In the next chapter we will lay out the framework for community action in promoting exercise, and we will present brief case studies of some plans turned into action—in the workplace, in homes, in schools, and in the community. Basically, we will try to answer these questions: (1) What can be done to promote exercise? (2) Who can help do it? (3) Who stands to benefit most from it? (4) Where can it be done? (5) How can it be done? (6) Who will help pay for it? (7) Can the results be measured?

Chapter 8

Exercise and Health: Mobilizing Community Resources

A framework for community action to promote exercise includes (1) defining the range of potential actions; (2) cataloguing community resources; (3) targeting population groups; (4) choosing a setting or a locale; (5) devising a plan of action; (6) searching for funding sources; (7) setting the plan into action; and (8) attempting to evaluate the results. This general framework will be useful for those working at the community level in Departments of Public Health, in Departments of Parks and Recreation, in health care or social service settings, in voluntary and community action groups, in local school districts, in colleges or universities, or in occupational health or medical departments of private businesses or industries. It also may be useful to primary care physicians, nurses, and other health professionals interested in stimulating the development of community-based exercise programs.

The Range of Action

A wide range of possibilities are open to those seeking to promote exercise. In *Promoting Health/Preventing Disease: Objectives for the Nation,* the report of a conference sponsored by the Department of Health, Education, and Welfare in Atlanta, Georgia, in June 1979, five potential measures to promote physical fitness and exercise were identified: exercise education and information; exercise services, programs and events; exercise and recreation facility development; legislative and regulatory measures; and economic measures.[1]

Together these measures constitute a broad-based strategy aimed at getting people interested in exercise; informing them and teaching them about exercise; providing opportunities, places, and facilities for exercise; and providing incentives for people to exercise as well as for private and public employers and others to sponsor exercise programs and to develop and maintain exercise and recreational facilities. This range of action is necessary to modify psychological, social and environmental factors contributing to physical inactivity. People's desire and ability to modify their personal habits and to initiate and sustain an active and regular program of exercise are influenced strongly by social and environmental factors. As Blackburn points out:

> Elevated cardiovascular risk factors in both patients and normal individuals are mass phenomena in American society. . . . Because of the widely established community mores and inducements that lead to *mass* elevations of multiple risk factors, a mass multiple strategy is required for their reduction and prevention. . . . Mass public education is probably required for individuals and communities to become aware of and to change risk behavior. Community supports are required for motivated individuals to improve their risk behavior.[2]

Exercise Education and Information. These activities range from mass media campaigns in major news weeklies—such as the one launched in the fall of 1978 by the American Medical Association with the theme "Exercise is something you can get your heart into"—to the publication of booklets and brochures about exercise for the general public, patients, physicians, and employers, to the airing of public service announcements enticing people to exercise. The Blue Cross and Blue Shield Associations recently joined with the President's Council on Physical Fitness and Sports as well as the American Association of Fitness Directors in Business and Industry to produce a guide for corporation executives entitled *Building a Healthier Company*.[3] The Blue Cross Association also has a mass media campaign promoting fitness with the theme "Five miles a day keeps the doctor away." The Connecticut Mutual Life Insurance Company has teamed with the American Heart Association and the President's Council to conduct a nationwide "Run for Life" campaign featuring clinics on running, instructional and motivational films, booklets, and public service announcements. Both the American Heart Association and the American Medical Association have produced instructional materials for patients and physicians, including *Risk Factors and Coronary Disease: A Statement for Physicians; Exercise Testing and Training of Apparently Healthy Individuals: A Handbook for Physicians; A Guide to Prescribing Exercise Programs; Basic Bodywork for Fitness and Health;* and, *Why Risk Heart Attack: Six Ways to Guard Your Heart. Guidelines for Physical Fitness Programs in Business and Industry* is a joint statement of the President's Council on Physical Fitness and Sports and the American Medical Association's Committee on Exercise and Physical Fitness.[5] Individual authors and their book publishers also have done their share.

Millions of people have read bestselling books on aerobic exercise by Cooper[6] and on running by Fixx[7] for guidance in carrying out their own exercise programs or in designing cooperative programs. Another very popular book has been the *Royal Canadian Air Force Exercise Plan for Physical Fitness.*[8]

One of the most successful promotional campaigns on exercise has been launched in Canada by PARTICIPaction . . . The Canadian Movement for Personal Fitness.[9] Not a part of the government, PARTICIPaction operates independently with a volunteer board of directors comprising men and women from various walks of life. Supported with an annual operating grant from the Fitness and Amateur Sport Branch of the Canadian Department of National Health and Welfare, the group has borrowed heavily from the marketing techniques of free enterprise. Among these marketing tools are: (1) public service advertising in cooperation with a variety of media; (2) corporate sponsorship, whereby large companies are shown the merits of spending advertising dollars on fitness promotion; (3) booklets, posters, and films; and (4) community and regionally based demonstration projects. The PARTICIPaction experiment, which began in 1971, has met with an unusual degree of success. Surveys indicate that a majority of people of all ages—over 70 percent of all Canadians—are familiar with PARTICIPaction's message and logos.[10] The President's Council on Physical Fitness and Sports in the United States has used some of these same tools, in particular public service television announcements and magazine advertisements.

There is a need today in the United States for the development of more specialized fitness messages for the public. Television, radio, magazine, and newspaper messages might be used to instruct people on the need for regular, not just weekend, physical activity, as well as on the differences between dynamic aerobic exercise and low-intensity exercise. Messages also need to be targeted to low-income populations, the elderly, women, and children.

Dissemination of information to the health care community is another special need. As noted in the Final Report of the Wisconsin Advisory Commission on Prevention and Wellness:

> A concept cannot be integrated into a system without the support and understanding [of] the system's major actors. For the concepts of health promotion and prevention to become more prominent in the health care system, the actors—physicians, non-physician practitioners, nurses, pharmacists, administrators, and professionals—must understand the concepts. The Commission believes that the opportunity exists for increasing levels of awareness of prevention and wellness through professional education and continuing education.[11]

Health professionals seem to concur that there is a need for such information about exercise. A popular way for health professionals to provide this information is through courses in continuing education.[12] However, the medical literature is still probably the most common source of information for physicians. The problem is that much of the valuable information about exercise for primary care physicians appears in specialty journals, such as *The Physician and Sportsmedicine, Circulation*, the *American Journal of Sports Medicine, Medicine and Science in Sports*, and the *American Journal of Epidemiology*, as well as in books or monographs of particular interest to cardiologists or epidemiologists. The same problem exists for the public health generalist, except that even less information about exercise and health appears in most public health journals. Integrating intruction about exercise into medical and other health professions' school curricula is more difficult; few faculty members are qualified to teach about exercise, and in most medical schools there is no central focus of interest in exercise. Special funds might be sought to support faculty positions, as has been done in other areas such as nutrition and geriatrics. Modules on exercise could be taught in physiology, epidemiology, preventive medicine, primary care, cardiology, sports medicine, and rehabilitation courses. More undergraduate courses for students majoring in human biology, physical education, and recreation also would be useful, as would more advanced courses for physical education faculty.[13] The Report of the Community Health Task Force, Division of Physical Health, Department of Human Resources of the State of Georgia suggests that "a physical fitness analyst specialty [be developed] at the graduate level in colleges and universities to prepare qualified persons to direct and staff private and public recreational programs."[14]

Education and information measures in promoting exercise include effectively using the mass media, school-based programs, health care delivery systems, community service agencies, parks and recreation departments, and other public and private agencies. The experience of cardiac rehabilitation and cardiovascular disease prevention can be helpful in the design and execution of community exercise education programs.[15] The experience of the Stanford Heart Disease Prevention Program is particularly instructive because these investigators have evaluated the impact of screening examinations combined with mass media and both of these interventions supplemented by personal contact.[16] It is important in programs of information and education to stress the need for individual goals and programs to meet these goals, and not to create unrealistic expectations—everyone need not, indeed cannot, become a long-distance or marathon runner.

Exercise Services, Programs, and Events. These include the high-visibility running races in some of the nation's largest cities—the Boston

Marathon, the San Francisco Bay-to-Breakers Race, and the Women's Mini-Marathon in New York's Central Park—as well as physician and nurse services in support of these events. The Honolulu Marathon Clinic, directed by cardiologist Jack Scaff and his colleagues, has demonstrated the value of medical leadership. Dr. Scaff or one of his associates gives a motivational talk and holds a recreational distance run every Sunday morning for nine months of the year. Attracting up to 1800 participants, the clinic has received much of the credit for Hawaii's number-one national rank in the numbers of runners and joggers per 100,000 population. An example of lay leadership in community-based programs is the pilot program to promote year-round fitness for the half-million senior citizens who live in Los Angeles County. This program, a joint venture of Senior Sports International Inc. (a private nonprofit corporation that sponsors the Senior Olympic Games) and the Los Angeles Parks and Recreation Department, is called "Maintenance of Vitality Through Physical Fitness."[17] Volunteers from the Senior Olympic staff lead classes in five county parks on easy-to-moderate exercises. A 30-page instructional booklet, which has been endorsed by the President's Council on Physical Fitness and Sports, is distributed free to all participants so that they can exercise at home as well as in the parks. The booklet cautions participants to see a physician before starting strenuous new activities, then diagrams arm extensions, shoulder shrugs, knee pulls, side bends, and other stretching exercises.

School-based programs provide the opportunity to reach more people than all the well-publicized marathons, jogs, and related community-based programs. The schools, unfortunately, are not doing the job that needs to be done, either for students or for adults who could make excellent use of many school facilities. Although thousands of public and private schools conduct sports and recreation programs, few emphasize dynamic aerobic exercise or reach out to students who are overweight or others who might benefit from regular exercise. A federal grant of $1800 launched a 20-week experimental cardiovascular-fitness program for fifth-grade students of the John F. Kennedy Elementary School in West Babylon, New York. The idea was conceived by the school's principal after he had suffered a heart attack, in conjunction with his cardiologist and two physical education teachers.[18] Three days a week 10 youngsters, chosen from among 100 classmates because they were overweight, had above-normal blood pressure, and lacked energy, are bused to school at 8:00 A.M. for an hour of running and stationary bicycle use. For at least 30 minutes of the hour, they exercise hard enough to keep their heart rates at a recommended training level. Each checks his or her own rate by inserting a finger in a pulsemeter while running. When their hour is up, the children record their achievement on a chart, go to the cafeteria for breakfast, and start classes. In Fort Worth, Texas, the school board adopted an aerobic exercise program in place of their standard program, and substantial benefits were realized by those who participated.[19] Several other school districts have sponsored innovative exercise programs.[20]

Programs in the workplace provide yet another opportunity to promote exercise. These programs are usually designed to meet the needs of employees of the particular company or of the government agency conducting the program. Too often, however, programs and exercise facilities have been available only to executives, when all employees can benefit from exercise. The Xerox Corporation has a highly regarded physical fitness program, which the President's Council on Physical Fitness and Sports recently rated as the top corporate health plan in the nation.[21] This plan, now being marketed for sale to corporations throughout the country, is open to Xerox employees as well as to families and friends. The plan is based on the concept that an individual must manage his or her own health and decide whether to make changes in lifestyle. Each employee is given a fitness test and views a film on health care. He or she is then asked to fill out a three-month goal sheet and is given a booklet containing exercise programs for such goals as losing weight, controlling stress, or just feeling better, physically and mentally. Upon completion of the three-month program, the employee receives a t-shirt with the inscription "I'm taking charge of my life." The director of the health management program at Xerox's Santa Clara, California, facility sees both tangible and intangible results of the program: "The tangible results include increased productivity, lower medical costs, and lower absenteeism. The intangible results include an improved self-image and feeling and looking better and a closer family relationship."[22] Nationally, Xerox has seven exercise facilities, each equipped with an exercise gym, sauna, volleyball court, universal gym, swimming pool, and several tennis courts. The facilities are worth $5 million; the annual operating cost is $2 million. Without such exercise facilities, the Santa Clara Xerox health plan offers dance classes, exercise classes, running groups, biking groups, and Red Cross cardiopulmonary resuscitation classes.

The federal government provides a variety of exercise programs for its employees. The Congress has extensive facilities for swimming, jogging, and stretching and strengthening exercises, but these facilities are limited to the members of the Congress. The Department of Health and Human Services is initiating a health-promotion program for its employees in seven of its Washington, D.C., facilities, but funds, staff, and space for a department-wide program that would include its 10 regional offices have not yet been made available. The Department of Defense, particularly the armed forces, has the most extensive fitness programs of any federal department. In addition to the programs that directly involve members of the armed forces, organized sports on military bases attract a great many family members, particularly children.

Some states have developed imaginative, low-cost exercise programs for the general public. The *Plus* (Program to Lower Utilization of Services) Program of the State of Kansas Health Department is an example of a public health agency's involvement in fitness.[23] The program is designed for people of all ages, and it uses the facilities of workplaces, schools, "Ys," community senior centers, 4-H clubs, and similar organizations. With the theme, "Add Plus to Your Life," the program aims to provide information, assess individual fitness, and develop improvement plans on the basis of seven health risks. The fitness component is particularly well planned, emphasizing individually paced aerobic exercise such as walking–running, cycling, swimming, and rope skipping. Participants compete against themselves to earn a minimum target number of points per week over a 16-week period. The key to the program's success is reported to be effective community networking, a relatively low budget, and a high rate of volunteerism.

Exercise services and programs in the workplace, at home, in schools, and in the community need to be increased substantially. (Case studies of several more innovative programs designed for each of these settings are presented at the conclusion of this chapter.)

Exercise and Recreation Facility Development. Many community programs can be launched with existing facilities in parks, in schools, and in the workplace. Others will require an increase in the number and the availability of both natural and man-made recreational facilities. Natural facilities include parks, hiking trails, fresh water swimming facilities, ski trails, skating areas, tobogganing hills, camping areas, canoe and rafting streams and rivers, and fitness trails. These recreational facilities can be developed at relatively low cost, and they also represent simple, intensive-use facilities. The need for the development of such facilities is great, especially in areas close to urban centers and in inner cities. Man-made recreational facilities include swimming pools, gymnasiums, arenas, playing fields for soccer, baseball, football, and running (often best located on school grounds), facilities for court games, Parcourses, and, in some cases, bicycle paths. Lalonde's conviction that expanded development of "fitness trails, nature trails, ski trails, facilities for court games, playing fields, bicycle paths, and skating rinks" is needed in Canada applies also to the United States.[24] Fox, Naughton, and Gorman have commented on the lack of "attractive, well-equipped, and appropriately staffed facilities at reasonable cost within easy access for most of our citizens." They go on to say, "Heart associations, community planners, medical societies, regional medical programs, academic institutions, and other elements of our complex society all have responsibilities in helping individuals find rewarding activities."[25]

The Department of Health of the State of Rhode Island agrees. In the

Lifestyle Goal Statements of its preliminary State Health Plan, the department recommended the expansion of exercise facilities:

> The Department of Environmental Management should increase the number of miles of hiking trails, the number of state fresh water swimming facilities near urban centers, and the number of miles of jogging paths and bicycle paths on state lands. Each city and town in Rhode Island should construct jogging paths, bicycle paths, swimming pools, tennis courts, and gymnasiums adequate to the needs of their population.
>
> Some federal funding is available for outdoor recreational facility development. The state should provide matching funds for outdoor facilities.
>
> All new facilities should be designed and staffed to ensure that the capacity of each facility is fully utilized and that exercise activities are pursued safely. More extensive use should be made of existing facilities by the employment of personnel to staff facilities and provide recreation programming. Exercise facilities open to the public should be widely advertised.
>
> All employers should establish physical fitness and weight control programs for their employees and construct exercise facilities or make arrangements for the use of public or privately owned facilities by their employees.[26]

As a first step in implementing this ambitious plan, the Department of Health recommended that a statewide inventory be taken of "the existence, current utilization, and potential capacity of all exercise facilities which can be used by the public to promote fitness and weight control."[27] The Rhode Island Department of Environmental Management and the Rhode Island Department of Health were to undertake this inventory with the cooperation of city and town governments, the Rhode Island school districts, and organizations such as the scouts, the YMCA, and exercise clubs. The projected cost of the inventory was $7500.

States need to examine the role of exercise more seriously as part of long-range plans and programs for health promotion and disease prevention. The State Health Plan provides a particularly useful vehicle because it would, of necessity, have to involve grass-roots planning through the Health Systems Agencies within the state.

Public schools have been moving gradually to make their exercise facilities available to the adult population in some communities. In other communities, fiscal crises have reversed this trend. The trend to open gymnasiums, pools, and playing fields for youth and adult use on nights, weekends, and during the summer months should be accelerated. High school swimming pools, in particular, could be better utilized. Instead of being used solely during the afternoon for high school swimming teams, pool facilities could be used for physical education classes and programs for adults during the morning, evening, or weekend hours. Most pools are heated and maintained during the winter for team practices and games; little extra energy would be required to allow others to use the facilities in off-hours. In addition to opening pools, gyms, and other facilities for adult use, regular exercise and sport programs and instruction are needed for optimum use of these facilities. Adult fitness classes could be an integral part of the general adult education program.

Several European countries have developed extensive community-based exercise and recreational facilities to support their fitness movements. Sweden has relied on the Training Track as the chief facility for its exercise movement. The Training Track consists of hundreds of kilometers of fitness trails—woodland trails covered with a natural spongy surface such as wood chips or sawdust.

Switzerland and several other countries have used the Parcourse for community-based programs. A concept introduced and brought to reality by a Swiss insurance company, Parcourses are laid out over a 2- to 3-kilometer trail with exercise stations located about every 300 yards. Virtually every community in Switzerland now has its own Parcourse, funded either through public or private sources. Since its introduction to the United States in 1973, the Parcourse idea has attracted widespread support. An estimated 740 Parcourses are currently in use throughout the country.[28] The best location for Parcourses may be in community or neighborhood parks.[29] A Parcourse can do much to convert scenic grassy areas for picnicking into areas for walking, jogging, exercising, and picnicking. Installation costs are surprisingly low, often less than $5000 for a two-mile course.[30]

In Norway, cross-country skiing and swimming are the major modalities in a nationwide fitness campaign. Expanding swimming instruction in the schools and building many public pools have greatly increased the number of swimmers in the country.[31]

Exercise and recreation facility development includes increasing the availability of existing facilities and promoting the development of new facilities by public agencies, private companies, and community groups.[32] Building codes and improvements in the design of workplaces also can promote the development of exercise programs.[33]

Legislative and Regulatory Measures. Examples of such measures to promote exercise include the State of Oregon's allocation of 1 percent of its highway funds for the construction of bikeways and footpaths;[34] the vote of residents of Davis, California, in 1966 to establish bicycle lanes, paths, and bicycle parking lots;[35] and the decision of numbers of communities to ban automobile traffic from downtown areas. Also included in this category would be the legal requirement to install sidewalks in all urban residential areas or to require developers not only to build wide streets and to install curbs and gutters in new housing tracts, but also to provide off-street bike trails as well. Legislative and regulatory measures to promote exercise also can be used to encourage resource sharing, to increase the number of school-mandated physical education programs, to develop and operate state and national park facilities that can be used for physical activities in urban areas, and to establish state and local councils on physical fitness.[36]

Economic Measures. Economic measures to promote exercise, which might necessitate legislative action, include the development of tax incentives for the private sector to develop and maintain physical fitness facilities and programs and the development of personal incentives for beginning and continuing a program of regular vigorous physical activity through reduced health and life insurance premiums. We do not agree with the latter approach, although the idea is popular. Dr. Jonathan Fielding, former Commissioner of the Commonwealth of Massachusetts Department of Public Health and present Co-Director of the Center for Health Enhancement, Education, and Research at the University of California, Los Angeles, and others have suggested that life insurance premiums should reflect self-imposed risks, and that lower rates should be given to individuals who maintain cardiovascular fitness through regular exercise.[37] Several life insurance companies offer reduced insurance premiums to adult nonsmokers; the count in 1976 was 30 companies.[38] Recently, several firms have begun to offer reduced premiums to regular exercisers as well. Among these firms are the Manhattan Life Insurance Company, Unity Mutual of Syracuse, New York (which is licensed in the District of Columbia and 19 states), and Occidental of Raleigh, North Carolina, whose discounts are available nationwide, except in New York and Hawaii, under its newly formed affiliate, Financial Fitness, Inc.[39] To obtain a Manhattan Life physical fitness discount (the physical fitness and nonsmoker discounts are about 15 percent each), the applicant must participate in some aerobic exercise for not less than 20 minutes per day, four times a week. The company "reserves the right to request a confirmation letter from a YMCA or YWCA or from the applicant's doctor."[40] Unity Mutual offers a discount up to 8.9 percent for the physically fit on its "whole life" policies. The applicant must give evidence that exercise is a part of his or her lifestyle, must see a doctor regularly for examination, and must not smoke. Verification is usually through a background investigation.[41] Occidental of Raleigh, North Carolina, offers discounts of up to 20 percent on "whole life" policies and 25 percent on "term" policies. Applicants must jog or complete other aerobic exercise for 20 minutes per day, three times a week for a year in order to become eligible for the policy.

Tax and insurance premium incentives, relatively new ideas in health promotion and disease prevention, deserve a thorough evaluation. Our opposition to premium incentives is based on the view that those with greater risks to their health, those in high-risk occupations, the poor, and minorities, can do relatively little as individuals to alter the social or physical environments in which they live and work. These environments, in turn, often promote unhealthy lifestyles.

CATALOGUING COMMUNITY RESOURCES

Community resources vary with the size and location of the community. Large cities often provide a rich array of resources; rural areas have fewer resources, but these resources—4-H clubs, agricultural extension bureaus, granges, schools, and churches—may be a more integral part of family life and of the lives of individual community members. Compiling a list of potential community resources is a useful step in planning an exercise initiative in any community. A model Community Resource Inventory was developed in the North Karelia Project in Finland, a comprehensive community program directed toward the primary and secondary prevention of cardiovascular diseases.[43] Potential community resources include:

government agencies (federal, state, regional, county, and municipal), particularly health-related agencies, including health planning agencies, education and social agencies, parks and recreation agencies, and transportation agencies;

businesses and industries, particularly the largest employers in the community and others with a special interest, such as health and life insurance companies and sports equipment and apparel manufacturers and their wholesale and retail outlets;

schools (private and public grade schools, intermediate schools, and high schools; trade and vocational schools; schools for the handicapped; junior colleges; colleges; universities, including institutions with schools of medicine, nursing, and public health);

hospitals, medical groups, health maintenance organizations, neighborhood health centers, free clinics, nursing homes, and other long-term care facilities;

voluntary health organizations (American Heart Association, American Lung Association, American Diabetes Association, American Cancer Society);

professional health and education organizations, particularly state or

local medical, nursing, public health, sports medicine, and physical
education associations;

social service and welfare organizations (Urban League, Catholic Social
Services, Meals on Wheels, National Council on Aging, United Way);

civic, service, and fraternal organizations (Lions Club, Kiwanis Club,
Chamber of Commerce, Big Brothers and Big Sisters);

trade associations, including business organizations and union groups;

churches and religious organizations

exercise clubs/athletic organizations;

youth organizations and centers (Girl Scouts, Boy Scouts, 4-H clubs,
YMCA, YWCA, YMHA, YWHA);

senior citizens' services, organizations, centers;

smoking cessation clinics (profit and nonprofit);

weight reduction clinics (profit and nonprofit);

health clubs, private exercise facilities, spas;

women's organizations;

foundations;

community leaders and key individuals (mayor, sports figures);

physicians, nurses, health educators, occupational health specialists,
and physical therapists.

A systematic effort to inventory these and other sources—including the
type, location, and availability of exercise and recreational facilities in the
community—may be helpful in moving toward a community plan of
action to promote exercise. The inventory is useful if a number of organizations are involved in promoting exercise to coordinate the efforts
of multiple organizations in meeting the needs of the general population
and of special groups.

TARGETING POPULATION
GROUPS

Each community comprises population groups with special
health needs—the elderly, children and adolescents, the handicapped, and
racial and ethnic minorities—and those with special health risks—
smokers, hypertensives, the obese, diabetics, sedentary workers, and those
with multiple cardiovascular disease risk factors. Besides these groups,
which can be identified to some extent demographically, epidemiological-
ly, or clinically, others—women at home, patients with mental illness who
may be at risk because of social isolation—are not so easily identifiable. An
exercise program of some type could be targeted to any of these groups and
probably produce physical, psychological, or social benefits.

It is difficult to answer the question: "Who stands to benefit most from exercise?" In terms of future benefits or lifetime benefits, children clearly stand to gain the most from exercise, especially from dynamic aerobic exercise, stretching, and muscle strengthening. Cardiologists seem almost unanimous on this point. Dr. John Bergfeld, director of sports medicine at the Cleveland Clinic, says, "If we are really to make progress, we'll have to start with the kids, because with people 30 and older you're playing catch-up. You want people to develop good exercise habits the same way you want them to develop good study habits."[44] Dr. John Naughton, dean of the medical school at the State University of New York in Buffalo, New York, agrees. He studied 400 men at a local YMCA in Oklahoma in the 1960s; men who had taken part in exercise programs earlier in their lives remained throughout the study while others tended to drop out.[45] Canadian studies show that children in that country do not have very high fitness levels and that those levels decline with age.[46] Fitness levels of American children also are below optimal levels. If choices must be made, this is clearly the place to begin.

CHOOSING THE SETTING

The setting or locale for an initiative to promote exercise depends on the population(s) to be targeted as well as on the feasibility of a particular strategy or strategies—an education and information strategy, a program or service strategy, a facility development strategy, a legislative or regulatory strategy, or an economic incentive strategy—in the community. Basically, there are four places to promote exercise: the home, the workplace, schools, and the community. The home may be the logical place to reach certain high-risk groups, such as the elderly, the handicapped, or others who may be homebound. The school and the workplace are well suited to reach special populations. The primary advantage of a community-based program is the abundance of natural settings and institutional resources, including parks, recreational centers, and hospitals. A community-based program also provides greater choice for a wide range of people who want to undertake regular exercise programs.

THE PLAN OF ACTION

A plan of action to promote exercise in the community should first include the development of community support, preferably in all sectors of the community—political, professional, business, labor, consumer, and voluntary. No plan advances far without enlisting the support of appropriate organizations and potential participants. People do like to be consulted and included, especially when they have special interests (e.g., the elderly, the handicapped), special skills (e.g., coaching, sports medicine, particular sports), or special plans or programs of their own to mobilize community support to promote exercise. After the informal or formal assistance of participants and sponsors has been marshaled, it is useful to consider how these people could work together to design and implement a program (e.g., volunteering as coaches for a basketball team for handicapped children, providing assistance in preparing legislation). A variety of skills are usually required even in the simplest of enterprises. A plan of action includes (1) goals and objectives, expected outcomes; (2) a description of the population to be served and the specific needs of the population that the plan will address; (3) a detailed listing of resources required to set the plan in motion (e.g., time, staff, support of other cooperating agencies or institutions, space, facilities, and a budget); and (4) when appropriate, a plan to evaluate the results.

Exercise programs can be initiated on a modest or large scale. For example, Gregory S. Thomas, one of the coauthors of this book, developed a running clinic (described in greater detail later in this chapter) for members of the University of California, San Francisco, campus community and the public. This effort required a small group to plan and carry out the program, which provided an opportunity both to instruct beginners and to stimulate reluctant runners. News of the program spread by word of mouth and by campus announcements. The program began with only a few devoted runners, but it now supervises exercise for hundreds. On a much larger scale, events such as the Bay-to-Breakers Race in San Francisco have grown to such an extent that the cooperation of many organizations, public and private, is essential for the program's success. Small or modest exercise programs can sometimes be built into existing neighborhood or community-based health programs.

SEARCHING FOR FUNDING SOURCES

In the interest of saving time, money, and effort as well as of maximizing chances for support, the search for whatever funding is required should begin "close to home"—in the community or locale in which the plan is to be set into motion. Local institutions, such as banks, businesses, and industries, are often more interested in, and more sympathetic to, local programs. Private foundations often earmark funds for particular populations (e.g., the elderly or children), for particular geographic areas, and for particular activities. The most recent edition of the *Foundation Directory* is a useful guide to the funding priorities, addresses, telephone numbers, and names of executive officers of foundations.[47]

Public health departments, public schools, and park and recreation departments are government agencies that are potential sources for program planning, organization, implementation, and funding. However, these agencies must often turn to state or federal agencies for help for new or expanded programs. At this time it is not an exaggeration to say that public funds for health and human services are jeopardized at all levels of government. Limited revenues have meant eliminating services, decreasing levels of services, and not supporting services unless they are mandated by law. Obtaining funding for new projects, especially in health promotion and disease prevention, is therefore difficult. It requires a fairly intimate knowledge of legislation in health promotion and disease prevention, as well as of legislation in related areas (e.g., the National Parks and Recreation Act of 1978) and an understanding of congressional and state legislative authorizations and appropriations in support of specific programs. The *Catalog of Federal Domestic Assistance* is a helptul guide to potential sources of federal funding.[48]

MEASURING THE RESULTS

Can a community be mobilized to improve its health practices? Can improvement in these practices change individual health behavior? Can changes in individual health behavior affect risk factors for coronary heart disease and stroke? Can changes in risk factors reduce mortality and morbidity from these diseases? Can the results be achieved by cost-effective measures? All these questions were posed by Dr. Albert Stunkard, Professor of Psychiatry at University of Pennsylvania, to the U.S. House of Representatives Subcommittee on Health and Environment when he testified about a new health intervention project to be begun in Lycoming County, Pennsylvania.[49] Patterned on the North Karelia Project[50] and the Stanford Three Community Study,[51] the program does not cover fitness but will focus on three risk factors: smoking, high blood pressure, and elevated serum cholesterol levels. The answers to all the questions that Dr. Stunkard posed are still incomplete; we hope that the Lycoming County Project and other projects will help complete them. During the past two decades, we have witnessed increasing professional and public interest in preventive interventions of various types. As Dr. Blackburn reminds us, all these developments

> . . . have occurred in the absence of conclusive experimental evidence that changes in lifestyle, and their attendant reduction of risk factors, actually result in reduced disease rates among high-risk populations. Without such

definitive experiments, the consistent observations of the relationship between personal and cultural differences in risk factors and subsequent risk of vascular events serve to give strong and sufficient evidence that a hygienic lifestyle is good medical practice—and needed public health policy.[53]

PLANS INTO ACTION: EXERCISE IN THE WORKPLACE, AT HOME, IN SCHOOLS, AND IN THE COMMUNITY

The final section of this chapter is a series of case studies of exercise promotion in four settings: at work, at home, in schools, and in the community. Many of these case studies describe programs in the State of California and in the San Francisco Bay Area about which the authors have first-hand knowledge. Others are condensed descriptions of programs reported in the literature. Still others have been drawn from state and local health department planning documents and from personal discussions with program planners. These case studies are offered only as selected examples of efforts to promote exercise. We are aware that we have not included a nationwide sample of programs, and that we have overlooked innovative programs in dozens of states and localities. It is our hope that the samples that we have included will help others interested in promoting exercise to turn their plans into action.

Exercise in the Workplace

Through the encouragement of the President's Council on Physical Fitness and Sports and the enthusiasm of sports- and fitness-minded executives and employees, many private companies, as well as some public agencies, now provide exercise facilities and programs for their employees. The list of large American firms that presently sponsor employee programs includes Xerox, Arco, Rockwell, General Foods, Boeing, Kimberly-Clark, Employers Insurance of Wausau, and Lockheed. The President's Council may have a point when it says that such programs are "good business"; potential benefits include increased productivity, lower absenteeism, and strengthened morale. Dr. Jonathan Fielding, in a recent article entitled "Preventive Medicine and the Bottom Line," makes a strong case for industry involvement in preventive programs, including exercise and fitness programs: "Like it or not," he says, "industry bears a heavy share of the cost of [accidents, heart disease, cancer, and liver and lung diseases and many other causes of death and disability]. Industry first

ays by laying down the lion's share of the [health insurance] premium
ased on the health care experience of its employee group, and then pays
gain by bearing the burden of both acute and chronic illness through
mployee absenteeism, turnover, and premature retirement or death, or
oth."[54] Fielding goes on to cite cost savings to business and industry from
ealth screening and risk reduction, in-house medical departments, driver
raining, health "bonuses" and financial incentives for employees, and
xercise programs. He cites three studies of on-the-job exercise programs
hat show that adults who exercise regularly have reduced illness and
bsenteeism and improved attitudes toward work.[54]

1. In 1968, the National Aeronautics and Space Administration
   provided a three-times-a-week exercise program for 259 men aged 35
   to 55. After a year, participants completed a questionnaire and
   underwent a thorough medical examination. Half reported better
   job performance and better attitudes toward work. Eighty-nine
   percent reported improved stamina, and more than 40 percent
   reported sounder sleep. Many quit smoking or cut down, and more
   than 60 percent lost weight. The medical tests documented
   improved health status.[55]
2. A study in the Soviet Union found that working people who
   exercise regularly produce more, visit the doctor less, and are less
   prone to industrial accidents than they were prior to exercising.[56]
3. A five-year regular exercise program for 847 state employees in
   Albany, New York, also yielded positive results. Cardiac risk factors
   were reduced in the participants, health problems eased, and
   employee absenteeism reduced.[57]

Several general questions regarding health promotion and disease
revention in the workplace were outlined by participants in a conference
n health promotion sponsored by the State of Georgia's Department of
Iuman Resources, Division of Physical Health, Office of Heath
ducation and Training, in Atlanta in 1977.[58] This conference was
esigned to explore how different community settings can appropriately
romote health, how these efforts can be more effectively coordinated, and
hat methods should be developed to improve the health status of
eorgians by addressing their lifestyles. Questions relating to health
romotion and disease prevention in work settings include the following:

1. For what aspects of health promotion and maintenance should
   management be responsible? in plant? out of plant?
2. What role should labor unions play in health promotion and
   maintenance for their workers?
3. What aspects of work settings make it difficult to carry out
   programs of general health promotion during the working day?

4. How can health care programs in industry be coordinated mor effectively with other community health programs impinging o workers?

5. What arguments can be advanced both for and against th proposition that employers should grant time off, without loss c pay, for workers to obtain needed out-of-plant health and medica care services?

6. How can employee absenteeism and accident records be utilized i planning more effective health-promotion programs for workers

7. What evidence supports the value of general health-promotio programs carried on in work settings?

8. How should employers deal with the many health agencie requesting permission to reach workers on company time with variety of categorical health-promotion programs?[59]

These questions and others are useful to consider in planning exercis programs as well as other health-promotion and disease-preventio programs for the workplace.

Guidelines for physical fitness programs in business and industry hav been developed jointly by the President's Council on Physical Fitness an Sports and the American Medical Association's Committee on Exercis and Physical Fitness.[60] These guidelines encompass the purpose an beliefs undergirding such programs as well as medical provision administration, and facilities. The guidelines are reprinted in thei entirety in Appendix A.

Exercise programs in the workplace vary widely, as the following cas studies will show. Some employers have launched extensive programs a part of a broad-based health-promotion and disease-prevention effor these programs also feature an expensive array of exercise and spor facilities. Other employers have launched strong outdoor jogging an cycling programs simply by installing locker and shower facilities i basements or storerooms. Still other employers, who cannot afford th space or the money to construct exercise facilities, have been able to solv this problem by contracting with a local organization, such as the YMC or a private club, that has the necessary facilities and personnel.

Kimberly-Clark's Health Management Program. This program's goal i "to achieve a higher level of wellness among employees and thereb improve productivity and reduce absenteeism and health care costs." The program is available to all salaried employees in the Fox Valley area c Wisconsin. From entry-level health risk profiles, participating employee have an opportunity to examine and evaluate their own health risks, an data can be collected to serve as a basis for measuring the effectiveness of th program.

The principal program components are a computerized medical history and health hazard appraisal, multiphasic screening, a physical examination, an exercise test on a treadmill or bicycle ergometer, and a health review with recommendations. The aerobic exercise program offers jogging, swimming, stationary cycling, circuit training, aerobic dancing, rope jumping, water exercise, cardiac rehabilitation, and cross-country skiing. The exercise facility has lockers, showers, saunas, a whirlpool, and a lounge and dining area. Employees also may attend health education classes on a variety of topics: diet management, coronary risk factors, smoking control, cancer, breast self-examination, chemical dependence, high blood pressure, low-back pain, basic life support (cardiopulmonary resuscitation), and self-instruction classes on early warning symptoms of heart attack, relaxation skills, and understanding reactive depression. In addition, employees may enter the Employee Assistance Program for chemical dependency and other health problems.

The program staff includes 35 full-time and part-time employees, including 2 physicians, 1 nurse practitioner, 7 registered nurses, 7 technicians, and counselors, exercise specialists, secretaries, receptionists, and lifeguards. Community participants in the program include a six-member physician advisory council, family practitioners and internists, who help with exercise testing and physical examinations, and consulting cardiologists, radiologists, and dietitians.

The exercise prescription for an employee is based on his or her age, treadmill-estimated functional capacity, the presence of risk factors or known cardiovascular disease, and the presence of orthopedic abnormalities. A supervised exercise program for persons with known coronary heart disease, coronary bypass surgery, pulmonary disease, or persons at high risk for coronary events was begun in 1977. Exercises include jogging, stationary cycling, exercising in structured classes, aerobic dancing, treadmill jogging, rowing, circuit training, and swimming. A water exercise class also has been incorporated. Exercise sessions are conducted with a physician, registered nurse, and technician in attendance and defibrillilation equipment available. (A limited number of telemetry units and Holter monitors is available for use with persons with known cardiac rhythm abnormalities for 12 to 24 hours after exercise.)

What are the results of Kimberly-Clark's Health Management Program? Since the program has been in existence for only about two and a half years, no data on long-range cost benefits or risk factor reduction are yet available. However, in a first-time retesting, 25 employees who had been in the program for 12 to 18 months showed significant reductions in systolic and diastolic blood pressure and serum triglyceride levels.[62] They showed no significant changes in weight, percentage of body fat, total serum cholesterol, HDL cholesterol, or fasting blood sugar. When asked about one of the company's objectives—to reduce costs—the company's representatives had these comments:

> At the present, the staff participant ratio is 1/62 and our per capita expenditure is about $435, including the comprehensive medical examination. These figures compare favorably with other large-scale preventive efforts being conducted on a trial basis. Our projections indicate that the overall break-even point for our program will be about 9.5 years (three years for the Employee Assistance Program, and about 6.5 years for the risk factor reduction portion of the program). In about ten years significant annual savings should be achieved. In addition, the program has enhanced Kimberly-Clark's public reputation and has assisted in corporate recruiting efforts.[63]

In sum, preliminary results at Kimberly-Clark support the view that a program of regular physical exercise significantly improves a subjective sense of well-being and physical work capacity in people both with and without heart disease.[64] Exercise helped lower systolic and diastolic blood pressure and serum triglycerides, but it did not have much effect on total serum cholesterol.

Employers Insurance of Wausau Programs. Another Wisconsin-based company, Employers Insurance of Wausau, offers two independent programs.[65] One program, based on the idea of an individual practice association (IPA) health maintenance organization, has changed the incentives of most physicians serving Employers' employees.[66] The second program is an independent disease-prevention and health-promotion program. With a pre-employment physical evaluation as a baseline for the program, employees at all Employers Insurance of Wausau offices, coast to coast, have access to clinics screening for hypertension, hyperlipidemia, respiratory diseases, diabetes, cancer, stress, and mental and emotional problems. The company also offers an employee assistance program that deals with alcohol, drug, and mental health problems.

The exercise component of this program includes a Presidential Sports Award program and team sports for both men and women. YMCA memberships are given to some employees. Employers Insurance has experienced success with this program and has found that it is especially useful for personnel who work outside of a central office. The company is planning, however, to build a new training and educational center including a Parcourse with nine exercise stations and a physical fitness center for employees at the home office.

The Lockheed Employees Recreation Association (LERA). The LERA was incorporated in 1963 as a nonprofit organization.[67] The LERA facility located in Lockheed Aircraft's Sunnyvale, California plant, contains fully equipped meeting rooms for the association's 35 special-interest clubs. These rooms range from a complete indoor small-bore rifle and pistol range to a ceramic lab complete with kilns. All Lockheed employees and their families, who are automatically members of the LERA, are free to participate in the range of club activities. Two years ago, after a group of joggers and bikers decided that they wanted showers and raised money for the project on their own, support for athletic facilities grew among the plant's 20,000 employees. Today the LERA's Family Fitness Center, with locker and shower facilities for men and women and an exercise room, is nearly complete. A recreational administrator for the LERA says that the association hopes to have its own tennis courts, softball fields, and jogging tracks in the near future. "The average age among employees at Lockheed is 47 years. But this is beginning to change. We will use our new facilities as both a recruitment tool and a means of creating a healthier and more enjoyable working environment."[68]

New York State Department of Education Physical Fitness/Heart Disease Intervention Program. Employees were notified in 1972 of the initiation of an experimental heart disease intervention program.[69] The program was available to all employees regardless of age, sex, salary, position, or physical health. At a preprogram orientation, prospective participants were informed of the potential objectives and benefits of the program, time requirements, cost commitments, and general format. Participation time—1¼ hours per day, three days per week during lunch hour for 15 weeks—was arranged by each participant with his or her supervisor and negotiated within the framework of the department's flexible hours policy. Employees who could meet this time commitment, as well as pay a $25 matriculation fee, were asked to register for a three-phase medical evaluation. Employees unable to make this commitment were placed with the pool of uninterested employees to form a group for later consideration as a control group.

Phases I and II of the three-part medical appraisal were completed at the Department of Civil Service Health Clinic. Phase I examination included a medical history questionnaire and a comprehensive clinical evaluation (blood and urine chemistry, chest x ray, pulmonary function tests, resting electrocardiogram, blood pressure, visual acuity, and audiometric examinations). After the clinical examination, each participant consulted with an exercise physiologist, who documented an exercise history and determined percent fat and lean body weight. In Phase II of the screening, conducted two weeks later, a clinic physician reviewed the medical history questionnaire, interpreted the Phase I clinical test data, and performed a complete physical examination. After correlating these results, the physician determined the cardiovascular risk factor status of the employee and counseled him or her on risk factor modification. Subjects at high risk of cardiovascular disease, under physician care, or with a past history of cardiovascular disease were classed as provisional participants and referred to their personal physicians for written consent to participate in further program testing. In the final phase, Phase III, the subject is given a resting electrocardiogram and then is tested on an exercise treadmill.

The Physical Fitness/Heart Disease Intervention Program was a two-part intervention: a formal exercise program and a classroom educational program. The exercise program was conducted at a state armory within five minutes' walking distance of the State Education Building. A formal 15-week beginner or primary activities program consisted of a 10-minute warm-up period, a 25- to 30-minute regimen of jog–walk intervals, and a 5-minute period of instruction in relaxation techniques. Supervised activity programs were conducted on four weekdays. All subjects were taught to monitor their own heart rates by palpating their radial or carotid artery for a 15-second count. The education program included biweekly classroom seminars on (1) principles of cardiorespiratory health and fitness; (2) exercise and cardiovascular dynamics; (3) tension/hypertension: stress and high blood pressure; (4) nutritional fundamentals; (5) weight control: diet/calorie expenditure; (6) cholesterol, triglycerides, and fats; (7) aerobics and respiration; and (8) motivation: self-directed lifestyle intervention. Employees were required to attend a minimum of half of these seminars to qualify for "graduation" to secondary program status as well as for a refund of $10 of the $25 matriculation deposit. The seminars were presented by volunteer health professionals from the community.

Employees completing the 15-week primary intervention program were reevaluated, and information from the retest was compared with preprogram data and used to motivate participants and redefine their secondary or ongoing program. Employees completing one year of participation were given the same comprehensive health evaluation that they received at entry. Employees wanting to continue to participate were assessed a $15 annual membership fee; health appraisals were conducted annually for these employees.

Over 800 employees—about one-third of the Department of Education staff—participated in the 15-week primary intervention program during the five-year period from 1972 through 1977. A study of the outcome of the first eight primary intervention programs, in which 719 employees participated, revealed several interesting results.[70] Program retention on an average was 80 percent. Mean sick leave for participants during their program (46.5 hours) was substantially below the mean sick leave for all New York State employees for the same year (73.5 hours). Significant reductions in serum cholesterol levels, body weight, tobacco consumption and both systolic and diastolic blood pressure contributed to overall reductions in risk factors for program participants. Significant improvements in both physical work capacity and predicted maximal oxygen uptake also were demonstrated.

Madison, Wisconsin, Police Department Fitness Program. The city of Madison's police department has developed a fitness program to improve the health of its 292 commissioned officers as well as its 77-member civilian staff.[71] In the beginning, the only employee was a part-time physical fitness coordinator. In 1978, when the Wisconsin State Legislature endorsed the creation of a 37-member Commission on Prevention and Wellness and appropriated $980,000 to stimulate program development, local public agencies, profit and nonprofit organizations, and individuals were encouraged to apply for incentive grants.[72] Over 301 applications for grants were received, one of which was a proposal from the Madison Police Department to expand its fitness program. The department indicated that grant funds would be used to continue the fitness coordinator's employment, to add the services of a registered dietitian, and to purchase additional equipment. The department's overall program goal is

. . . the improved fitness of Department employees. A minimum of 20% of the employees are expected to participate during the first year. Each participating employee will exhibit increased cardiovascular endurance, muscle strength, and flexibility, and will receive education on good nutrition practices. . . . Increases in cardiovascular endurance will be recorded by measuring functional capacity for each participant at six month intervals; similarly, every six months individual flexibility ranges will be measured using a flexometer. Increases in muscular strength will be evaluated through records of weight lifting.[73]

The project was funded for $13,700 to support the first year of a proposed three-year effort. Three reasons were given by the Wisconsin Department of Health and Social Services for funding the project: (1) the project population is a unique and needy target population; (2) the potential for interesting data is high; and (3) objectives and tasks are well-developed.[74] Wisconsin's Department of Health and Social Services funded 29 projects in health promotion and disease prevention throughout the state during 1979 in meeting its legislative mandate to disburse the nearly $1 million in incentive grants.

The Alexandria, Virginia, Fire Department Fitness Program. Today, administrators in many of the country's police and fire departments are grappling with the problems of on-duty injury and off-duty illness by instituting fitness and conditioning programs for their personnel.[75] Both the Los Angeles Fire Department and the Dallas Police Department were pioneers in establishing fitness programs. The smaller Alexandria, Virginia, Fire Department also has taken an innovative approach to fitness.

The program includes a compulsory exercise program comprising 10 minutes of flexibility and warm-up exercises, 30 minutes of cardiovascular endurance exercises, and 20 minutes of strength-building exercises on each duty day.[76] The department also bans the hiring of smokers. A longitudinal study of fitness levels within the department was begun about four years ago. Each member of the department receives an entry-level workup—response to exercises, blood studies, and motor fitness—which is repeated every year. Data on 145 firemen have revealed two categories of disability time users. Those in one category tended to be "heterogeneous, to be injured more seriously in chance happenings, and use their disability time in large blocks."[77] Those in the other category tended to be "smokers, preobese or obese, and weaker; they had multiple minor injuries and used several short blocks of disability time."[78] Alexandria's fire chief is convinced that the department's policy has benefits. Overall neuromuscular strength and coordination have improved, sick leave has dropped, and the department has lost "one ton of fat" since the program was adopted. "I don't know how you can put a price tag on the health benefits," the chief concludes. "For us, it is the best investment we can make in the men on the force."[79]

The Connecticut State Department of Health Model for Prevention Programs at the Worksite.[80] Based on a multiple risk factor approach to cardiovascular disease, the model includes short-term and long-term goals for primary prevention, secondary prevention, and tertiary prevention, as well as examples of specific plans of action in four areas: hypertension, smoking, nutrition, and exercise. The exercise model is presented in Appendix B.

This model of primary, secondary, and tertiary prevention activities centered in exercise at the worksite, as well as the case studies of exercise programs tailored to different types of workers in different settings, suggests the broad gamut of plans to promote exercise that can be set into motion. As Jonathan Fielding reminds us:

> In some countries exercise at the work station is considered a normal part of daily life. . . . [M]ore companies should consider providing facilities and encouragement for employees to be able to perform vigorous exercise of the kind that seems to be useful in improving the heart's ability to withstand the effects of heart attack. While some companies have elaborate gymnasium and track facilities, a beneficial program can be established at a much lower cost. The provision of lockers and shower facilities, for example, would allow

those that jog to run at lunch time or after work. It would also encourage employees to take their bicycles to work or even to jog to work. If companies have fairly extensive grounds, they can develop, for a very small investment, jogging trails or "life" trails where people can walk briskly as a way of getting exercise. For companies willing to make a larger investment, racquetball, handball, basketball, or squash courts might be considered. An indoor track may be a good investment because of the large numbers of employees that can use it simultaneously.[81]

Exercise promotion can mean different things to different companies and public agencies, depending on the nature of their work force, their size, their location, and their willingness to make an investment in their workers' health, fitness, and morale.

Exercise in the Home

The home presents opportunities for physical activity that could be more fully exploited, especially for high-risk groups—those with chronic health problems, the elderly, and the disabled. More importantly, the home is a place to learn about physical activity and to establish patterns of physical activity that will last for a lifetime. As the Canadians point out, most people have newspapers, magazines, books, records, radios, and televisions in their homes; these media could be much more fully exploited to present information about physical activity. "These include programs and articles that explain the nature of physical fitness and the importance and benefits of physical activity. . . . [D]etailed information on the availability of local physical activities could be presented through the media. . . . [T]elevision could be used more extensively to present exercise programs for specific population segments such as children, elderly persons and housewives."[82]

Lifetime exercise habits, like other habits (including eating habits), begin at home. Parents have a strong influence both on their children's daily exercise habits and on their attitudes toward exercising throughout their lives. There are several ways for parents to foster good exercise habits and attitudes:

1. For the health of both mother and child, physical activity programs should be followed during and after pregnancy. Education materials for pregnant women should stress the importance of physical activity not only during pregnancy, but, throughout life.
2. Parents have an important exemplar role to play. If parents are physically active, their children are likely to be physically active.
3. Physically active family outings—hiking, skiing, canoeing, swimming—are important activities in shaping lifelong habits.

4. Parents should encourage children to participate in sports, in games, or in other physical activity with other children. This activity should emphasize participation and enjoyment rather than competition. Competition should receive less emphasis among children, particularly among younger children.[83]

Women at home, especially mothers with young children, however, often find it difficult to participate in regular exercise or recreation programs outside the home. Programs designed specifically for such women, which include babysitting arrangements or activity programs to include both mothers and children, need to be designed.

The elderly have special needs and problems with regard to exercise. Both their opportunities and capacities for exercise may be limited. Lack of public and private transportation may leave them homebound and unable to participate in community exercise or recreation activities; health problems may further restrict their mobility. A plan of exercise for homebound elderly persons as well as exercise programs tailored to the elderly in neighborhood centers are two possible directions to take. The Rhode Island Department of Health has recommended that "all senior citizen centers should offer organized walks, jogging programs and indoor light exercise programs."[84] An awareness of the varying needs and capacities for exercise of different population groups as well as a recognition of the home as an important setting for exercise promotion led the Canadian government to develop a unique tool in its national fitness campaign.

The Fit-Kit, designed and distributed by the Fitness and Amateur Sport Branch of the Canadian Department of National Health and Welfare, is one component of the Department's "Operation Lifestyle."[85] This major health-promotion and disease-prevention program, which includes seven target areas—alcohol use, smoking, fitness, nutrition, drugs, safety, and general health—was launched after the publication of the Canadian government's policy document on health, *A New Perspective on the Health of Canadians.*[86] The idea for the Fit-Kit itself came out of a national conference on fitness and health in 1972. One of the conference recommendations was:

[that] Recreation Canada develop a safe, simple, self-administered fitness test, the purpose of which would be motivational rather than accurately to evaluate fitness. More specifically, the test should be designed for all age groups and fitness levels and should enable each participant to classify himself according to established norms by indicating the desirable levels of fitness to be achieved. The test could form the core of the educational and promotional program.[87]

The Fit-Kit contains eight items: (1) The Canadian Home Fitness Test;[88] (2) a long-playing record used to assess fitness level and to measure progress in a recommended physical activity program; (3) a Progress Chart; (4) a Fit-Tips Exercise wall chart; (5) a Walk-Run Distance calculator; (6) Rx for Physical Activity; (7) a booklet, "Health and Fitness," by Astrand;[89] and (8) an Advanced Fitness Test. The basic ingredient of the Fit-Kit is the phonograph record, which permits anyone between 15 and 69 years of age to conduct a test of cardiopulmonary fitness in his or her own home.[90] Entitled "The Canadian Home Fitness Test: 1, 2, 3 . . . Steps to Better Health," the record provides instructions on how to perform a two-step exercise test and how to relate the pulse rate to the three levels of fitness—undesirable, minimum, and recommended. The instructions accompanying the phonograph record direct the person to answer seven simple questions about his or her medical history before deciding to take the test. Studies of the test in 14,794 persons demonstrate the safety of the test.[91] A market survey of the Fit-Kit in two Canadian communities showed that 94 percent of people completing the test found the instructions simple and clear, that 54 percent actually took the test and that 96 percent had others in their homes take the test, and that 83 percent responded positively to the test.[92]

The Fit-Kit has been made available to the public through Government of Canada bookstores and organizations such as the YMCA. (The Fit-Kit can be obtained for $8.50 from the Department of Supply and Service, the Canadian Government Publishing Center, Hull, Quebec, Canada K1A0S9.)

Exercise in Schools

Public and private elementary (grade) schools, intermediate (junior high) schools, secondary (senior high) schools, junior colleges, colleges, and universities as well as trade and vocational schools and special schools for the handicapped all have a role to play with respect to exercise. Basically, schools have several well-defined areas of activity in promoting exercise. Schools provide a setting for instruction about exercise and about particular types of exercise and sports; schools provide opportunities to participate in exercise and sports; schools in most cases have both indoor and outdoor sports and exercise facilities (gynmasiums, swimming pools, lockers and showers, playing courts and fields).

Schools have a responsibility to serve students' interests as well as the interests of the community. The American Medical Association's Council on Scientific Affairs Panel on Exercise and Fitness comments that "schools have the same responsibility to provide a physical education as they have to provide an academic education. Schools need to consider the total educational process when planning budget expenditures for physical education and academic pursuits."[93] The Panel on Exercise and Fitness recently issued a statement strongly urging "school boards, school administrators and parents to provide physical education programs during elementary, junior high and senior high years. The programs should be conducted by qualified personnel, be designed to teach health habits and physical skills, and instill a desire in the student for physical fitness that will carry over into his adult life. Physical education must be considered as an integral part of the total educational process."[94] In 1978, the American Medical Association's House of Delegates adopted a resolution that called on the association (1) to continue to educate the medical profession about exercise, including continuing medical education courses and conferences on the role of exercise prescriptions in medical practice; (2) to help medical students receive instruction about the prescription of exercise; (3) to confirm its long-standing policy regarding the need for physical education instruction in the school system; and (4) to continue to educate the public about the benefits of exercise.[95]

Today a number of forces are conspiring to keep schools, especially public schools, from meeting their responsibility to educate "the whole student." Shrinking local tax revenues in some communities are forcing schools and school boards to look for places to slash "frills" from budgets. Team sports and physical education as well as exercise and recreational equipment and facilities have been considered "priority items" for budget cuts. The school curriculum also is changing. Physical education, once a required course in secondary schools and in colleges and universities, is now an elective. Many students pass through several years of school life as "nonparticipants" in exercise or fitness programs. As a recent staff paper of the President's Council on Physical Fitness and Sports point out, there has been "a decline in the number and quality of school physical education and sports programs."[96]

A recent study by the Canadian Association for Health and Physical Education and Recreation has identified a good elementary school physical education program as having the following elements:

daily instruction;
maximum activity participation;
wide range of movement experience;
total fitness activities;
qualified competent teachers;
adequate and appropriate facilities and equipment;
principles of child growth and development at its base;
opportunities to develop positive attitudes to activity; and suitable competition.[97]

These elements, the report noted, could also apply to secondary school programs. Unfortunately most school programs of physical education lack these elements.

A number of actions can be taken to reverse this trend. One plan is for State Departments of Education to adopt guidelines for a required comprehensive health education curriculum (K–12) that includes education and information about the health benefits of dynamic aerobic exercise as well as an emphasis on instruction and participation in lifetime sports. Another plan of action is to influence colleges and universities that train physical education teachers to alter their curricula to emphasize teaching about lifetime sports, aerobic exercise, and the physiology of exercise, including, as the Division of Health of the State of Georgia has recommended, "the critical role of humidity, barometric pressure, the physiological stress of heat to electrolyte depletion and the nutritional needs of athletes."[98] Since lifetime sports education and participation for children are critical, a plan to influence curriculum content both in schools and in colleges and universities will most likely have the greatest impact over the longest period of time of any plan to promote exercise. A background study to explore the need for such a plan for the State of California has been conducted by the Health Policy Program, University of California, San Francisco. This information will be represented in the form of a case study.

Physical Education Curriculum Content in the State of California. Like the content of all curricula of public elementary (grade), intermediate (junior high), and secondary (senior high) schools, the California curriculum content is determined by a process that begins at the Office of Curriculum Services in the State Department of Education and ends with the individual teacher. First, the State Department of Education develops guidelines for the curriculum content of virtually all courses taught in the school system. Then the local school board and its district staff develop rather detailed curriculum plans specifying the skills that children are to be taught and the textbooks that are to be used. To implement these plans, teacher guides and manuals, lesson plans, and lesson kits containing charts, pictures, and other audio-visual materials are disseminated to schools for distribution to teachers. The individual school and the department head (the head of the Department of Physical Education in this case) then decide the specific curriculum content to be taught. Because the structure of elementary schools does not include heads of departments of specific subjects, individual teachers (with guidance from the principal's office) take on the role of determining the specific curriculum. Information about curriculum content also is provided at regular meetings of all teachers in elementary schools and of teachers in a department in junior and senior high schools. With this guidance, the teacher develops lesson plans for day-to-day instruction.

In private schools, the curriculum is developed through a continuum descending from the central office to whom the school reports to the individual teacher. The State Department of Education has little impact on the curriculum of private schools.

Another factor that influences curriculum content in both public and private schools is the instruction that teachers themselves receive in their college and graduate school education courses. Elementary teachers are required to take one course on methods in children's physical education. According to a recent graduate of one of these programs, the concept of dynamic aerobic exercise and the principles of exercising 20 to 30 minutes three times per week are generally not introduced in this course.[99] In intermediate and secondary schools, physical education courses are generally taught by full-time physical education teachers who have completed college and graduate course work as physical education majors. As physical education majors, these teachers have taken numerous courses on physical education teaching methods, but such courses give little emphasis to dynamic aerobic sports that can be carried on for a lifetime.

Teachers in both public and private institutions also are constrained in the sports and activities that they can teach by the facilities available at the school. The activity area of most elementary schools consists of a rather small, blacktop playground. Because a substantial number of children must be accommodated on such playgrounds at any given time, teachers must rely on team sports, which by their nature generally revolve around one ball that stays in a rather small area, for example, kickball or dodgeball. Individual sports, such as jogging and swimming, or two-persons sports, such as handball, generally require more room and, in the case of swimming, more extensive facilities. Interventions to alter the physical education curriculum content could be made at any level—in the development of an improved curriculum, in the education of teachers, or in the development of facilities available for use by teachers and students.

A lifetime sports education curriculum has two distinct components: (1) teaching the need for lifetime dynamic aerobic exercise activity, including the frequency and duration of exercise required to improve cardiovascular fitness; and (2) instruction in one- and two-participant aerobic sports that can be carried on for a lifetime. Sports and activities can be divided into those that require two or more participants, those that require at least two participants, and those that require only one participant. Some sports that require more than two persons, the so-called team sports, are aerobic in nature (Table 8.1). This group includes basketball and soccer, two sports frequently taught in the schools. However, both sports require the participation of a large number of players, 6 to 10 in basketball and approximately 20 in soccer. Teams are easily formed in a school physical education course, but gathering such a large group of adults on a regular basis is difficult. Dynamic aerobic sports requiring one or two persons are more appropriate for lifetime participation. Of the one- and two-participant sports listed in Table 8.1, dancing, jogging, swimming, handball, platform tennis, regular tennis, racquetball, and squash are appropriate at various times as the child's motor skills improve with age. Of these, dancing, jogging, handball, regular tennis, racquetball, and squash are the least costly in terms of facilities and equipment.

Most children do not have the motor skills necessary to play many of the one- and two-person sports, such as racquetball, until they reach the end of elementary school. Elementary school facilities also generally do not meet the space requirements of one- and two-person aerobic sports. However, team sports that are aerobic can be emphasized at the elementary school level; examples are soccer, basketball, and volleyball. Elementary school teachers also have the opportunity to reinforce the sentiment already held by many children that exercise is really play and that, as such, it is fun. Teachers can also generally introduce the concept that exercise is of value to the children's current and future health status and physical abilities.

By the time students reach junior high school, they are intellectually capable of understanding how exercise can benefit their health and what type, intensity, frequency, and duration of exercise are needed to achieve these benefits. However, because children and adolescents are more concerned with their present physical appearance and physical skills than with their future health, the concept of dynamic aerobic exercise is best presented with an emphasis on how it will improve their present status (e.g., allow them to lose weight or improve their disabilities in other sports, such as football). Lifetime sports also could be taught much more frequently than they are now in junior high school. Physical education instruction currently focuses on major American spectator sports—football, baseball, and basketball—rather than on sports that can be carried on for a lifetime. It appears that schools are preparing children to become sports spectators rather than sports participants.

It is not until senior high school that the guidelines developed by the California State Department of Education in its *Physical Education Framework* call for the inclusion in the curriculum of:

> Opportunities for continued development, maintenance, and understanding of physical fitness by developing programs which aid the student in demonstrating knowledge of the relation of exercise and nutrition to a feeling of well-being; *demonstrating knowledge of the need for adult fitness; developing individual exercise program to fit individual requirements;* participating in vigorous running, swimming, dancing, or jumping activities . . .[100]

Thus, the California State Department of Education does call for some aspects of lifetime sports education to be included in the curriculum, but not until students reach senior high school. This is too late for the following reasons: (1) fewer and fewer senior high schools require their students to take courses in physical education; (2) many adolescents already dislike and are "turned off" to exercise by the time that they reach senior high school; and (3) many senior high school students participate in interscholastic sports or related activities such as the band or cheerleading team, which replace regular physical education instruction, resulting in their missing an education in lifetime sports. Thus, classes in aerobic exercise principles and lifetime sports should be offered in high school, but they also should be offered as part of the junior high school curriculum.

The role of physical education as it is currently taught is: (1) to teach children about their bodies; (2) to provide instruction that allows the development of motor skills; and (3) to develop children's social skills by placing them in situations in which they must work cooperatively toward a goal and by teaching them the values of sportsmanship.[101]

Team sports are the generally accepted means to meet these goals. Individual and two-person sports, however, can meet all these goals except working cooperatively with others. When these sports are combined with the introduction of the concept of aerobic fitness, they do a better job than team sports in teaching children about their bodies. Finally, these sports allow for the accomplishment of a goal that we believe should be added to the physical education curriculum: they allow for the development of skills in sports that can be played for a lifetime and that can influence health and well-being over a lifetime. A number of approaches might be taken to move schools in the direction of lifetime sports education. We will discuss three alternative approaches that policymakers and program managers at the state level of government might consider.

The first approach is based on incentives generated by the state to bring about a voluntary change in the curricula of local school districts. First, the governor would announce a "Lifetime Sports Week." Each school interested in participating in the Lifetime Sports Week would have made available the following items: (1) suggested sports activities to be carried out during the week; (2) teaching modules that physical education and health education instructors could use to teach students about the fundamentals and benefits of dynamic aerobic exercise and lifetime sports; and (3) Governor's Lifetime Sports Award badges for all students who would participate in the week's activities. Suggested activities for the week would include tennis and racquetball tournaments; running, cycling, and swimming races; aerobic dancing parties; and sessions or competitions in other lifetime sports. To overcome the facility limitations of participating schools, community park and college facilities could be utilized. To avoid overlapping use of community facilities that might occur when several neighboring schools participated, each school could designate a "Lifetime Sports Day" during Lifetime Sports Week. Parents could be invited to all the activities. Teaching modules could be jointly developed by the State Departments of Education and Health. The expertise of the American Heart Association affiliates in the state and State Medical Association Committees on Exercise could be drawn to provide technical assistance in the development of this material. Lifetime Sports Award badges might encourage participation by children in participating schools and increase the visibility of the state in the program. Funding for the state's role in the program could be provided by state funds or by project grants from the federal government. Such grants are to be made available under Title V of Public Law 95-626, the Health Services and Centers Amendments of 1978. This approach would not mandate school participation in the program either by regulation or by law. Each school would go through its established decisionmaking channels to determine its level of involvement, if any. If a school did participate, the school, or perhaps individual teachers within the school, would determine what percentage of the school year they would like to devote to the use of the lifetime sports teaching modules. Teaching modules could be developed so that if a school desired, the entire year-long curriculum in each grade level could be based on the teaching of the fundamentals and health benefits of dynamic aerobic exercise and lifetime sports. Private schools could be encouraged to participate in all aspects of the program.

The second approach would involve the adoption of guidelines for lifetime sports education programs as part of State Department of Education guidelines for schools and the development of a television program on lifetime sports suitable for junior and senior high school students. The State Departments of Education and Health could work jointly to develop the guidelines, along with specific lesson plans or modules, in conjunction with available medical and physical education resource groups. These same groups also could act as advisors for a television program (or miniseries) for junior and senior high school students about the fundamentals and benefits of lifetime sports and dynamic aerobic exercise. The program could be shown on educational and public television stations. In communities where no such station is available, the program could be made available to commercial stations as suitable for their public service contribution. After its airing on television, a film of the show could be made available for future classroom use. While private schools would not be required to participate in the program, all materials pertaining to the program could be made available to interested schools.

A third and more long-range approach would be to alter the state educational requirements necessary to obtain a teacher's certificate to include education in the teaching of lifetime sports.

A variety of other approaches might, of course, be considered. Exercise promotion in schools extends past changes in public and private elementary, intermediate, and secondary schools to include colleges and universities. The next two case studies focus on the promotion of exercise in a medical school and in a trade–technical college.

The University of California, San Francisco, Running Clinic. The running clinic began in 1978 with two goals: (1) to educate the public about the value of exercise as a health maintenance measure and to teach people how to integrate running into their lifestyles by beginning slowly and easily; and (2) to educate medical students as well as other health-profession students about the value and use of exercise in medical practice. The public consisted of the population of the San Francisco Bay Area. Participants were encouraged to come as often as they wanted—once or twice to have their questions answered or every week to run with a group and meet new running partners and friends. The running clinic has been conducted every Saturday from November through May for two seasons, 1978–1979 and 1979–1980. The format for the clinic includes:

1. A question-and-answer period with questions asked by clinic participants and answered by volunteer health professions' student staff. All volunteer staff are veteran runners with some interest in sports medicine. Questions commonly deal with running injuries, diet, and running form.
2. A stretching session led by volunteer student staff.
3. Group runs of varying distances, each led by a volunteer staff member, that usually include a 1-mile walk/jog for beginners, a 2-mile jog, a 3-mile run, and a 5- to 7-mile run. While on the run, participants are encouraged to ask questions of the volunteer staff members, who provide information and support to individual participants and to the running group as a whole.

Once a month or sometimes more frequently, a guest expert is invited to present a brief lecture on a topic of special concern. Such topics have included "Preventing Rape on the Run," "Nutrition, Exercise, and Carbohydrate Loading," "Running After 40," "Smoking, Alcohol, and Exercise," "Fitness and Heart Disease Prevention," "Women Running," and "Why Run and How to Get Started." The clinic also has featured a health hazard appraisal in cooperation with the San Francisco Department of Public Health, Bureau of Health Promotion and Education. It is estimated that over 1000 people have made at least one visit to the clinic; participants were predominantly women aged 20 through 50.

The University of California, San Francisco (UCSF) Running Clinic is free to all participants. Volunteer staff members include students in several health professional schools—medicine, nursing, dentistry, and physical therapy. The budget, not including volunteer staff time, was $150 for the 1978–1979 season and $300 for the 1979–1980 season. Cosponsors of the clinic have been the UCSF Chapter of the American Medical Students Association, the San Francisco Department of Public Health, Outdoors Unlimited, the San Francisco Recreation and Parks Department, the Millberry Student Union, UCSF, and Public Service Programs, UCSF.

The Be-Fit Program of Los Angeles Trade–Technical College (LATTC). This program grew out of a need for an exercise program for a multicultural mix of students, whose average age is 30 and who are commuters to a large inner-city school with limited recreational and physical education facilities.[102] The program's objectives are:

to operate a health awareness and physical activity program that will involve 10 percent of the LATTC student body and staff (approximately 1900) within a nine-month period;

to involve members of each student support service department and the instructional Department of Physical and Health Education in the program;

to operate the program with limited staff, budget, and facilities; and

to provide a "model physical fitness program" for the other colleges and business, industrial, and governmental agencies.

The Be-Fit Program, which has borrowed heavily from the "Fit to Live" Program,* is individualized and focuses on both fitness awareness and fitness training. Initially, awareness comes about through a physical examination and the completion of a personal health and exercise inventory, which informs a person of his or her physical "condition" and where he or she is placed on a national normative fitness scale. The fitness training becomes progressively more strenuous. A point system places values on a broad spectrum of activities, including household, outdoor recreational, indoor recreational, sports, and exercise activities, which range from gardening to dancing, from cleaning house to marathons. Through a nine-week period, with three-week improvement blocks, a person can reach a level of physical fitness and exercise that he or she can maintain and improve. Posters, program descriptions handed to students at registration, special announcements, and letters are used to promote the program. Another effective promotional method is the wearing of "Los Angeles Trade–Technical College Be-Fit" t-shirts. Enrollment stations for the "Be-Fit" Program are located in the Physical and Health Education

*Copyright by Dawson College, Montreal, Quebec.

offices, the Counseling Center, the Career Guidance Center, and the Health Office. The program requires a half-time coordinator and a full-time clerk typist. All other assistance is provided by student assistants, existing staff, and volunteers. The budget for the program is in the range of $10,000 to $20,000.

Exercise in the Community

A community embraces a geographic area, some form of local government, a mix of population groups (identifiable by age, sex, marital status, socioeconomic status, racial and ethnic characteristics), several political constituencies, a more or less self-contained system of mass media, a system of mass transportation, a range of business and industries, a network of service and community organizations, and institutions such as schools, churches, and hospitals.

Communities have been the target for and the base of systematic campaigns to identify and to reduce cardiovascular risk factors during the past decade. The Stanford Three Community Study, conducted in the semi-rural communities of Gilroy, Watsonville, and Tracy, California, is the most well-known effort to "unsell heart disease" in this country.[103] The North Karelia Project in Finland is a comprehensive community project involving both primary and secondary preventive measures to reduce risks in a population with reportedly the highest incidence of cardiovascular disease in the world.[104] And the Ontario Ministry of Culture and Recreation has launched what is probably the most ambitious fitness program in Canada. In the Ontario program, seven mobile testing laboratories, each staffed by five individuals trained to implement a sophisticated version of the Canadian Home Fitness Test, are made available to communities in the province. The assessment and consultation part of the program is only one facet of a larger program, which includes a promotional campaign, a training program for instructors, and the provision of financial assistance to various community motivation projects. There is little doubt that this province places cardiovascular fitness high on its list of priorities in the prevention of heart disease.[105]

Institutions within communities, such as hospitals, also have been active in reaching out into the community to provide programs for those who want to assess and to improve their current level of fitness. Peralta Hospital's East Bay Sports Medicine Program provides a health and exercise program (P.E.P.) for San Francisco Bay Area executives as well as preseason physical performance evaluations and exercise prescriptions for professional athletes.[106]

Finally, communities themselves have been instrumental in conducting formal or informal experiments in changing behavior and in changing environments in which behavior occurs. Davis, California, known as "Bike City, U.S.A.," is an example of a city whose citizens chose to create a local transportation system that emphasizes bicycle transportation.[107] These community-wide interventions and decisions have the potential to change the context of both individual and group health behavior. Indeed, the community context may well be an ideal context in which to work to effect long-term changes in behavior.

Communities are now being encouraged to develop "an organized approach to risk reduction" to qualify for health education/risk-reduction grants available through the Center for Disease Control, Public Health Service, U.S. Department of Health and Human Services. In March 1980, the Center for Disease Control issued guidelines describing the steps that agencies or organizations (e.g., Departments of Public Health) should take in developing an organized approach to reduction of risk in seven areas: (1) smoking; (2) alcohol use; (3) obesity; (4) exercise (physical inactivity); (5) stress; (6) hypertension; and (7) accident prevention and injury control.[108] The guidelines summarize the importance of physical inactivity as a risk factor and outline steps to develop an organized, community-wide approach to risk reduction:

1. Provide a brief description of the community—a community is definable as a geographic area (e.g., a county or counties, town, city, health district, Indian reservation, federation of natives).
2. List participating organizations in the community and the lead agency.
3. Determine the prevalence of risk factors for the population in the community (e.g., by estimates or projections from existing data, a sample survey, a planned survey).
4. Establish objectives to reduce the prevalence of risk factors in the community—agreed on by multiple agencies and organizations interested in reducing risk in the community.
5. Describe each current activity or commitment to reduce the prevalence of risks in the community.
6. Schedule an annual reassessment of the status of risk factors within the community.[109]

A community-based approach to risk reduction also is recommended in revised draft national guidelines and goals for health planning issued by the Health Resources Administration of the Department of Health and Human Services in July 1979. One of the goals delineated is that "health promotion and preventive health services should be an integral component of care provided by health care and other community institutions."[110] To achieve this goal, agencies with major health responsibilities, as well as educational, occupational, and social agencies, are encouraged to include health promotion and preventive health services in their respective programs. "Wherever they are located," the guidelines read, "prevention programs should typically be aimed at changing knowledge, attitudes, and behaviors of the community toward improved health status and appropriate utilization of existing health services."[111]

Six convincing arguments have been given for developing community-based models of lifestyle intervention by Dr. John Farquhar, Director of the Stanford Heart Disease Prevention Program:

1. to develop methods of risk reduction that are applicable to the real environments in which people live;
2. to increase the power of interventions through diffusion in the community and social support;
3. to test the effectiveness of programs that are more generalizable than those of clinic-based trials;
4. to provide public policymakers with evidence of the feasibility and effectiveness of public health programs;
5. to eliminate some of the ethical problems of individual randomization;
6. to reduce the cost of trials.[112]

The Stanford Three Community Study. The Stanford study was a field experiment conducted between 1972 and 1975 in three Northern California agricultural communities—Gilroy, Watsonville, and Tracy—each with a population of approximately 15,000, to study the modification of cardiovascular disease risk factors through community education.[113] A joint effort of the Stanford Heart Disease Prevention Program within the School of Medicine and of the Institute for Communication Research of Stanford University, the study involved baseline studies as well as three annual follow-up surveys to assess the effects of the campaign in a random sample of individuals between the ages of 35 and 59. In Gilroy and Watsonville, an extensive bilingual (English and Spanish) mass media health education campaign was conducted for two years and maintained at a lower level of intensity during a third year. A broad range of media materials was utilized, including over 150 radio and television spots, several hours of radio and television programming, weekly newspaper columns, newspaper advertisements and stories, billboards, bus posters, and printed material sent via direct mail to people in the random samples selected for the surveys. In Watsonville, this media campaign was supplemented with "change agent" risk reduction administered to a randomly selected two-thirds of the top quartile at risk in the random sample. The instruction took place primarily during the final four months of the first-year campaign effort and consisted of 10 one- to three-hour groups or home instruction classes related to dietary modification, weight loss, smoking cessation, and increase of physical activity. This type of instruction was maintained at a lower level during the second year of campaigning. In the third community, Tracy, no campaign was conducted.

Results of the Stanford Three Community Study included (1) changes in knowledge about risk factors; (2) changes in dietary habits and dietary risk factors; (3) changes in cigarette smoking; (4) changes in blood pressure; and (5) changes in the risk of coronary heart disease as measured by changes in the multiple logistic function of risk factors.[114] Increases in risk appeared in the control group, Tracy, even though members of this group had yearly examinations in which their risk factors were reported to them and to their physicians. In contrast, reductions in risks occurred during the first year in the two "treatment" groups; these changes were not only maintained but improved during the second year. It also was evident that groups in Watsonville, in which some face-to-face instruction was provided, showed a greater decrease than the "media-only" groups at the end of the first year. By the end of the second year, the groups exposed only to media showed substantial further gains and the difference between media and media plus face-to-face instruction was diminished and no longer was statistically significant. There was a close parallel relationship between the two media groups in Gilroy and Watsonville. This provides evidence for the similarity of the media campaigns and for their effects on risk in the two treatment communities. As the program directors noted:

> The results of the Three-Community Study in which the intensively instructed individuals did show considerable change in risk [are] an example of an effect of combined treatment. Although it is not surprising that a combination of treatments is more successful than a single treatment, the more relevant question is whether or not a community setting offers opportunities for diffusion of health innovations and if so how one might best harness these opportunities for diffusion in a way that would enhance the effectiveness of any treatment input into that community. One method of achieving accelerated diffusion of health information and health habit innovations is to create a cadre of individuals who possess extra knowledge and who have begun changes in health practices in their own lives. If one could scatter such individuals throughout a community, they might serve to catalyze the effect of general health information put into the community through mass media; these "early adopters" may be recognized by the average citizen of the community as peers who are respected for their innovations. . . .[115]

In our opinion, such people are already scattered throughout communities in the United States and are making significant progress in changing national, community, and individual profiles of health.

Table 8.1. Dynamic Aerobic Sports and Activities

Requiring only one participant
Bicycling (briskly)
Cross-country skiing
Dancing (briskly)
Ice skating (briskly)
Jogging/running
Rollerskating (briskly)
Swimming
Walking (briskly)

Requiring at least two participants
Badminton
Basketball
Fencing
Football
Handball
Platform tennis
Racquetball
Soccer
Squash
Tennis
Volleyball

Requiring two participants or more
Basketball
Football
Soccer
Volleyball

Appendix A

Guidelines for Physical Fitness Programs in Business and Industry

A JOINT STATEMENT OF THE PRESIDENT'S COUNCIL ON PHYSICAL FITNESS AND SPORTS AND THE AMERICAN MEDICAL ASSOCIATION'S COMMITTEE ON EXERCISE AND PHYSICAL FITNESS

Research indicates that programs of regular exercise can promote increased physical fitness and health, provided the exercise prescribed is appropriate to the physical capacity and needs of the individual. Many companies concerned with the health of their employees are initiating physical exercise programs to assist in the promotion of optimal health, reduce absenteeism from work due to illness, and increase production and morale.

The President's Council on Physical Fitness and Sports and the American Medical Association's Committee on Exercise and Physical Fitness support company-sponsored exercise programs that are developed in accordance with current scientific and medical knowledge. The following guidelines are presented to assist companies in determining the policies they will follow in the administration and management of these programs:

PURPOSE AND BELIEFS

1. Company-sponsored physical fitness programs should be conducted as an adjunct to the company's medical program. Policies pertaining to the development and management of the program should receive medical endorsement. In companies not having their own medical director, operating policies should be developed in consultation with appropriate medical and physical fitness authorities.
2. Individuals vary in their exercise needs. Therefore, consideration should be given to programs of physical fitness education,

rehabilitiation and training, and maintenance.

3. At least a portion, if not all, of the physical fitness program should be conducted on company time for purposes of motivation and supervision. Many participants will engage in a prescribed program for a specified period of time, and at the completion of that period, progress to other physical activities outside the company.

4. A qualified physical education instructor, e.g., exercise physiologist or scientist, should supervise the program under the overall direction of the company's medical policy.

5. Health education programs, such as consultation and seminars on smoking, obesity, and alcoholism, should be included in programs where appropriate.

6. All participants should understand the specific benefits of the program that is prescribed for them.

7. Participants should attempt to improve their individual fitness levels. They should not be placed in competition with each other for effort expended, goals obtained, or strength increased.

8. All programs should be designed with the goal of physical fitness for adults, both men and women, in mind. Activities will be suggested and/or planned that will develop adequate levels of muscular strength and endurance, cardiovascular endurance, flexibility, coordination, and balance.

MEDICAL PROVISIONS

1. All candidates for a company-sponsored physical fitness program should obtain medical clearance for physical activity. In some instances, modified exercise programs will be recommended based on medical evaluation. "Evaluation for Exercise Participation" is a joint statement prepared by the Committee and the Council to assist physicians in evaluating the apparently healthy individual who wishes to begin a vigorous exercise program. Suggestions are made relative to whom should have a special evaluation before undertaking an exercise program; tests and examinations to determine who can be classified as "out of condition;" and recommendations for the intensity and duration of beginning exercise programs. The statement can be obtained by contacting either the Committee or the Council.

2. Medical emergency procedures should be established for the fitness program under the supervision of the medical department or consultant.

3. Results of the participant's progress in the exercise program should be sent to the medical director on a periodic schedule.

ADMINISTRATION

1. A written set of operational procedures and objectives should be developed for all programs.
2. Definite hours of operation of the facility should be established.
3. Participants should be required to make a commitment to an established set of goals before entering the program. These goals should be expressed in terms of length of time in the program; number of days to be spent per week in the program; and physiological accomplishments such as weight loss, cardiovascular improvement, and strength development.
4. Participants should receive a specific training program to follow.
5. Evaluation of the participant's progress should be noted by the fitness director prior to each training session and related to the participant in terms of increased or decreased work output or change of conditioning routine.
6. Motivational devices in the form of awards for progress and/or completion should be developed.
7. Strict safety rules should be developed in regard to use of equipment and adherence to conditioning routines.
8. Dress codes should be established commensurate with the degree of program sophistication.
9. Research and evaluation studies should be conducted to determine the effect of the program in meeting stated objectives.

FACILITIES

1. All physical fitness facilities must be kept in above average hygienic conditions for health as well as motivational purposes.
2. Adequate locker room, dressing area, and shower facilities should be provided.
3. Towels, soap, and uniforms should be provided whenever possible. Cleanliness of the facility is eased when participants do not have to bring towels and uniforms with them on each visit.
4. Where possible, wall-to-wall carpeting, background music, sauna baths, steam baths, special uniforms, and attractive decor should be provided to aid the motivational quality of the facility.
5. A bulletin board should be maintained that posts current articles relative to health and exercise.

Lifestyle at the Worksite: a Model Exercise Program

PRIMARY PREVENTION

Short-term Goal: To promote work-associated aerobic activity by encouraging physical exertion as an alternative to a sedentary routine.

Install bicycle racks by worksite entrances with posted signs at these sites that encourage travel from home on bicycles.

Arrange with neighborhood shops for group discounts on new (sports and recreational equipment and apparel) purchases.

Organize seasonal regular short- or long-distance bike races.

Post signs at every floor that encourage the use of staircases in place of an elevator.

Organize seasonal weekly recreation meets on the grounds after work. Suggested activities are volleyball, badminton, round robin softball, horseshoes, and archery.

Long-term Goal: To develop plans whereby employees may enjoy physical activity and grow into a fitness regimen at the worksite and/or at nearby existing facilities.

Develop a fitness parcourse modeled after one of the many succesful existing parcourses in New England. Stations in the parcourse would include signs with easy instructions and be designed to work different groups of muscles, to exercise, and to develop the entire body. Guidelines would promote a gradual process of working up to more demanding routines. Equipment would be designed for both low cost and durability and would be for people of various abilities. A "buddy system" would be developed for individual incentive and for safety.

Build a worksite fitness facility that would include a universal gym, outdoor running/jogging track, calisthenics clinic with a group leader and locker and shower facilities.

Source: State of Connecticut, Department of Health, 79 Elm Street, Hartford, Connecticut 06115.

Provide access to group membership in one of several commercial fitness centers and health spas with possible organization of group activities at the site, i.e., competition racquetball, basketball, a calisthenics clinic, and swimming.

SECONDARY PREVENTION

Short-term Goal: Exercise with physician approval will promote rehabilitation of cardiac patients and will safeguard them from further episodes. Provide either of the following exercise stress tests to both cardiac patients and healthy employees under the supervision of appropriate medical personnel.

The Harvard Step Test for employees periodically at minimal cost.
The Treadmill Stress Test, whereby individual's heart rate, blood pressure, and EKG are all monitored.

Long-term Goal: To establish an in-house system of monitoring recently identified employees with coronary disease in order to reduce the risk of second infarction.

Develop with physician–individualized exercise regimen for cardiac patients.

TERTIARY PREVENTION

Short-term Goal: To provide methods for reintegration of returning cardiac patients into the work force through renewed involvement in physical activity.

Evaluate performance capabilities (test of aerobic power) through physical exertion followed by monitoring of heart rate and repetition.
Educate employee about posture, respiration, energy expenditures, and orthopedic problems.

Long-term Goal: To develop a follow-up program for returning cardiac patients to the workplace.
Share with hospital-based setting the primary rehabilitation functions of exercise education.
Provide leader/education for all rehabilitation activities.

Notes

CHAPTER 1
PATTERNS OF
EXERCISE IN THE
AMERICAN
POPULATION

1. U.S. Department of Health, Education, and Welfare, Public Health Service, Center for Disease Control, *Health Education Risk Reduction Grants Interim Guidelines*, March 18, 1980.
2. Ralph S. Paffenbarger, Jr., "Countercurrents of Physical Activity and Heart Attack Trends," in *Proceedings of the Conference on the Decline of Coronary Heart Disease Mortality*, National Institutes of Health, DHEW Publication No. (NIH) 79-1610 Washington, D.C.: U.S. Government Printing Office, May 1979), pp. 298–311.
3. Ibid.
4. Personal communication, Verle Nicholson, President's Council on Physical Fitness and Sports, Washington, D.C., August 26, 1980.
5. Wilson Riles, "Foreword," in *Physical Education Framework* (Sacramento, Calif.: California State Department of Education, 1973), p. iv.
6. Personal communication, J. R. Fisher, National Council, YMCA, New York, September 1978.
7. Personal communication, S. Fonger, National Board, YWCA, New York, September 1978.
8. Personal communication, A. S. Gordon, Sierra Club, San Francisco, September 1978.
9. Gregory S. Thomas, Patricia E. Franks, Philip R. Lee, and Ralph S. Paffenbarger, Jr., "Exercise and Health: The Evidence and the Policy Implications," Health Policy Program Discussion Paper, University of California, San Francisco, May 1979.
10. William J. Bowerman and W. E. Harris, *Jogging* (New York: Grosset and Dunlap, 1967).
11. Kenneth H. Cooper, *Aerobics* (New York: Bantam Books, 1968).
12. Kenneth H. Cooper, *The New Aerobics* (New York: Bantam Books, 1970); Kenneth H. Cooper and M. Cooper, *Aerobics for Women* (New York: Bantam Books, 1970); Kenneth H. Cooper, *The Aerobics Way* (New York: M. Evans and Company, 1977).
13. Joe Henderson, *Long Slow Distance: The Humane Way to Train* (Mountain View, Calif.: World Publications, 1969).
14. Joan Ullyot, *Women's Running* (Mountain View, Calif.: World Publications, 1976).
15. George A. Sheehan, *Dr. Sheehan on Running* (Mountain View, Calif.: World Publications, 1976).
16. James F. Fixx, *The Complete Book of Running* (New York: Random House, 1977).
17. Diana Jones, "Fixed at Random," *The Runner* (January 1980), p. 12.
18. Jane Leavy and Susan Okie, "The Runner: Study Tells a Lot About the Man on the

Run," *The Atlanta Journal and Constitution* (November 18, 1979), p. 13-D.

19. "Running Books Surpassed Sex Manuals," *The Physician and Sportsmedicine* 7(5):24 (1979).
20. James F. Fixx, *Jim Fixx's Second Book of Running* (New York: Random House, 1980).
21. Joan Ullyot, *Running Free: A Book for Women Runners and Their Friends* (New York: G. P. Putnam's Sons, 1980).
22. Peter D. Wood, *Run to Health* (New York: Charter, 1980).
23. Colman McCarthy, "Americans Flash Physical Fitness," *The Philadelphia Inquirer* (January 5, 1979).
24. Leavy and Okie, "The Runner."
25. Glenn Kramon, "The Compleat Guide to the Craziest Race in the World," *San Francisco Sunday Examiner and Chronicle* (May 11, 1980), p. C5.
26. "Unofficial Count of 24,000 in Bay to Breakers," *San Francisco Examiner* (May 19, 1980), p. 60.
27. "The World Is Going Marathon Crazy," *The Washington Post* (April 16, 1978), p. D1.
28. John R. Sutton, Letter to the editor: "Heat Stroke from Running," *Journal of the American Medical Association* 243(19):1896 (1980).
29. "Jogging—Italian Style," *Jogging Magazine* 1(6):43 (1979).
30. J. D. Cantwell, "Coronary Prevention and Rehabilitation in Selected Countries," in Michael L. Pollock and Donald H. Schmidt, eds., *Heart Disease and Rehabilitation* (Boston: Houghton Mifflin, 1979), pp. 496–505.
31. Sol Stern, "The New Wave in Swimming," *The New York Times Magazine* (June 1, 1980), pp. 84–86, 92–93.
32. Ibid.
33. U.S. Department of Health, Education, and Welfare, President's Council on Physical Fitness and Sports, "Aquadynamics: Physical Conditioning Through Water Exercises," 1977.
34. Marianne Brems, *Swim for Fitness* (San Francisco: Chronicle Books, 1979).
35. Harvey S. Wiener, *Total Swimming* (New York: Simon and Schuster, 1980).
36. "Comes the Revolution," *Time* (June 26, 1978), pp. 54–60.
37. "A Question of Nomenclature," *Sports Illustrated* (October 1, 1979), p. 16.
38. Ibid.
39. P. S. Wood, "The Emerging Woman Athlete," *San Francisco Chronicle* (May 25, 1980), p. 5.
40. "A Question of Nomenclature."
41. "Running Battle," *Time* (February 5, 1979), p. 140.
42. George Gallup, "All Out Fitness Craze," *San Francisco Chronicle* (October 6, 1977), p. 36.
43. Ibid.
44. U. S. Department of Health, Education, and Welfare, Public Health Service, National Center for Health Statistics, "Exercise and Participation in Sports Among Persons 20 Years of Age and Over: United States, 1975," *Advancedata*, Vital and Health Statistics, DHEW Publication No. (PHS) 78-1250 (Washington, D.C.: U.S. Government Printing Office, 1978).
45. Pacific Mutual Life Insurance Company, *Health Maintenance* (San Francisco, November 1978), pp. 24–30.
46. Grace Wyshak, George A. Lamb, Robert S. Lawrence, and William J. Curran, "A Profile of the Health-Promoting Behaviors of Physicians and Lawyers," *The New England Journal of Medicine* 303:104–107 (July 10, 1980).
47. Gallup, "All Out Fitness Craze."
48. U.S. Department of Health, Education, and Welfare, National Center for Health Statistics, "Exercise and Participation in Sports Among Persons 20 Years of Age and Over: United States, 1975."
49. Leavy and Okie, "The Runner."

50. Ibid.
51. Ibid.
52. Mike Tymn, "Turning on the Hawaiians," *Runners World* 12(2):45–48 (1977).
53. Leavy and Okie, "The Runner."
54. Pacific Mutual Insurance Company, p. 26.
55. Ibid., p. 68.
56. Ibid., p. 26.
57. Ibid., pp. 27–28.
58. Ibid., p. 29.
59. "Situation Report on Exercise in U.S.," *President's Council on Physical Fitness and Sports Newsletter* (Washington, D.C.: U.S. Department of Health, Education and Welfare, October 1979), p. 4.
60. K. H. Cooper and A. Zechner, "Physical Fitness in United States and Austrian Military Personnel," *Journal of the American Medical Association* 215:931–934 (February 8, 1971).
61. McCarthy, "Americans Flash Physical Fitness."
62. Ibid.

CHAPTER 2
EXERCISE, PHYSICAL FITNESS, AND HEALTH

1. J. P. Clausen, "Circulatory Adjustments to Dynamic Exercise and Effect of Physical Training in Normal Subjects and in Patients with Coronary Artery Disease," *Progress in Cardiovascular Diseases* 18:459–495 (May/June 1976); D. T. Lowenthal, K. Bharadwaja, and W. W. Oaks, eds., *Therapeutics Through Exercise* (New York: Grune and Stratton, 1979), p. 222; W. C. Adams, M. M. McHenry, and E. M. Bernauer, "Long-Term Physiological Adaptations to Exercise with Special Reference to Performance and Cardiorespiratory Function in Health and Disease," in M. L. Pollock and D. H. Schmidt, eds., *Heart Disease and Rehabilitation* (Boston: Houghton Mifflin, 1979), pp. 322–343; L. D. Segal, "Myocardial Adaptations to Physical Condition," in Pollock and Schmidt, *Heart Disease and Rehabilitation*, pp. 95–107.
2. Clausen, "Circulatory Adjustments"; Adams, McHenry, and Bernauer, "Long-Term Physiological Adaptations."
3. Adams, McHenry, and Bernauer, "Long-Term Physiological Adaptations," p. 330–332.
4. D. A. Cunningham, K. J. Ingram, and P. A. Rechnitzer, "The Effect of Training: Physiological Responses," *Medicine and Science in Sports* 11:379–381 (1979).
5. A. A. Bove, "Heart and Circulatory Function in Exercise," in Lowenthal, Bharadwaja, and Oaks, *Therapeutics Through Exercise*, pp. 21-31.
6. Clausen, "Circulatory Adjustments."
7. Cunningham, Ingram, and Rechnitzer, "The Effect of Training."
8. Clausen, "Circulatory Adjustments."
9. P. Felig and V. Koivisto, "The Metabolic Response to Exercise: Implications for Diabetes," in Lowenthal, Bharadwaja, and Oaks, *Therapeutics Through Exercise*, pp. 3–20.
10. F. Heinzelmann and R. W. Bagley, "Response to Physical Activity Programs and Their Effects on Health Behavior," *Public Health Reports* 85905–911 (October 1970); J. F. Massie and R. J. Shephard, "Physiological and Psychological Effects of Training," *Medicine and Science in Sports* 3:110–117 (Fall 1971).
11. Stephen Havas, *Exercise and Your Heart*, draft June 19, 1980, U.S. Department of Health

and Human Services, National Institutes of Health, National Heart, Lung, and Blood Institute (Bethesda, Md., in press).

CHAPTER 3
EXERCISE AND CORONARY
HEART DISEASE

1. G. F. Fletcher and J. D. Cantwell, *Exercise and Coronary Heart Disease* (Springfield, Ill.: Charles C. Thomas, 1979), p. 47.
2. William B. Kannel, "Some Lessons in Cardiovascular Epidemiology from Framingham," *American Journal of Cardiology* 37:269–282 (February 1976).
3. Abdel R. Omran, "The Epidemiologic Transition: A Theory of the Epidemiology of Population Change," *Milbank Memorial Fund Quarterly* 49(2):509–538 (1971).
4. U.S. Department of Health, Education, and Welfare, Public Health Service, Office of the Assistant Secretary for Health and Surgeon General, *Healthy People: The Surgeon General's Report on Health Promotion and Disease Prevention, 1979*, DHEW Publication No. (PHS) 79-55071 (Washington, D.C.: U.S. Government Printing Office, 1979), p. 6-6.
5. D. P. Rice, J. J. Feldman, and K. L. White, *The Current Burden of Illness in the United States* (Washington, D.C.: Institute of Medicine/National Academy of Sciences, 1977), p. 36.
6. U.S. Department of Health, Education, and Welfare, Public Health Service, National Center for Health Statistics, *Facts of Life and Death*, DHEW Publication No. (PHS) 79-1222 (Washington, D.C.: U.S. Government Printing Office, 1978).
7. U.S. Department of Health, Education, and Welfare, Public Health Service, Office of Health Research, Statistics, and Technology, *Health United States: 1979*, DHEW Publication No. (PHS) 80-1232 (Washington, D.C.: U.S. Government Printing Office, 1980), pp. 100–103.
8. Kannel, "Some Lessons," p. 271.
9. U.S. Department of Health, Education, and Welfare, *Healthy People.*
10. U.S. Department of Health, Education, and Welfare, *Facts of Life and Death*, p. 13.
11. Brian MacMahon and Thomas F. Pugh, *Epidemiology: Principles and Practice* (Boston: Little, Brown and Company, 1970), pp. 40–41.
12. Kannel, "Some Lessons."
13. William B. Kannel, "Habitual Level and Risk of Coronary Heart Disease: The Framingham Study," *Canadian Medical Association Journal* 96:811–812 (March 25, 1967).
14. MacMahon and Pugh, *Epidemiology*, p. 232.
15. Ibid., p. 233.
16. Ibid., p. 234.
17. Ibid., p. 22.
18. "The Multiple Risk Factor Intervention Trial (MRFIT): A National Study of Primary Prevention of Coronary Heart Disease," *Journal of the American Medical Association* 235:825–828 (1976).
19. A. L. McAlister, J. W. Farquhar, C. E. Thoresen, and N. Maccoby, "Behavioral Science Applied to Cardiovascular Health: Progress and Research Needs in Modification of Risk-Taking Habits in Adult Populations," *Health Education Monographs* 4:45–74 (1976).
20. University of North Carolina at Chapel Hill, Division of Health Sciences, School of Public Health, Department of Biostatistics, Central Patient Registry and Coordinating Center, *Lipid Research Clinics Program*, 1976.
21. V. F. Froehlicher, "The Effects of Chronic Exercise on the Heart and on Coronary Athero-

sclerotic Heart Disease," in A. Brest, ed., *Cardiovascular Clinic* (Philadelphia: F. A. Davis Co., 1976).

22. S. M. Fox, III and J. P. Naughton, "Physical Activity and the Prevention of Coronary Heart Disease," *Preventive Medicine* 1:92–120 (1972); S. M. Fox, III, "Relationship of Activity Habits to Coronary Heart Disease," in J. Naughton and H. K. Hellerstein, eds., *Exercise Testing and Exercise Training in Coronary Heart Disease* (New York: Academic Press, 1973); R. A. Bruce, "The Benefits of Physical Training for Patients with Coronary Heart Disease," in F. J. Ingelfinger, R. V. Ebert, M. Finland, and A. S. Relman, eds., *Controversies in Internal Medicine II* (Philadelphia: W. B. Saunders Company, 1974), pp. 145–161; K. S. Brown and P. Milvy, "A Critique of Several Epidemiological Studies of Physical Activity and Its Relationship in Aging, Health and Mortality," *Annals of the New York Academy of Sciences* 301:703–719 (1977); J. A. Bonanno, "Coronary Risk Factor Modification by Chronic Physical Exercise," in E. A. Amsterdam, J. H. Wilmore, and A. N. DeMaria, eds., *Exercise in Cardiovascular Health and Disease* (New York: Yorke Medical Books, 1977), pp. 274–279; G. F. Fletcher and J. D. Cantwell, *Exercise and Coronary Heart Disease* (Springfield, Ill.: Charles C. Thomas, 1979), pp. 47–71; M. A. Greenberg, S. Arbeit, and I. L. Rubin, "The Role of Physical Training in Patients With Coronary Disease," *American Heart Journal* 97:527–534 (1979).

23. J. N. Morris, J. A. Heady, P. A. B. Raffle, C. G. Roberts, and J. W. Parks, "Coronary Heart-Disease and Physical Activity of Work," *The Lancet* 2:1053–1057 and 1111–1120 (November 21 and 28, 1953); J. N. Morris, A. Kagan, D. C. Pattison, M. J. Gardner, and P. A. B. Raffle, "Incidence and Prediction of Ischaemic Heart-Disease in London Busmen" *The Lancet* 2:553–559 (September 10, 1966); J. N. Morris, *Uses of Epidemiology* (New York: Churchill Livingstone, 1975), pp. 163–165.

24. J. N. Morris, S. P. W. Chave, C. Adam, C. Sirey, L. Epstein, and D. J. Sheehan, "Vigorous Exercise in Leisure-Time and the Incidence of Coronary Heart-Disease," *The Lancet* 1:333–339 (February 17, 1973).

25. Harold A. Kahn, "The Relationship of Reported Coronary Heart Disease Mortality to Physical Activity of Work," *American Journal of Public Health* 53(7):1058–1067 (July 1963).

26. William J. Zukel, Robert H. Lewis, Philip E. Enterline, Robert C. Painter, Lloyd S. Ralston, Robert M. Fawcett, Alla P. Meredith, and Beatrice Peterson, "A Short-Term Community Study of the Epidemiology of Coronary Heart Disease: A Preliminary Report on the North Dakota Study," *American Journal of Public Health* 49(12):1630–1639 (December 1959).

27. D. Brunner, G. Manelis, M. Modan, and S. Levin, "Physical Activity at Work and the Incidence of Myocardial Infarction, Angina Pectoris and Death Due to Ischemic Heart Disease: An Epidemiological Study in Israeli Collective Settlements (Kibbutzim)," *Journal of Chronic Diseases* 27:217–233 (1974).

28. Henry L. Taylor, Ernest Klepetar, Ancel Keys, Willis Parlin, Henry Blackburn, and Thomas Puchner, "Death Rates Among Physically Active and Sedentary Employees of the Railroad Industry," *American Journal of Public Health* 52(10):1697–1707 (October 1962).

29. R. S. Paffenbarger, Jr., M.E. Laughlin, A. S. Gima, and R. A. Black, "Work Activity of Longshoremen as Related to Death from Coronary Heart Disease and Stroke," *The New England Journal of Medicine* 282(20):1109–1114 (May 14, 1970).

30. J. M. Chapman and F. J. Massey, Jr., "The Interrelationship of Serum Cholesterol, Hypertension, Body Weight, and Risk of Coronary Disease," *Journal of Chronic Diseases* 17:933–949 (1964).

31. J. Stamler, H. A. Lindberg, D. M. Berkson, A. Shaffer, W. Miller, and A. Poindexter, "Prevalence and Incidence of Coronary Heart Disease in Strata of the Labor Force of a Chicago Industrial Corporation," *Journal of Chronic Diseases* 11(4):405–420 (April 1960);

Oglesby Paul, Mark H. Lepper, William H. Phelan, G. Wesley Dupertuis, Anne MacMillan, Harley McKean, and Heebok Park, "A Longitudinal Study of Coronary Heart Disease," *Circulation* 28:20–31 (July 1963).

32. Samuel M. Fox, III and William L. Haskell, "Physical Activity and the Prevention of Coronary Heart Disease," *Bulletin of the New York Academy of Medicine* 44(8):950–967 (August 1968).

33. Ansel Keys, et al., *Seven Countries: A Multivariate Analysis of Deaths and Coronary Heart Disease* (Cambridge, Mass.: Harvard University Press, 1980).

34. Paffenbarger, Laughlin, Gima, and Black, "Work Activity of Longshoremen"; R. S. Paffenbarger, Jr., and W. E. Hale, "Work Activity and Coronary Heart Mortality," *The New England Journal of Medicine* 292(11):545–550 (March 13, 1975); R. S. Paffenbarger, Jr., "Physical Activity and Fatal Heart Attack: Protection or Selection," in E. A. Amsterdam, J. H. Wilmore, and A. N. DiMaria, eds., *Exercise in Cardiovascular Health and Disease* (New York: Yorke Medical Books, 1977), pp. 35–49; R. S. Paffenbarger, Jr., W. E. Hale, R. J. Brand, and R. T. Hyde, "Work-Energy Level, Personal Characteristics, and Fatal Heart Attack: A Birth-Cohort Effect," *American Journal of Epidemiology* 105(3):200–213(1977); R. J. Brand, R. S. Paffenbarger, Jr., R. I. Sholtz, and J. B. Kampert, "Work Activity and Fatal Heart Attack Studied by Multiple Logistic Risk Analysis," *American Journal of Epidemiology* 110:52–62 (1979); R. S. Paffenbarger, Jr., R. J. Brand, R. I. Sholtz, and D. L. Jung, "Energy Expenditure, Cigarette Smoking, and Blood Pressure Level as Related to Death from Specific Diseases," *American Journal of Epidemiology* 108(1):12–18 (1978).

35. S. P. W. Chave, J. N. Morris, S. Moss, and A. M. Semmence, "Vigorous Exercise in Leisure Time and the Death Rate: A Study of Male Civil Servants," *Journal of Epidemiology and Community Health* 32:239–243 (1978).

36. John Cassel, Siegfried Heyden, Alan G. Bartel, Berton H. Kaplan, Herman A. Tyroler, Joan C. Cornoni, and Curtis G. Hames, "Occupation and Physical Activity and Coronary Heart Disease," *Archives of Internal Medicine* 128:920–928 (December 1971).

37. W. B. Kannel, "Habitual Level of Physical Activity and Risk of Coronary Heart Disease: The Framingham Study," *Canadian Medical Association Journal* 96:811–812 (March 25, 1967).

38. Sam Shapiro, Eve Weinblatt, Charles W. Frank, and Robert V. Sager, "Incidence of Coronary Heart Disease in a Population Insured for Medical Care (HIP): Myocardial Infarction, Angina Pectoris, and Possible Myocardial Infarction," *American Journal of Public Health* 59(6):1–101 (June 1969).

39. Chapman and Massey, "Interrelationship."

40. R. S. Paffenbarger, Jr., P. A. Wolf, J. Notkin, and M. C. Thorne, "Chronic Disease in Former College Students: I. Early Precursors of Fatal Coronary Heart Disease," *American Journal of Epidemiology* 83(2):314–328 (1966).

41. R. S. Paffenbarger, Jr., A. L. Wing, and R. T. Hyde, "Physical Activity as an Index of Heart Attack Risk in College Alumni," *American Journal of Epidemiology* 108(3):161–175 (September 1978).

42. Paffenbarger and Hale, "Work Activity."

43. Chave, Morris, Moss, and Semmence, "Vigorous Exercise."

44. L. Wilhelmsen, H. Sanne, D. Elmfeldt, G. Grimby, G. Tibblin, and H. Wedel, "A Controlled Trial of Physical Training After Myocardial Infarction," *Preventive Medicine* 4:491–508 (1975).

45. Peter A. Rechnitzer, H. A. Pickard, A. U. Paivio, M. S. Yuhasz, and D. Cunningham, "Long-Term Follow-up Study of Survival and Recurrence Rates Following Myocardial Infarction in Exercising and Control Subjects," *Circulation* 45:853–857 (April 1972).

46. Paffenbarger, Wolf, Notkin, and Thorne, "Chronic Disease"; Paffenbarger, Wing, and Hyde, "Physical Activity."

47. Paffenbarger, Hale, Brand, and Hyde, "Work-Energy Level"; Paffenbarger, Wing, and

Hyde, "Physical Activity"; Chave, Morris, Moss, and Semmence, "Vigorous Exercise."
48. P. D. Wood and W. L. Haskell, "The Effect of Exercise on Plasma High Density Lipoproteins," *Lipids* 14(4):417–427 (1979).
49. R. S. Williams, E. E. Logue, J. L. Lewis, T. Barton, N. W. Stead, A. G. Wallace, and S. V. Pizzo, "Physical Conditioning Augments the Fibrinolytic Response to Venous Occlusion in Healthy Adults," *The New England Journal of Medicine* 302(18): 987–991 (May 1, 1980); R. S. Paffenbarger, Jr., and R. T. Hyde, "Exercise as Protection Against Heart Attack," *The New England Journal of Medicine* 302:1026–1027 (May 1, 1980).
50. P-O. Astrand and K. Rodhal, *Textbook of Work Physiology* (New York: McGraw-Hill, 1970).
51. O. Peterson, H. Beck-Nielson, and L. Heding, "Increased Insulin Receptors After Exercise in Patients with Insulin-Dependent Diabetes Mellitus," *The New England Journal of Medicine* 302:886–892 (April 17, 1980).

CHAPTER 4
EXERCISE AND OTHER HEALTH PROBLEMS: HYPERTENSION, OBESITY, DIABETES MELLITUS, ANXIETY, DEPRESSION, AND ASTHMA

1. Mladen Vranic and Michael Berger, "Exercise and Diabetes," *Diabetes* 28:147–167 (February 1979).
2. D. T. Lowenthal, K. Bharadwaja, and W. W. Oaks, eds., *Therepeutics Through Exercise* (New York: Grune and Stratton, 1979), p 222.
3. U. S. Department of Health, Education, and Welfare, Public Health Service, National Center for Health Statistics: "National Ambulatory Medical Care Survey of Visits to General and Family Practitioners, January-December, 1975," *Advancedata from Vital and Health Statistics* (Hyattsville, Md.: U.S. Department of Health, Education, and Welfare), No. 15, DHEW Publication No. (PHS) 78-1250 (December 14, 1977).
4. U.S. Department of Health, Education, and Welfare, Public Health Service, National Center for Health Statistics: "Office Visits to Internists: National Ambulatory Medical Care Survey, United States, 1975," *Advancedata from Vital and Health Statistics* (Hyattsville, Md.: U.S. Department of Health, Education, and Welfare), No. 16, DHEW Publication No. (PHS) 78-1250 (February 7, 1978).
5. U. S. Department of Health, Education, and Welfare, Public Health Service, Office of Health Research, Statistics and Technology, *Health United States: 1979* (Washington, D.C.: U.S. Government Printing Office), DHEW Publication No. (PHS) 80-1232, p. 33.
6. U.S. Department of Health, Education, and Welfare, "Office Visits to Internists," p. 5; U.S. Department of Health, Education, and Welfare, "National Ambulatory Medical Care Survey," p. 5.
7. Asa Kibom, L. H. Hartley, B. Saltin, G. Grimby, and Irma Astrand, "Physical Training in Sedentary Middle-Aged and Older Men. I. Medical Evaluation," *Scandinavian Journal of Clinical and Laboratory Investigation* 24:315–322 (December 1969); D. M. Berkson, I. T. Whipple, W. E. Sime, H. Lerner, I. Bernstein, W. MacIntyre, and J. Stamler, "Experience With a Long-Term Supervised Ergometric Exercise Program for Middle-Aged Sedentary American Men" (Abstract), *Circulation* (Suppl. 2) 36:67 (October 1967); J. Naughton, K. Shanbour, R. Armstrong, J. McCoy, and M. T. Lategola, "Cardiovascular Responses to Exercise Following Myocardial Infarction," *Archives of Internal Medicine* 117:541–595 (April 1966); G. V. Mann, H. L. Garret, A. Farhi, H.

Murray, and F. T. Billings, "Exercise to Prevent Coronary Heart Disease: An Experimental Study of the Effects of Training on Risk Factors for Coronary Disease in Men," *American Journal of Medicine* 46:12–27 (January 1969); W. Miall and P. D. Oldham, "Factors Influencing Arterial Blood Pressure in the General Population," *Clinical Science* 17:409–444 (1958); K. H. Cooper, M. L. Pollock, R. P. Martin, S. R. White, A. C. Linnerud, and A. Jackson, "Physical Fitness Levels vs. Selected Coronary Risk Factors," *Journal of the American Medical Association* 235:166–169 (July 12, 1976); G. F. Fletcher and J. D. Cantwell, *Exercise and Coronary Heart Disease* (Springfield, Ill.: Charles C. Thomas, 1979).

8. J. N. Morris and M. J. Crawford, "Coronary Heart Disease and Physical Activity of Work," *British Medical Journal* 2:1485–1496 (1958).

9. J. L. Boyer and F. W. Kasch, "Exercise Therapy in Hypertensive Men," *Journal of the American Medical Association* 211:1668–1671 (March 9, 1970).

10. S. E. Strauzenberg, I. Goetz, L. Dietrich, R. Mueller, and H. Brende, "On the Significance of Physical Conditioning in the Prophylaxis of Cardiovascular and Metabolic Disorders," *Proceedings of the 20th World Congress in Sports Medicine*, Melbourne, Australia, 1974, pp. 224–230.

11. G. Choquette and R. J. Ferguson, "Blood Pressure Reduction in 'Borderline' Hypertensives Following Physical Training," *Canadian Medical Association Journal* 108:699–703 (March 17, 1973).

12. Boyer and Kasch, "Exercise Therapy."

13. J. A. Bonanno and J. E. Lies, "Effects of Physical Training on Coronary Risk Factors," *American Journal of Cardiology* 33:760–764 (May 20, 1974).

14. G. H. Williams, P. I. Jagger, and E. Braunwald, "Hypertensive Vascular Disease," in K. J. Isslebacher, R. D. Adams, E. Braunwald, R. F. Petersdorf, and J. D. Wilson, eds., *Harrison's Principles of Internal Medicine* (New York: McGraw-Hill, 1980), p. 1173.

15. H. R. Black, "Non-Pharmacologic Therapy for Hypertension," *American Journal of Medicine* 66:837–842 (May 1979).

16. J. Scheuer and C. M. Tipton, "Cardiovascular Adaptation to Physical Exercise," *Annual Review of Physiology* 39:221 (1976).

17. U.S. Department of Health, Education, and Welfare, *Health United States: 1979*, p. 33.

18. Ibid.

19. J. F. Fixx, *The Complete Book of Running* (New York: Random House, 1977), p. 79.

20. Stephen Havas, *Exercise and Your Heart*, draft, June 19, 1980 (U.S. Department of Health and Human Services, National Institutes of Health, National Heart, Lung, and Blood Institute (Bethesda, Md., in press).

21. M. L. Johnson, B. S. Burke, and J. Mayer, "Relative Importance of Inactivity and Overeating in the Energy Balance of Obese High School Girls," *American Journal of Clinical Nutrition* 4(1):37–44 (January–February 1956).

22. M. E. Thomson and F. M. Cruickshank, "Survey into the Eating and Exercise Habits of New Zealand Pre-Adolescents in Relation to Overweight and Obesity," *New Zealand Medical Journal* 89:7–9 (January 10, 1979).

23. L. Balabanski, "Diet and Physical Performance in the Rehabilitation of Obesity," *Bibliotheca Nutritio et Dieta* 27:33–40 (1979).

24. J. Sonka, "Effects of Diet and Diet and Exercise in Weight Reducing Regimens," in Jana Parizkova and V. A. Rogozkin, eds., *Nutrition, Physical Fitness, and Health* (Baltimore: University Park Press, 1978), pp. 239–248.

25. S. Lewis, W. L. Haskell, P. D. Wood, N. Manoogian, J. E. Bailey, and M. B. Periera, "Effects of Physical Activity on Weight Reduction in Obese Middle-Aged Women," *The American Journal of Clinical Nutrition* 29:151–156 (February 1976).

26. P. M. Stalonas, W. G. Johnson, and M. Christ, "Behavior Modification for Obesity: The Evaluation of Exercise, Contingency Management, and Program Adherence," *Con-*

sulting and Clinical Psychology 46(3):463–469 (1978).

27. Stauzenberg et al., "On the Significance of Physical Conditioning," pp. 224–230.

28. L. B. Oscai and B. T. Williams, "Effects of Exercise on Overweight Middle-Aged Males," *Journal of the American Geriatrics Society* 16(7):794–797 (July 1968).

29. G. Gwinup, "Effect of Exercise Alone on the Weight of Obese Women," *Archives of Internal Medicine* 135:676–680 (May 1975).

30. P. Bjorntorp, "Physical Training in the Treatment of Obesity," *International Journal of Obesity* 2: 149–151 (1978).

31. M. Jette, W. Barry, and L. Pearlman, "The Effects of an Extracurricular Physical Activity Program on Obese Adolescents," *Canadian Journal of Public Health* 68:39–42 (January–February 1977).

32. American Diabetic Association, "What Is the American Diabetic Association?" (New York, n.d.)

33. U.S. Department of Health, Education, and Welfare, *Health United States: 1979,* p. 36.

34. M. Berger and P. Berchtold, "The Role of Physical Exercise and Training in the Management of Diabetes Mellitus," *Bibliotheca Nutritio et Dieta* 27:41–54 (1979).

35. Ibid.

36. M. Vranic and M. Berger, "Exercise and Diabetes Mellitus," *Diabetes* 28:147–163 (February 1979).

37. H. L. Minuk, M. Vranic, and B. Zinman, "Glucoregulation During Exercise in Not-Insulin Dependent Diabetes Mellitus" (abstract), *Diabetes* 28:424 (Program, 39th Annual Meeting, 1979).

38. B. Zinman, "Diabetes and Exercise" (guest editorial), *Postgraduate Medicine* 66(5):81–82 (November 1979).

39. V. A. Koivisto and R. S. Sherwin, "Exercise in Diabetes: Therapeutic Implications," *Postgraduate Medicine* 66(5):87–96 (November 1979); Vranic and Berger, "Exercise and Diabetes Mellitus."

40. O. Pedersen, H. Beck-Nielsen, and L. Heding, "Increased Insulin Receptors after Exercise in Patients with Insulin-Dependent Diabetes Mellitus," *The New England Journal of Medicine* 302:886–892 (April 17, 1980).

41. P. Bjorntorp, G. Holm, B. Jacobson, K. Schiller-de Jounge, P. -A. Lundberg, L. Sjostron, U. Smith, and L. Sullivan, "Physical Training in Human Hyperplastic Obesity. IV. Effects on the Hormonal Status," *Metabolism* 26(3):319–328.

42. J. S. Skinner, "Longevity, General Health, and Exercise," in H. B. Falls, ed., *Exercise Physiology* (New York: Academic Press, 1968), pp. 219–238.

43. Pedersen, Beck-Nielsen, and Heding, "Increased Insulin Receptors."

44. N. B. Ruderman, O. P. Ganda, and K. Johansen, "The Effect of Physical Training on Glucose Tolerance and Plasma Lipids in Maturity-Onset Diabetes," *Diabetes* (Suppl. 1) 28:89–92 (January 1979).

45. B. Saltin, F. Lindgarde, M. Houston, R. Horlin, E. Nygard, and P. Gad, "Physical Training and Glucose Tolerance in Middle-Aged Men With Chemical Diabetes," *Diabetes* (Suppl. 1) 28:30–31 (January 1979).

46 Ruderman, Ganda, and Johansen, "Effect of Physical Training."

47. Ibid.

48. J. Engerbretson, "The Effects of Exercise on Diabetic Control," *Journal of the Association of Physical and Mental Rehabilitation* 19:74–78 (1965).

49. Berger and Berchtold, "Role of Physical Exercise."

50. K. Berg, "The Insulin-Dependent Diabetic Runner," *The Physician and Sportsmedicine* 7(11):71–79 (1979).

51. D. E. McMillan, "Exercise and Diabetic Microangiopathy," *Diabetes* (Suppl. 1) 28:103–106 (January 1979).

52. C. H. Folkins, S. Lynch, and M. M. Gardner, "Psychological Fitness as a Function of

Physical Fitness," Archives of Physical Medicine and Rehabilitation 53(2):503–508 (November 1972).

53. E. M. Layman, "Psychological Effects of Physical Activity," *Exercise and Sports Science Reviews* 2:33–70 (1974).

54. C. H. Folkins, "Effects of Physical Training on Mood," *Journal of Clinical Psychology* 32:385–388 (April 1976).

55. Ibid.

56. B. D. McPherson, A. Pavio, M. S. Yuhasz, P. A. Rechnitzer, H. A. Pickard, and N. M. Lefcoe, "Psychological Effects of an Exercise Program for Post-Infarct and Normal Adult Men," *Journal of Sports Medicine and Physical Fitness* 7:95–102 (June 1967).

57. L. S. Lion, "Psychological Effects of Jogging: A Preliminary Study," *Perceptual and Motor Skills* 47:1215–1218 (December 1978).

58. C. H. Folkins and E. A. Amsterdam, "Control and Modification of Stress Emotions Through Chronic Exercise," in E. A. Amsterdam, J. H. Wilmore, and A. N. DeMaria, eds., *Exercise in Cardiovascular Health and Disease*, (New York: Yorke Medical Books, 1977), pp. 280–294.

59. Folkins, Lynch, and Gardner, "Psychological Fitness"; Folkins, "Effects of Physical Training on Mood."

60. J. Naughton, J. G. Bruhn, and M. T. Lategola, "Effects of Physical Training on Physiologic and Behavioral Characteristics of Cardiac Patients," *Archives of Physical Medicine and Rehabilitation* 49:131–137 (March 1968).

61. T. Kavanagh, R. J. Shephard, J. A. Tuck, and S. Aureshi, "Depression Following Myocardial Infarction: The Effects of Distance Running," *Annals of the New York Academy of Science* 301:1029–1038 (1977).

62. "Ready, Set . . . Sweat!" *Time* (June 6, 1977), pp. 83–90.

63. W. P. Morgan, J. A. Roberts, F. R. Brand, and A. D. Feinerman, "Psychological Effect of Chronic Physical Activity," *Medicine and Science in Sports* 2(4):213–217 (Winter 1970).

64. J. H. Greist, M. H. Klein, R. R. Eischens, J. Faris, A. S. Gurman, and W. P. Morgan, Running for Treatment of Depression," *Comprehensive Psychiatry* 20:41–54 (January–February, 1979).

65. Ibid, pp. 41–54.

66. Kenneth D. Fitch, "Effects of Exercise on Asthma," *Australian Family Physician* 6:592–597 (1977).

67. H. Herxheimer, "Hyperventilation Asthma," *The Lancet* 1:83–87 (January 19, 1946); R. S. McNeil, J. R. Narin, J. S. Millar, and C. G. Ingram, "Exercise-Induced Asthma," *Quarterly Journal of Medicine* 35:55–67 (January 1966).

68. R. H. Strauss, E. R. McFadden, Jr., R. H. Ingram, Jr., and J. J. Jaeger, "Enhancement of Exercise-Induced Asthma by Cold Air," *The New England Journal of Medicine* 297: 743–747 (October 6, 1977).

69. O. Bar-Or, I. Neuman, and R. Dotan, "Effects of Dry and Humid Climates on Exercise-Induced Asthma in Children and Adolescents," *Journal of Allergy and Clinical Immunology* 60:163–168 (1977).

70. S. Godfrey, "Exercise Induced Asthma," *Allergy* 33:229–237 (1978).

71. L. Kawabori, W. E. Pierson, L. L. Conquest, and C. W. Bierman, "Incidence of Exercise Induced Asthma in Children," *Journal of Allergy and Clinical Immunology* 58:447–455 (1976); P. A. Eggleston, and J. L. Guerrant, "A Standardized Method of Evaluating Exercise Induced Asthma," *Journal of Allergy and Clinical Immunology* 58:414–425 (1976).

72. Godfrey, "Exercise Induced Asthma," pp. 231–234.

73. Fitch, "Effects of Exercise on Asthma"; W. P. Marley, "Asthma and Exercise, a Review," *American Corrective Therapy Journal* 31(4):95–102 (1977).

74. L. Strick, "Breathing and Physical Fitness Exercises for Asthmatic Children," *Pediatric Clinics of North America* 16(1):31–42 (February 1969).
75. G. J. A. Croop, "Exercise Induced Asthma," *Pediatric Clinics of North America* 22(1): 63–76 (February 1975). .
76. K. D. Fitch, "Comparative Aspects of Available Exercise Systems," *Pediatrics* (Suppl.) 56:904–907 (November 1975).
77. Fitch, "Effects of Exercise on Asthma," pp. 592–597.
78. J. S. Hyde and C. L. Swarts, "Effect of an Exercise Program on the Perenially Asthmatic Child," *American Journal of Diseases of Children* 116:383-396 (October 1968); K. H. Peterson and T. R. McElhenny, "Effects of a Physical Fitness Program Upon Asthmatic Boys," *Pediatrics* 35:295–299 (February 1965).
79. American Academy of Pediatrics, Committee on Children with Handicaps, "The Asthmatic Child and His Participation in Sports and Physical Education," *Pediatrics* 45:150–151 (January 1970); J. P. Winnink, "Physical Activity and the Asthmatic Child," *American Correctiver Therapy Journal* 31(5):148–151 (1977).
80. Marley, "Asthma and Exercise."
81. S. Oseid and K. Aas, "Exercise Induced Asthma" (editorial), *Allergy* 33:227–228 (1978).

CHAPTER 5
THE PRESCRIPTION FOR EXERCISE

1. "Cooper Credits Increased Exercise with Fatal Heart Attack Decline," *President's Council on Physical Fitness and Sports Newsletter* (Washington, D.C.: U.S. Department of Health, Education, and Welfare, March 1977), p. 6.
2. J. Cantwell, *Stay Young at Heart* (Chicago: Nelson-Hall, 1975), p. xi.
3. Pacific Mutual Life Insurace Company, *Health Maintenance* (San Francisco, November 1978), p. 27.
4. S. M. Fox, III, "Physical Activity and Coronary Heart Disease," in E. Chung, ed., *Controversy in Cardiology: The Practical Clinical Approach* (New York: Springer-Verlag, 1976), pp. 201–219; R. A. Bruce, "The Benefits of Physical Training for Patients with Coronary Heart Disease," in F. J. Ingelfinger, R. V. Ebert, M. Finland, and A. S. Relman, eds., *Controversies of Internal Medicine II*, (Philadelphia: W. B. Saunders Company, 1974), pp. 145–161; F. Hatch, "Atherosclerosis Calls for a New Kind of Preventive Medicine," *California Medicine* 109:134–145 (1968); K. H. Cooper, *Aerobics* (New York: Bantam, 1968), pp. 135–136.
5. American Medical Association, *Proceedings* (American Medical Association House of Delegates, December 1977).
6. American Heart Association, *Exercise Testing and Training of Apparently Healthy Individuals: A Handbook for Physicians* (New York, 1972).
7. American College of Sports Medicine, "Position Statement on Recommended Quantity and Quality of Exercise for Developing and Maintaining Fitness in Healthy Adults," *Medicine in Science and Sports* 10:vii–xi (1978); American College of Sports Medicine, *Guidelines for Graded Exercise Testing and Exercise Prescription* (Philadelphia: Lea & Febiger, 1975).
8. H. K. Hellerstein and A. B. Ford, "Rehabilitation of the Cardiac Patient," *Journal of the American Medical Association* 164:225–231 (1957).
9. H. K. Hellerstein, E. Z. Hirsch, R. Ader, N. Greenblott, and M. Siegel, "Principles of Exercise Prescription for Normal and Cardiac Subjects," in J. P. Naughton and H. K.

Hellerstein, eds., *Exercise Testing and Exercise Training in Coronary Heart Disease* (New York: Academic Press, 1973), pp. 129–167; E. A. Amsterdam, J. H. Wilmore, and A. N. DiMaria, eds., *Exercise in Cardiovascular Health and Disease* (New York: Yorke Medical Books, 1977); M. L. Pollock and D. H. Schmidt, eds., *Heart and Rehabilitation* (Boston: Houghton Mifflin, 1979), p. 725; G. F. Fletcher and J. D. Cantwell, *Exercise and Coronary Heart Disease* (Springfield, Ill.: Charles C. Thomas, 1979).

10. F. Heinzelman, "Social and Psychological Factors That Influence the Effectiveness of Exercise Programs," in J. P. Naughton and H. K. Hellertstein, eds., *Exercise Testing and Exercise Training in Coronary Heart Disease* (New York: Academic Press, 1973), pp. 275–287; I.M. Rosenstock, "Why People Use Health Services," *Milbank Memorial Fund Quarterly* 44:94–124 (1966); M. H. Becker, "Sociobehavioral Determinants of Compliance," in D. L. Sackett and R. B. Haynes, eds., *Compliance with Therapeutic Regimens* (Baltimore: Johns Hopkins Press, 1976), pp. 40–50.

11. D. M. Chisholm, M. L. Collis, L. L. Kulak, W. Davenport, and N. Gruber, "Physical Activity Readiness," *British Columbia Medical Journal* 17:375–378 (November 1975).

12. Ibid.

13. R. R. J. Lauzon, "Fit Kit for Fat Cats" (editorial), *Canadian Journal of Public Health* 67:95–97 (March/April 1976).

14. Chisholm et al., "Physical Activity Readiness," p. 378.

15. Ibid, p. 376.

16. D. A. E. Shephard, "Home Testing of Fitness of Canadians," *Canadian Medical Association Journal* 114:662–663 (1976).

17. M. Jette, J. Campbell, J. Mongeon, and R. Routhier, "The Canadian Home Fitness Test as a Predictor of Aerobic Capacity," *Canadian Medical Association Journal* 114:680–682 (1976).

18. M. Jette, "An Exercise Prescription Program for Use in Conjunction with the Canadian Home Fitness Test," *Canadian Journal of Public Health* 66:461–464 (1975).

19. R. J. Jones, "Bayes Theorem, the Exercise ECG and Coronary Artery Disease," *Journal of the American Medical Association* 242:1067–1068 (1979).

20. Alan G. Bartel, Victor S. Behar, Robert H. Peter, Edward S. Organ, and Yihang Kong, "Graded Exercise Stress Tests in Angiographically Documented Coronary Artery Disease," *Circulation* 49:348–356 (February 1974).

21. D. Thompson, M. P. Stern, P. Williams, K. Duncan, W. L. Haskell, and P. D. Wood, "Death During Jogging or Running," *Journal of the American Medical Association* 242(12):1265–1267 (1979).

22. Jones, "Bayes Theorem."

23. R. R. Rynearson, J. W. Roberts, and W. L. Stewart, "Do Physicians Believe in Pre-Exercise Examinations and Stress Tests?" *The New England Journal of Medicine* 301(14):792–793 (1979).

24. E. K. Chung, "Exercise ECG Testing," *Archives of Internal Medicine* 140:895–896 (July 1980).

25. Hellerstein et al., "Principles of Exercise Prescription," pp. 131–132; H. R. Pyfer "Safety Precautions and Procedures in Cardiac Exercise Rehabilitation Programs," in M. L. Pollock and D. H. Schmidt, eds., *Heart Disease and Rehabilitation* (Boston: Houghton Mifflin, 1979), pp. 630–639; American College of Sports Medicine, *Guidelines*; American Heart Association, *Exercise Testing and Training of Apparently Healthy Individuals*; American Heart Association, *Exercise Testing and Training for Individuals with Heart Disease or at High Risk for Its Development: A Handbook for Physicians* (Dallas, 1975); C. G. Blomquist and J. H. Mitchell, "Exercise Testing and Electrocardiographic Interpretation," in M. L. Pollock and D. H. Schmidt, eds., *Heart Disease and Rehabilitation* (Boston: Houghton Mifflin, 1979), pp. 140–156; L. R. Zohman, "Principles of Performance Testing," in L. R. Zohman and R. E. Phillips, eds.,

Medical Aspects of Exercise Testing and Training (New York: Intercontinental Medical Book Corporation, 1973), pp. 39-55.

26. Hellerstein et al., "Principles of Exercise Prescription," p. 131.
27. Blomquist and Mitchell, "Exercise Testing," p. 141.
28. Ibid., p. 142.
29. Ibid, pp. 140-156.
30. Hellerstein et al., "Principles of Exercise Prescription," p. 138.
31. Ibid, p. 142.
32. W. S. Bowerman and W. E. Harris, *Jogging* (New York: Grosset and Dulap, 1967).
33. M. L. Rendle, "A Comparison of a Walk/Jog Sequence with Jogging to Determine Minimum Exercise Levels," *Proceedings of the 20th World Congress in Sportsmedicine* (Melbourne, Australia, 1974), pp. 145-148.
34. Thompson et al, "Death During Jogging or Running."
35. Fletcher and Cantwell, *Exercise and Coronary Heart Disease*, p. 340.
36. J. H. Wilmore, "Individual Exercise Prescription," in E. A. Amsterdam, J. H. Wilmore, and A. N. DiMaria, eds., *Exercise in Cardiovascular Health and Disease* (New York: Yorke Medical Books, 1979), pp. 267-273.
37. American College of Sports Medicine, "Position Statement."
38. J. F. Fixx, *Jim Fixx's Second Book of Running* (New York: Random House, 1980); Peter D. Wood, *Run to Health* (New York: Charter, 1980); J. Ullyot, *Women's Running* (Mountain View, Calif.: World Publications, 1976); K. H. Cooper, *The Aerobic Way* (New York: M. Evans and Company, 1977); B. Gale, *The Wonderful World of Walking* (New York: William Morrow, 1979); D. L. Smith and E. A. Gaston, *Get Fit With Bicycling* (Emmaus, Pa.: Rodale Press, 1979); J. Sorensen, *Aerobic Dancing* (New York: Rawson Wade, 1979); D. Gould, *Tennis Everyone*, 3rd ed. (Palo Alto, Calif.: Mayfield, 1978); J. Counsilman, *The Science of Swimming* (Englewood Cliffs, N.J.: Prentice-Hall, Inc., 1968); Marianne Brems, *Swim for Fitness* (San Francisco: Chronicle Books, 1979); Harvey S. Wiener, *Total Swimming* (New York: Simon and Schuster, 1980); B. Verner and D. Skowrup, *Racquetball* (Palo Alto, Calif.: Mayfield, 1977).
39. Fletcher and Cantwell, *Exercise and Coronary Heart Disease*, pp. 250-288.
40. Ibid.
41. Ibid.
42. D. C. Durbeck, F. Heinzelmann, J. Schacter, W. L. Haskell, G. H. Payne, R. T. Moxley, M. Nemiroff, D. C. Limoncelli, L. B. Arnoldi, and S. M. Fox, "The National Aeronautics and Space Administration-U.S. Public Health Service Evaluation and Enhancement Program," *American Journal of Cardiology* 30:784-790 (November 20, 1972).
43. L. Pratt, "The Relationship of Socioeconomic Status to Health," *American Journal of Public Health* 61:281-291 (February 1971).
44. M. Mackie, "Perceptions of Beneficial Health Behavior: Smoking and Exercise," *Canadian Journal of Public Health* 66:481-487 (November/December 1975).
45. G. V. Mann, H. L. Garrett, A. Farhi, H. Murray, and F. T. Billings, "Exercise to Prevent Coronary Heart Disease," *American Journal of Medicine* 46:12-26 (January 1969); J. F. Massie and R. J. Shephard, "Physiological and Psychological Effects of Training—A Comparison of Individual and Gymnasium Programs, With a Characterization of the Exercise Drop-Out," *Medicine and Science in Sports* 3(3):110-117 (Fall 1971); T. Kavanagh, R. J. Shephard, H. Doney, and V. Pandit, "Intensive Exercise in Coronary Rehabilitation," *Medicine and Science in Sports* 5(1):34-39 (1973); H. L. Taylor, E. R. Buskirk, and R. D. Remington, "Exercise in Controlled Trials for the Prevention of Coronary Heart Disease," *Federation Proceedings* 32(5):1624-1627 (May 1973); P. Oja, P. Teraslinna, T. Partanen, and R. Karava, "Feasibility of an 18 Months' Physical Fitness Training Program for Middle-Aged Men and Its Effect on Physical

Fitness," *American Journal of Public Health* 64(5):459–465 (May 1974); E. R. Nye and W. T. Poulsen, "An Activity Programme for Coronary Patients: A Review of Morbidity, Mortality and Adherence After Five Years," *New Zealand Medical Journal* 79:1010–1013 June 13, 1974); L. Wilhelmsen, H. Sanne, D. Elmfeldt, G. Grimby, G. Tibblin, and H. Wedel, "A Controlled Trial of Physical Training after Myocardial Infarction: Effects on Risk Factors, Nonfatal Reinfarction, and Death," *Preventive Medicine* 4:491–508 (1975); E. Kentala, "Physical Fitness and Feasibility of Rehabilitation after Myocardial Infarction in Men of Working Age," *Annals of Clinical Research* 4(Suppl. 9):1–84 (1972); E. Bruce, R. Frederick, R. A. Bruce, and L. D. Fisher, "Comparison of Active Participants and Dropouts in CAPRI Cardiopulmonary Rehabilitation Programs," *American Journal of Cardiology* 37:53–60 (January 1976); E. L. Reid and R. W. Morgan, "Exercise Prescription: A Clinical Trial," *American Journal of Public Health* 69(6):591–595 (June 1979); N. B. Oldridge, "Compliance of Post-Myocardial Infarction Patients to Exercise," *Medicine and Science in Sports* 11(4):373–375 (1979); G. M. Andrew and J. O. Parker, "Factors Related to Dropout of Post-Myocardial Infarction Patients from Exercise Programs," *Medicine and Science in Sports* 11(4):376–378 (1979); N. B. Oldridge, "Compliance with Exercise Programs," in M. L. Pollock and D. H. Schmidt, eds., *Heart Disease and Cardiac Rehabilitation* (Boston: Houghton Mifflin, 1979).

46. Oldridge, "Compliance of Post-Myocardial Infarction Patients to Exercise"; Andrew and Parker, "Factors Related to Dropout"; Oldridge, "Compliance with Exercise Programs"; Bruce, Frederick, Bruce, and Fisher, "Comparison of Active Participants."

47. Oldridge, "Compliance of Post-Myocardial Infarction Patients to Exercise," p. 375.

48. Taylor, Buskirk, and Remington, "Exercise in Controlled Trials."

49. Massie and Shephard, "Physiological and Psychological Effects."

50. I. M. Rosenstock, "Patients' Compliance with Health Regimens," *Journal of the American Medical Association* 234(4):402–403 (1975).

51. R. B. Haynes, "A Critical Review of the 'Determinants' of Patient Compliance with Therapeutic Regimens," in D. L. Sackett and R. B. Haynes, eds., *Compliance with Therapeutic Regimens* (Baltimore: The Johns Hopkins University Press, 1976), pp. 26–39.

52. Heinzelmann, "Social and Psychological Factors."

53. R. F. Gillium and A. J. Barkey, "Diagnosis and Management of Patient Noncompliance," *Journal of the American Medical Association* 228:1563–1567 (June 17, 1974).

54. Durbeck et al., "National Aeronautics and Space Administration."

55. Haynes, "A Critical Review," p. 36.

56. Rosenstock, "Why People Use Health Services"; S. V. Kasl and S. Cobb, "Health Behavior, Illness Behavior and Sick Role Behavior," *Archives of Enviornmental Health* 12:246–266 (February 1966).

57. Rosenstock, "Patients' Compliance with Health Regimens"; Kasl and Cobb, "Health Behavior."

58. Becker, "Sociobehavioral Determinants."

59. B. L. Svarstad and H. L. Lipton, "Informing Parents about Mental Retardation: A Study of Professional Communication and Parent Acceptance," *Social Science and Medicine* 11:645–651 (1977); B. L. Svarstad, "Physician-Parent Communication and Patient Conformity with Medical Advice," in David Mechanic, ed., *The Growth of Bureaucratic Medicine* (New York: Wiley InterScience, 1974), pp. 220–235.

60. Hellerstein et al., "Principles of Exercise Prescription"; M. M. Dehn, D. G. Pansegrau, and J. H. Mitchell, "Exercise Training after Acute Myocardial Infarction," *Cardiovascular Clinics* 9(3):117–132 (1978).

CHAPTER 6
RISKS OF EXERCISE

1. G. F. Fletcher and J. D. Cantwell, *Exercise and Coronary Heart Disease* (Springfield, Ill.: Charles C. Thomas, 1979), pp. 215–224.

2. P. Rochmis and H. Blackburn, "Exercise Tests: A Survey of Procedures, Safety and Litigation Exerience in Approximately 170,000 Tests," *Journal of the American Medical Association* 217:1061–1066 (1971).

3. S. N. Morris and P. L. McHenry, "Cardiac Arrhythmias During Exercise Testing and Exercise Conditioning," *Cardiovascular Clinics* 9(3):57–68 (1978).

4. W. L. Haskell, "Physical Activity Following Myocardial Infarction," in M. L. Pollock and D. H. Schmidt, eds., *Heart Disease and Rehabilitation* (Boston: Houghton Mifflin, 1979), pp. 344–363; R. J. Shephard, "Current Status and Prospects for Post Coronary Exercise Multicenter Studies," *Medicine and Science in Sports* 11:383–385 (1979).

5. Haskell, "Physical Activity," pp. 356–357.

6. Morris and McHenry, "Cardiac Arrhythmias."

7. T. G. Pickering, "Jogging, Marathon Running and the Heart," *The American Journal of Medicine* 60:718 (May 1979).

8. P. D. Thompson, M. P. Stern, P. Williams, K. Duncan, W. L. Haskell, and P. D. Wood, "Death During Jogging and Running," *Journal of the American Medical Association* 242:1265–1267 (September 1979).

9. M. H. Crawford and R. A. O'Rourke, "The Athlete's Heart," in G. H. Stollerman, W. S. Harrington, J. B. Kirscher, C. E. Kossman, and M. Siperstein, eds., *Advances in Internal Medicine* (Vol 24) (Chicago: Year Book Publisher, 1979), pp. 311–329; S. Zoneraich, J. J. Rhee, O. Zoneraich, D. Jordan, and J. Appel, "Assessment of Cardiac Function in Marathon Runners by Graphic Noninvasive Techniques," *Annals New York Academy of Sciences* 301:900–917 (1977); J. Morganroth, "The Athlete's Heart Syndrome: A New Perspective," *Annals New York Academy of Sciences* 301:931-941 (1977).

10. Crawford and O'Rourke, "The Athlete's Heart"; Morganroth, "The Athlete's Heart Syndrome."

11. C. H. Wyndham, "Heat Stroke and Hyperthermia in Marathon Runners," *Annals New York Academy of Sciences* 301:128–138 (1977).

12. Ibid, p. 137.

13. A. P. Freedman, "Climate and Exercise," in D. T. Lowenthal, K. Bharadwaja, and W. W. Oaks, eds., *Therapeutics Through Exercise* (New York: Grune and Stratton, 1979), pp. 81–87.

14. A. J. Siegel, C. H. Hennekeus, H. S. Soloman, and B. Van Boeckel, "Exercise Related Hematuria," *Journal of the American Medical Association* 241:391–392 (January 26, 1979).

15. N. J. Blacklock, "Bladder Trauma in the Long Distance Runner," *The American Journal of Sports Medicine* 7:239–241 (1979).

16. "The Haematuria of the Long Distance Runner" (editorial) *British Medical Journal* (6183):159 (July 21, 1979).

17. G. E. Burch, "Of Jogging," *American Heart Journal* 97:407 (1979).

18. P. Milvy, Letter to the Editor: on "Of Jogging," *American Heart Journal* 98:136 (1979).

19. Lyle J. Micheli, "Low Back Pain in the Adolescent: Differential Diagnosis," *American Journal of Sports Medicine* 7:362-364 (November/December 1979).

20. Richard B. Chambers, "Orthopedic Injuries in Athletes (Ages 6 to 17)," *American Journal of Sports Medicine* 7:195–197 (May/June 1979).

21. Robert A. Jacobs and Eugene L. Miller, "Skateboard Accidents," *Pediatrics* 59:939 (June

1977); Cynthia M. Illingworth, Ann Jay, Dilys Noble, and Mary Collick, "225 Skateboard Injuries in Children," *Clinical Pediatrics* 17:781–789 (October 1978).

22. James W. Pritchett, "High Cost of High School Football Injuries," *American Journal of Sports Medicine* 8:197–199 (May/June 1980).

23. Joseph S. Torg, Theodore C. Quedenfeld, Albert Burstein, Alan Spealman, and Claude Nichols III, "National Football Head Injury and Neck Injury Registry: Report on Cervical Quadriplegia, 1971 to 1975," *American Journal of Sports Medicine* 7:127–132 (March/April 1979).

24. Peter Fowler, "Swimmer Problems," *American Journal of Sports Medicine* 8:141-142 March/April 1979.

25. Allen B. Richardson, Frank W. Jobe, and H. Royer Collins, "The Shoulder in Competitive Swimming," *American Journal of Sports Medicine* 8:159–163 (May/June 1980).

26. S. David Stulberg, Keith Shulman, Steven Stuart, and Peggy Culp, "Breaststroker's Knee: Pathology, Etiology and Treatment," *American Journal of Sports Medicine* 8:164-170 (May/June 1980).

27. Peter D. Wood, *Run to Health* (New York: Charter, 1980), pp. 89–101 and 41–71.

28. David N. Kurland, Frank C. McCue, David A. Rockwell, and Joe H. Gieck, "Tennis Injuries: Prevention and Treatment," *American Journal of Sports Medicine* 7:249–253 (July/August 1979).

29. Kenneth G. Campbell, *Playing Tennis When It Hurts* (Millbrae, Calif.: Celestial Arts, 1976).

30. Robert J. Johnson, Carl F. Ettlinger, Robert J. Campbell, and Malcolm H. Pope, "Trends in Skiing Injuries. Analysis of a 6-Year Study (1972 to 1978)," *American Journal of Sports Medicine* 8:106–112 (March/April 1980).

31. Paul C. Williams, *The Lumbosacral Spine: Emphasizing Conservative Management* (New York: Blakiston Division, McGraw-Hill, 1965), p. 200.

32. Robert A. Anderson, *Stretching* (Fullerton, Calif.: Shelter Publications, 1977).

33. Wood, *Run to Health*, pp. 54–56 and 89–100.

34. Ibid, pp. 73–81.

CHAPTER 7
EXERCISE AND PUBLIC POLICY

1. Marc Lalonde, *A New Perspective on the Health of Canadians* (Ottawa: Information Service, 1975).

2. Ibid, p. 66.

3. D. A. Bailey, R. J. Shephard, and R. L. Mirwald, "Validation of a Self-Administered Home Test of Cardio-respiratory Fitness," *Canadian Journal of Applied Sports Science,* 1:67–68 (1976); R. J. Shephard, D. A. Bailey, and R. L. Mirwald, "Development of the Canadian Home Fitness Test," *Canadian Medical Association Journal* 114:675–679 (April 17, 1976); R. R. J. Lauzon, "Fit Kit for Fat Cats " (editorial), *Canadian Journal of Public Health* 67:95–97 (March/April 1976); T. Kavanagh, "Intervention Studies in Canada: Primary and Secondary Intervention," in M. L. Pollock and D. H. Schmidt, eds. *Heart Disease and Rehabilitation* (Boston: Houghton Mifflin), pp. 317–329; D. M Chisholm, M. L. Collis, L. L. Kulak, W. Davenport, and N. Gruber, "Physical Activity Readiness,"*British Columbia Medical Journal* 17:375–378 (November 1975).

4. Victor Fuchs, *Who Shall Live? Health, Economics, and Social Choice* (New York: Basic Books, 1974); Ivan Illich, *Medical Nemesis: The Expropriation of Health* (New York Pantheon, 1976); Rick J. Carlson, *The End of Medicine* (New York: John Wiley and Sons 1975); Thomas McKeown, *The Role of Medicine: Dream, Mirage, or Nemesis?* (London

The Nuffield Provincial Hospitals Trust, 1976); Kerr L. White, ed., *Life and Death and Medicine* (San Francisco: W. H. Freeman, A Scientific American Book, 1973); Robert F. Rushmer, *Humanizing Health Care: Alternative Futures for Medicine* (Cambridge, Mass.: MIT Press, 1975); Ann R. Somers, ed., *Promoting Health: Consumer Education and National Policy* (Germantown, Md.: Aspen, 1976); Henrik L. Blum, *Expanding Health Care Horizons* (Oakland, Calif.: Third Party Associates, 1976); Eric J. Cassell, *The Healer's Art: A New Approach to the Doctor–Patient Relationship* (Philadelphia: J. B. Lippincott, 1976); Lewis Thomas, *Lives of a Cell: Notes of a Biology Watcher* (New York: Viking Press, 1974); A. L. Cochrane, *Effectiveness and Efficiency: Random Reflections on Health Service* (London: The Nuffield Provincial Hospitals Trust, 1972); *Doing Better and Feeling Worse: Health in the United States, Daedalus* 106(1): 1–281 (Winter 1977).

5. *Conference Report*, Conference on Future Directions in Health Care: The Dimensions of Medicine, Sponsored by the Rockefeller Foundation, the Blue Cross Association, and Health Policy Program, Universtiy of California, San Francisco (New York, December 10–11, 1975).

6. See Rick J. Carlson and Robert Cunningham, eds., *Future Directions in Health Care: A New Public Policy*, A Report of a Conference Sponsored by the Blue Cross Association, the Health Policy Program at the University of California Medical School at San Francisco, the Institute of Medicine, and the Rockefeller Foundation (Cambridge, Mass.: Ballinger Publishing Company, 1978).

7. See *Preventive Medicine, U.S.A.*, A Task Force Report sponsored by the John E. Fogarty Center for Advanced Study in the Health Sciences, National Institutes of Health, and the American College of Preventive Medicine (New York: Prodist, 1976).

8. John H. Knowles, "The Responsibility of the Individual," *Daedalus* 106(1):57–80 (Winter 1977).

9. Nedra B. Belloc, "Relationship of Health Practices and Mortality," *Preventive Medicine* 2:67–81 (1973).

10. Lester Breslow and James E. Enstrom, "Persistence of Health Habits and Their Relationship to Mortality," *Preventive Medicine* 9(4):469–483 (July 1980).

11. James A. Wiley and Terry C. Camacho, "Lifestyle and Future Health: Evidence From the Alameda County Study," *Preventive Medicine* 9:1–21 (1980).

12. Lisa F. Berkman and S. Leonard Syme, "Social Networks, Host Resistance and Mortality: A Nine-year Follow-up Study of Alameda County Residents," *American Journal of Epidemiology* 109(2):186–204 (1979).

13. Robert Crawford, "You Are Dangerous to Your Health: The Ideology and Politics of Victim Blaming," *International Journal of Health Services* 7(4):663–679 (1977).

14. Patricia E. Franks, "A Summary of Federal Activities Related to Prevention Outside of the Department of Health, Education, and Welfare," A Technical Assistance Report to the Deputy Assistant Secretary for Health (Special Health Initiatives), Office of the Assistant Secretary for Health, U.S. Department of Health, Education, and Welfare, April 19, 1978, unpublished. A shorter version of this report appears in: U.S. Department of Health, Education, and Welfare, Public Health Service, Office of the Assistant Secretary for Health, *Disease Prevention & Health Promotion: Federal Programs and Prospects*, DHEW Publication No. (PHS) 79-55071B (Washington, D.C.: U.S. Government Printing Office, 1979), pp. 138–165.

15. U.S. Department of Health, Education, and Welfare, Public Health Service, Health Resources Administration, *Papers on the National Health Guidelines: Baselines for Setting Health Goals and Standards*, DHEW Publication No. (HRA) 76-640 (Washington, D.C.: U.S. Government Printing Office, 1976), p. 6.

16. Ibid., p. viii.

17. "Promotion Rates High in Plans," *Health Planning Newsletter* 10:1–2 (May, 1980).

18. C. Wayne Higgins, B. W. Philips, and John G. Bruhn, "A National Survey of Health Promotion Activities in Health Systems Agencies," *Preventive Medicine* 9:150–158 (1980).

19. Personal communication, Marilyn Logan, Bureau of Health Planning. Health Resources Administration, U.S. Department of Health and Human Services, July 31, 1980.

20. *Preventive Medicine, U.S.A.*

21. See National Academy of Sciences, Institute of Medicine, *Perspectives on Health Promotion and Disease Prevention in the United States: A Staff Paper* (Washington, D.C., January 1978); National Academy of Sciences, Institute of Medicine, Division of Health Promotion and Disease Prevention, *Final Report: Summary Conference on Health Promotion and Disease Prevention* (Washington, D.C., March 27, 1978).

22. U.S. Department of Health, Education, and Welfare, Public Health Service, Office of the Assistant Secretary for Health and Surgeon General, *Healthy People: The Surgeon General's Report on Health Promotion and Disease Prevention, 1979*, DHEW Publication No. (PHS) 79-55071 (Washington D.C.: U.S. Government Printing Office, 1979).

23. U.S. Department of Health, Education, and Welfare, Public Health Service, Office of the Assistant Secretary for Health and Surgeon General, *Healthy People: The Surgeon General's Report on · Health Promotion and Disease Prevention: Background Papers, 1979*, Report to the Surgeon General on Health Promotion and Disease Prevention by the Institute of Medicine, National Academy of Sciences, DHEW Publication No. (PHS) 79-55071A (Washington D.C.: U.S. Government Printing Office, 1979).

24. U.S. Department of Health, Education, and Welfare, Public Health Service, Office of the Assistant Secretary for Health, *Disease Prevention & Health Promotion: Federal Programs and Prospects*, Report of the Departmental Task Force on Prevention, September 1978, DHEW Publication No. (PHS) 79-55071B (Washington D.C.: U.S. Government Printing Office, 1979).

25. Philip R. Lee and Patricia E. Franks, "Primary Prevention and the Executive Branch of the Federal Government," *Preventive Medicine* 6:209–226 (1977).

26. U.S. Department of Health, Education, and Welfare, Public Health Service, Office of the Assistant Secretary for Health and Surgeon General, *Promoting Health/Preventing Disease: Objectives for the Nation* (Washington D.C.: U.S. Government Printing Office, 1979).

27. Suzanne Stenmark, Peggy McManus, Philip Lee, and Pat Franks, "In Search of Federal Exercise Policy: Six Federal Agencies' Policies on Exercise and Health," Technical Assistance Report to the Deputy Assistant Secretary for Disease Prevention and Health Promotion, Office of the Assistant Secretary for Health, U.S. Department of Health and Human Services (San Francisco: University of California, San Francisco, Health Policy Program, November 3, 1980).

28. U.S. Department of Health, Education, and Welfare, *Promoting Health/Preventing Disease*, pp. 99–104.

29. Stephen Havas, *Exercise and Your Health*, draft June 19, 1980, U.S. Department of Health and Human Services, National Institutes of Health, National Heart, Lung, and Blood Institute (Bethesda, Md., in press).

30. Carroll L. Estes, *The Aging Enterprise* (San Francisco: Jossey-Bass, 1979), pp. 124–126.

31. J. Pressman and A. Wildavsky, *Implementation* (Berkeley: University of California Press, 1973), p. 134.

32. T.R. Marmor and E. A. Kutza, *An Analysis of Federal Regulations Related to Aging: Legislative Barriers to Coordination Under Title III* (Chicago: University of Chicago, 1975).

33. Estes, *The Aging Enterprise*, p. 156.

34. Ibid., p. 56.

35. J. W. Farquhar, P. D. Wood, H. Breitrose, et al., "Community Education for Cardio-vascular Health," *The Lancet* 1:1192-1195 (June 4, 1977); K. Koskella, P. Puska, and J. Tuomilehto, "The North Karelia Project: A First Evaluation," *International Journal of Health Education* 19:59-65 (1976).

36. Lalonde, *A New Perspective*, 36-37 and 67-68.

37. U.S. Department of Health, Education, and Welfare, Public Health Service, Office of the Assistant Secretary for Health, *Forward Plan for Health, Fiscal Years 1978-82* (Washington D.C.: U.S. Government Printing Office, 1976), p. 83.

38. R. Beggs and E. Boyer, "Joint Management-Union Anaylsis of Employee Physical Fitness Program Questionnaire," Report of the Department of Health, Education, and Welfare, Region IX, August 1978.

39. U.S. Department of Health and Human Services, Public Health Service, Office of Health Information, Health Promotion, and Physical Fitness and Sports Medicine, "Department of Health and Human Services Employee Health Promotion Program," March 5, 1980.

40. D. C. Durbeck, F. Heinzelmann, J. Schacter, W. L. Haskell, C. H. Payne, R. T. Moxley, M. Nemiroff, P. D. Limoncelli, L. B. Arnoldi, and S. M. Fox, "The National Aeronautics and Space Administration-U.S. Public Health Service Evaluation and Enhancement Program," *The American Journal of Cardiology* 30:784-790 (November 20, 1972).

41. U.S. Department of Health, Education, and Welfare, Public Health Service, Office of Assistant Secretary for Health, *A Task Force Report on Disease Prevention and Health Promotion* (Washington, D.C.: U.S. Government Printing Office, 1978), pp. 190-191.

42. S. Fox, J. Naughton, and W. Haskell, "Physical Activity and the Prevention of Coronary Heart Disease," *Annals of Clinical Research* 3:404-432 (1971); J. N. Morris, A. Kagan, D. C. Pattison, et al., "Incidence and Prediction of Ischemic Heart Disease in London Busmen," *The Lancet* 2:553-559 (1966); G. Mann, "Sneakers and Supporters to Fight CHD," *The New England Journal of Medicine* 292:758 (1975).

43. Personal communication, Stephen Havas, M.D., Former Special Assistant to the Director, National Heart, Lung, and Blood Institute, National Institutes of Health, U.S. Department of Health and Human Services, July 31, 1980.

44. "Education Secretary to Review School Fitness Programs," *President's Council on Physical Fitness and Sports Newsletter* (Washington D.C.: Department of Health, Education, and Welfare, March 1980), p. 3.

45. Personal communication, Frank Turpan, Oregon Department of Transportation, February 28, 1979.

46. Jonathan Fielding, "Health Promotion—Some Notions in Search of a Constituency," *American Journal of Public Health* 67:1082-1085 (1977).

47. American Academy of Pediatrics, "Support for Circulatory-Respiratory Endurance Activities" (n.d.).

48. Henry Blackburn, "Preventive Cardiology in Practice," in Michael L. Pollock and Donald H. Schmidt, eds., *Heart Disease and Rehabilitation* (Boston: Houghton Mifflin, 1979), pp. 245-275.

49. Ibid., p. 246. Emphasis in original.

50. State of Rhode Island, Department of Health, Technical Report No. 5, "Health and Behavior Intervention in Rhode Island," September 1976, p. 65.

51. A. B. Morrison, "Prevention in the Canadian Health System," *Preventive Medicine* 7(4): 498-504 (1978).

CHAPTER 8
EXERCISE AND HEALTH:
MOBILIZING COMMUNITY
RESOURCES

1. U.S. Department of Health, Education, and Welfare, Public Health Service, Office of the Assistant Secretary for Health and Surgeon General, *Promoting Health/Preventing Disease: Objectives for the Nation* (Washington D.C.: U.S. Government Printing Office 1979).
2. Henry Blackburn, "Preventive Cardiology in Practice," in Michael L. Pollock and Donald H. Schmidt, eds., *Heart Disease and Rehabilitation* (Boston: Houghton Mifflin, 1979), pp. 245–275. Emphasis in original.
3. *Building a Healthier Company*, a publication of Blue Cross–Blue Shield, the President's Council on Physical Fitness and Sports, and the American Association of Fitness Directors in Business and Industry.
4. American Heart Association, *Risk Factors and Coronary Disease: A Statement for Physicians* (New York, 1968); American Heart Association, *Exercise Testing and Training of Apparently Healthy Individuals: A Handbook for Physicians* (New York 1972); American Medical Association, *A Guide to Prescribing Exercise Programs* (Chicago); American Medical Association, *Basic Bodywork for Fitness and Health* (Chicago); American Heart Association, *Why Risk Heart Attack: Six Ways to Guard Your Heart* (Dallas, 1968).
5. *Guidelines for Physical Fitness Programs in Business and Industry*, a joint statement of the President's Council on Physical Fitness and Sports and the American Medical Association's Committee on Exercise and Physical Fitness.
6. Kenneth H. Cooper, *Aerobics* (New York: Bantam Books, 1970); Kenneth H. Cooper, *The New Aerobics* (New York: Bantam Books, 1970); Kenneth H. Cooper and M. Cooper *Aerobics for Women* (New York: Bantam Books, 1970); Kenneth H. Cooper, *The Aerobics Way* (New York: M. Evans and Company, 1977).
7. J. F. Fixx, *The Complete Book of Running* (New York: Random House, 1977); J. F. Fixx, *Jim Fixx's Second Book of Running* (New York: Random House 1980).
8. *Royal Canadian Air Force Exercise Plan for Physical Fitness* (New York: Simon and Schuster, 1976).
9. Terence Kavanagh, "Intervention Studies in Canada: Primary and Secondary Intervention," in Michael L. Pollock and Donald H. Schmidt, eds., *Heart Disease and Rehabilitation* (Boston: Houghton Mifflin, 1979), pp. 317–329.
10. PARTICIPaction . . . The Canadian Movement for Personal Fitness. Montreal and Toronto: Sport Participation Canada.
11. State of Wisconsin, Department of Health and Social Service, Commission on Prevention and Wellness, *Final Report, Commission on Prevention and Wellness* (October 1979), p. 18.
12. Ibid.
13. State of Georgia, Department of Human Resources, Division of Health, Digest of the Report of the Community Task Force, *Georgia's New Health Outlook* (June 1976), p. 11.
14. Ibid.
15. Howard R. Pyfer, William F. Mead, Richard C. Frederick, and Belvin L. Docter, "Exercise Rehabilitation in Coronary Heart Disease: Community Group Programs,"

Archives of Physical Medicine and Rehabilitation 57:335–342. (July 1976); H. K. Hellerstein and A. B. Ford, "Rehabilitation of the Cardiac Patient," *Journal of the American Medical Association* 164:225–231 (1957).

16. A. L. McAlister, J. W. Farquhar, C. E. Thoresen, and N. Maccoby, "Behavioral Science Applied to Cardiovascular Health: Progress and Research Needs in Modification of Risk-Taking Habits in Adult Populations," *Health Education Monographs* 4:45–74 (1976); J. W. Farquhar, "The Community-Based Model of Life Style Intervention Trials," *American Journal of Epidemiology* 108(2):103–111 (1978); A. J. Meyer, J. D. Nash, A. L. McAlister, N. Maccoby, and J. W. Farquhar, "Skills Training in a Cardiovascular Health Education Campaign," *Journal of Consulting and Clinical Psychology* 48(2):129–142 (1980).

17. "Senior Olympics Shares Fitness," *The Physician and Sportsmedicine* 7(8)18–19 (August 1979).

18. "Reading, 'Riting and Running—Fitness Begins in School," *Medical World News*, February 5, 1979, pp. 54–55.

19. K. H. Cooper, J. G. Purdy, A. Friedman, K. L. Bohannon, R. A. Harris, and J. A. Arends, "An Aerobics Conditioning Program for the Fort Worth Texas School District," *The Research Quarterly* 46(3):345–350 (October 1975).

20. Michael L. Pollock, "Exercise—A Preventive Prescription," *The Journal of School Health*, 49(4):215–219 (April 1979).

21. Michael Myers, "Exercising For Fun and Profit," *City Sports*, March 1980, pp. 14–15.

22. Ibid., p. 15.

23. State of Wisconsin, *Final Report*, p. 15.

24. Marc Lalonde, *A New Perspective on the Health of Canadians* (Ottawa: Information Canada, 1975) pp. 36–37 and 67–68.

25. S. Fox, J. Naughton, and P. Gorman, "Physical Activity and Cardiovascular Health. The Exercise Prescription: Frequency and Types of Activity," *Modern Concepts of Caridovascular Disease* 61(6):25–30 (1972).

26. State of Rhode Island, Department of Health, Preliminary State Health System Plan, Goal Statements (Lifestyle), January 23, 1979.

27. State of Rhode Island, Department of Health, Preliminary Annual Implementation Plan (Lifestyle), July 11, 1979, p. 5.

28. Personal communication, Matthew Guidry, President's Council on Physical Fitness and Sports, March 7, 1979.

29. Matthew Guidry, "Programming for Physical Fitness," *Parks & Recreation* (August 1976), pp. 24–25, 48.

30. "Cost Information for Your Parcourse," Parcourse, Ltd., San Francisco.

31. "Swimming, a Way of Life for Most Norwegian Children," *President's Council on Physical Fitness and Sports Newsletter* (Washington, D.C.: Department of Health, Education, and Welfare, February 1977), p. 10.

32. U.S. Department of Health, Education, and Welfare, *Promoting Health/Preventing Disease*, p. 100.

33. Canadian Department of National Health and Welfare, Staff Papers, Long Range Health Planning, *Physical Activity in Canada* (July 1978), p. 57.

34. Personal communication, Frank Turpan, Oregon Department of Transportation, February 28, 1979.

35. Thomas Baake, "Bike City, USA: Life in the Slow Lanes," *The Physician and Sportsmedicine* 7(6):149–153 (June 1979).

36. U.S. Department of Health Education and Welfare, *Promoting Health/Preventing Disease*, p. 100.

37. J. Fielding, "Health Promotion: Some Notions in Search of a Constituency," *American Journal of Public Health* 67:1082–1085 (1977).

38. J. Fielding. "Preventive Medicine and the Bottom Line," *Journal of Occupational Medicine* 21(2):79–88 (February 1979).
39. James T. Yenkel, "Regular Exercise Can Reduce Insurance Premiums Too," *Los Angeles Times*, Part III, September 24, 1979, p. 22.
40. Ibid.
41. Ibid.
42. Ibid.
43. L. Neittaamaki, K. Koskela, P. Puska, et al., "Experiences with the Use of Lay Person in a Comprehensive Community Health Education Program," University of Kuopio Finland, 1978.
44. "Reading, 'Riting and Running—Fitness Begins at School," p. 56.
45. Ibid.
46. Canadian Department of National Health and Welfare, *Physical Activity in Canada* p. 31.
47. *The Foundation Directory: 7th Edition* (New York: The Foundation Center, 1979).
48. U.S. Executive Office of the President, Office of Management and Budget, *Catalog of Federal Domestic Assistance* (Washington, D.C.: U.S. Government Printing Office 1978).
49. Albert Stunkard, Statement to the U.S. House of Representatives Subcommittee on Health and Environment, March 21, 1979, p. 3.
50. K. Koskela, P. Puska, and J. Tuomilehto, "The North Karelia Project: A First Evaluation," *International Journal of Health Education* 19:59–65 (1976).
51. J. W. Farquhar, N. Maccoby, and P. Wood, "The Stanford Three-Community Study: A Multifactor Cardiovascular Risk Education Campaign," submitted to the Danish Heart Foundation for the Symposium on the Strategy of Postponement of Ischaemic Heart Disease (October 26, 1976), pp. 14-26.
52. Blackburn, "Preventive Cardiology," p. 245.
53. Fielding, "Preventive Medicine and the Bottom Line," p. 79.
54. Ibid, p. 82.
55. F. Heinzelmann and D. C. Durbeck, "Personal Benefits of a Health Evaluation and Enhancement Program," Heart Disease and Stroke Control Program, Regional Medical Programs, Health Services and Mental Health Administrations, 1971.
56. U. Pravosudov, "The Effects of Physical Exercise on Health and Economic Efficiency," Lesgaft State Institute of Physical Culture, Leningrad, USSR, 1975.
57. L. A. Bjurstrom and N. G. Alexiou, "A Program of Heart Disease Prevention for Public Employees: A Five-Year Report," *Journal of Occupational Medicine* 20(8):521-531 (August 1978).
58. State of Georgia, "Georgia's New Health Outlook," Proceedings of Georgia's Health Promotion Conference, Georgia State University, Atlanta, Georgia, January 12-13, 1977, Georgia Department of Human Resources, Division of Physical Health, Office of Health Education and Training, 47 Trinity Avenue, S.W., Atlanta, Georgia 30334 (July 1978).
59. Ibid., p. 34.
60. *Guidelines for Physical Fitness Programs in Business and Industry.*
61. State of Wisconsin, Department of Health and Social Services, Commission on Prevention and Wellness, *Final Report, Commission on Prevention and Wellness* Appendix B, "Survey of Employee Health Promotion Programs in Wisconsin," Report of the Business and Industry Committee, Commission on Prevention and Wellness (August 1979), p. 6; R. E. Dedmon, J. W. Gander, M. P. O'Conner, and A. C. Paschke "An Industry Health Management Program," *The Physician and Sportsmedicine* 7(11): 57-67 (November 1979).
62. Ibid., p. 65.

63. Ibid., pp. 65–66.
64. Ibid., p. 66.
65. State of Wisconsin, Appendix B., "Survey of Employee Health Promotion Programs in Wisconsin," p. 8.
66. Ibid.
67. Myers, "Exercising for Fun and Profit," pp. 14–15.
68. Ibid., p. 15.
69. Bjurstrom and Alexiou, "Program of Heart Disease Prevention, p. 521.
70. Ibid., p. 526.
71. State of Wisconsin, Department of Health and Social Services, Office of the Secretary, Memorandum to Chairpersons and Members Joint Committee on Finance, Assembly Committee on Health and Social Services and Senate Committee on Human Services from Donald E. Percy, "Report on 1979 Prevention and Health Promotion Grant Program and Projects Selected for Support," June 6, 1979 (unpaginated).
72. State of Wisconsin, Department of Health and Social Services, Office of the Secretary, Press Release, November 13, 1978.
73. State of Wisconsin, Department of Health and Social Services, Office of the Secretary, "Report on 1979 Prevention and Health Promotion Grant Program and Projects."
74. Ibid.
75. Michael Mealey, "New Fitness for Police and Fire Fighters," *The Physician and Sportsmedicine* 7(7):96–100 (July 1979).
76. Ibid., p. 100.
77. Ibid.
78. Ibid.
79. Ibid.
80. State of Connecticut, Department of Health, "Lifestyle at the Worksite: A Model for a Prevention Program," Connecticut State Department of Health, 79 Elm Street, Hartford, Connecticut 06115, September 1978 (unpaginated).
81. Fielding, "Preventive Medicine and the Bottom Line," p. 84.
82. Canadian Department of National Health and Welfare, p. 59.
83. Ibid., p. 59–60.
84. State of Rhode Island, Department of Health, Technical Report No. 5, "Health and Behavior Intervention in Rhode Island," p. 74.
85. D. D. Gelman, R. Lachaine, and M. M. Law, "The Canadian Approach to Health Policies and Programs," *Preventive Medicine* 6:265–275 (1977).
86. Lalonde, *A New Perspective*.
87. Richard R. J. Lauzon, "Fit Kit for Fat Cats?" *Canadian Journal of Public Health* 67:95–100 (March/April 1976).
88. D. A. Bailey, R. J. Shephard, and R. L. Mirwald, "Validation of a Self-Administered Home Test of Cardiorespiratory Fitness" (Ottawa: Department of National Health and Welfare, 1975).
89. P-O. Astrand, *Health and Fitness* (Stockholm, 1972).
90. D. A. E. Shephard, "Home Testing of Fitness of Canadians," *Canadian Medical Association Journal* 114:662–664 (April 17, 1976).
91. Ibid., p. 662.
92. *The Canadian Home Fitness Test: Summary of the Test Market Report* (Ottawa: Recreation Canada, 1975).
93. American Medical Association, Council on Scientific Affairs, Panel on Exercise and Fitness, Statement on Physical Fitness and Physical Education (March 1979).
94. Ibid.
95. Ibid.
96. U.S. Department of Health, Education, and Welfare, Staff of the President's Council on

Physical Fitness and Sports, "Physical Fitness and Exercise," A Draft Working Paper (n.d.), p. 15.

97. Canadian Department of National Health and Welfare, p. 63.

98. State of Georgia, Department of Human Resources, Division of Health, Digest of the Report of the Community Task Force, *Georgia's New Health Outlook*, p. 11.

99. Personal communication, Evelyn Sykora, fifth-grade teacher, Los Angeles Unified School District, May 1980.

100. State of California, Department of Education, *Physical Education Framework*, California State Department of Education, 721 Capitol Mall, Sacramento, California 95814, 1973, p. 33. Emphasis added.

101. Personal communication, Evelyn Sykora.

102. Personal communication, W. G. Thomas, Los Angeles Trade-Technical College, April 1980.

103. A. J. Meyer and J. B. Henderson, "Multiple Risk Factor Reduction in the Prevention of Cardiovascular Disease," *Preventive Medicine* 3:225–236 (1974); N. Maccoby and J. W. Farquhar, "Communication for Health: Unselling Heart Disease," *Journal of Communication* 25(3):114–126 (Summer 1975); J. W. Farquhar, N. Maccoby, P. D. Wood, and J. Alexander, et al., "Community Education for Cardiovascular Health," Stanford Heart Disease Prevention Program, Stanford University, Stanford, California 94305; N. Maccoby, J. W. Farquhar, P. D. Wood, and J. Alexander, "Reducing the Risk of Cardiovascular Disease: Effects of Community-Based Campaign on Knowledge and Behavior," *Journal of Community Health* 3(2):100–114 (Winter 1977).

104. Koskela, Puska, and Tuomilehto, "The North Karelia Project."

105. Kavanagh, "Intervention Studies in Canada," p. 324.

106. "Introducing P.E.P., an Approach to Health and Exercise That Really Makes Sense," Peralta Executive Program (P.E.P.), Peralta Hospital, 450 Thirtieth Street, Oakland, California 94609 (n.d.).

107. Baake, "Bike City, U.S.A.," p. 149.

108. U.S. Department of Health, Education, and Welfare, Public Health Service, Center for Disease Control, *Health Education/Risk Reduction Grants Interim Guidelines*, March 18, 1980.

109. Ibid.

110. U.S. Department of Health, Education, and Welfare, Health Resources Administration, *National Guidelines for Health Planning: Notice of Proposed Rulemaking*, July 6, 1979, p. 62.

111. Ibid.

112. Farquhar, "Community-Based Model," pp. 103–104.

113. A. J. Meyer, N. Maccoby, and J. W. Farquhar, "The Role of Opinion Leadership in a Cardiovascular Health Education Campaign," a paper presented at the 27th Annual Conference of the International Communication Association, Berlin, Germany (May 29–June 4, 1977).

114. Farquhar, Maccoby, and Wood, "The Stanford Three-Community Study."

115. Ibid., pp. 31–32.

Index

Activity type, in exercise prescription, 82. *See also* Complications; Tests
Acute exercise, in diabetics, 65
Advertising of exercise. *See* Fitness programs; Media
Aerobic capacity, 72, 82
Aerobic dancing, 86
Aerobic exercise, defined, 17. *See also* Dynamic aerobic exercise
Aerobic Way, The, 86
Agriculture, Department of, 121
Alameda County (California), life-expectancy survey: and community ties, 120; and health habits, 119
Alcohol consumption, as a predictor of health status, 119. *See also* Preventive health care
Alexandria, Virginia, Fire Department, fitness program, 174
Amateur Athletic Union, masters swim meets, 9
American Academy of Pediatrics: advice to schools, 146; asthma recommendations of, 72
American College of Preventive Medicine, 123
American College of Sports Medicine, 75
American Heart Association: *Exercise Testing and Training of Apparently Healthy Individuals: A Handbook for Physicians,* 75; media campaigns of, 8, 152; on physical examinations, 78
American Journal of Epidemiology, 154
American Journal of Sports Medicine, 154
American Medical Association: and fitness promotion, 8, 75, 139, 152; guidelines of for workplace fitness programs, 168; on physical education in schools, 146, 177–178
Anaerobic glycolysis, 18
Angina pectoris: and exercise training, 19. *See also* Complications; Coronary heart disease
Angiopathy, complications arising from, 67–68
Anxiety, assessment of, 68–69
Arco, 166
Arrhythmia, 99–101
Arthur, Dr. Ransom S., 9
Asthma, 3; effects of exercise on, 56, 70–72
Atherosclerosis, 41
Athlete's heart, 101
Athletes, exercise levels of in later life, 36, 38
Atkins diet, 62
Attributable risk, defined, 27
Automobile accidents: death rate from, 102; as hazard to joggers, 102
Autopsy, in study of hypertension, 57

Back problems, recommended exercises for, 108
Basic Bodywork for Fitness and Health, 152
Behavior modification, in obesity control, 63

Bergfeld, Dr. John, 163
Bicycling: and Dr. Paul Dudley White, 7–8; paths, 144–145, 159–160; stress test, 79, 81, 85
Blackburn, Dr. Henry, 146-147, 152
"Blaming the victim," 120–121
Blood glucose levels, 65–66. *See also* Diabetes mellitus
Blood lipid profile, 3; feedback, use of in obesity control, 64; relation of to coronary heart disease, 40–41
Blood pressure, relation of to exercise, 59–60. *See also* Hypertension
Blue Cross Association: conferences sponsored by, 117; and fitness promotion, 139; and promotion of running, 152
Body composition, 19
Body mass index, and hypertension, 56–57
Body weight: controlling factors, 61; in hypertension studies, 56–58; as predictor of health status, 119. *See also* Obesity
Boeing, 166
Books: about exercise activities, 9–10, 86; instructional, for physicians and patients, 152–153; about matters related to health policy, 117
Boston Marathon, 155
Bowerman, William J., and W. E. Harris, *Jogging,* 9
Brems, Marianne, *Swim for Fitness,* 10
British Columbia, fitness questionnaire, 77. *See also* Canada
Bronchoconstriction, 70–71
Budget cuts, effects of on physical education, 178
Bus conductors, study of heart disease risk in, 30
Building a Healthier Company, 152
Building codes, and exercise facilities, 159–160

California: physical education curriculum, proposed, 179–182; *Physical Education Framework,* 181–182
Caloric consumption, 61–62
Canada: children's fitness level in, 163; Department of National Health and Welfare, 153; fitness promotion by private groups, 153; government proposals on health care, 116–117; *A New Perspective on the Health of Canadians,* 116, 122, 126, 149
Cardiac exercise rehabilitation, 75–76, 140–141, 147; and research needs, 141–142. *See also* Complications; Coronary heart disease; Heart attack survivors
Cardiovascular disease: prevention program (Finland), 161; research and information dissemination, 132–133
Case-control studies, 26, 28
Causality, assumption of, 28
Chlorpropamide, 65
Cigarette smoking. *See* Smoking

221

About the Authors

Gregory S. Thomas, M.D., M.P.H., is a Research Fellow at the Health Policy Program, School of Medicine, University of California, San Francisco; Clinical Fellow in Medicine at the Harvard School of Medicine; and a resident at Massachusetts General Hospital.

Philip R. Lee, M.D., is Professor of Social Medicine and Director of the Health Policy Program at the School of Medicine, University of California, San Francisco.

Pat Franks is a Senior Research Associate at the Health Policy Program, School of Medicine, University of California, San Francisco.

Ralph S. Paffenbarger, Jr., M.D., Dr. P.H., is Professor of Epidemiology in the Department of Family, Community, and Preventive Medicine, School of Medicine, Stanford University.

KU-714-14

WITHDRA

PEOPLES
AND EMPIRES

Other titles in the Weidenfeld & Nicolson UNIVERSAL HISTORY series include:

Already published

Paul Johnson *The Renaissance*
Mark Mazower *The Balkans*
Karen Armstrong *Islam*
Michael Sturmer *The German Empire*

Forthcoming

Hans Kung *A History of the Catholic Church*
Robert Wistrich *The Holocaust*
John Ray *Ancient Egyptians*
Conor Cruise O'Brien *The French Revolution*
Bernard Williams *A History of Freedom*
Richard Pipes *A History of Communism*
Seamus Deane *The Irish*
Steven Weinberg *A Short History of Science*
R W Johnson *South Africa*
Keith Hopkins *Ancient Rome*
Gordon Wood *The American Revolution*
Felipe Fernández-Armesto *The Americas*
Patrick Collinson *The Reformation*
Joel Kotkin *The City*
Sunil Khilnani *Modern India*
Oswyn Murray *Ancient Greeks*
A N Wilson *A Short History of London*
Richard Fletcher *The Crescent and The Cross*
Colin Renfrew *Prehistory*
Ian Buruma *The Rise of Modern Japan*
Paul Fussell *The Second World War*
Chinua Achebe *A Short History of Africa*
James Davidson *The Golden Age of Athens*
James Word *A History of the Novel*

PEOPLES
AND EMPIRES

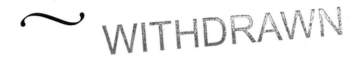

Anthony Pagden

Weidenfeld & Nicolson

LONDON

First published in Great Britain in 2001
by Weidenfeld & Nicolson

Copyright © Anthony Pagden 2001

The right of Anthony Pagden to be identified as the author of
this work has been asserted by him in accordance with the
Copyright, Designs and Patents Act of 1988.

A CIP catalogue record for this book is available
from the British Library.

ISBN 0 297 643703

Typeset by Selwood Systems, Midsomer Norton
Printed by Butler & Tanner Ltd, Frome and London

Weidenfeld & Nicolson

The Orion Publishing Group Ltd
Orion House
5 Upper Saint Martin's Lane
London WC2H 9EA

Contents

For Giulia

Prologue

This is a very short book on a very big subject – so big indeed that it could simply be described as the history of the world. It is the story of the transformation of groups of peoples into the massive states we call empires. However we choose to define the term – and it is, at best, a vague one – there have been empires in Africa, in Asia, in the Americas and in Europe. I am, however, largely concerned with the story of those empires of what is now called the West, from the rise of Alexander the Great to the collapse of the Soviet Union. I discuss China and Vijayanagara, or Safavid Iran only in so far as they touch upon that story. This is not because I imagine, as some do, that the Chinese or the Indians or the Iranians ultimately lacked the inventiveness, imaginative drive, or individuality which, supposedly, allowed the Europeans to dominate so much of the world. It is simply that since those other places have had their own histories, which have gone in sometimes quite different directions, it would require other books fully to tell them.

As with all books of this kind, which try to cover so much ground and so much historical time, I have relied on the goodwill of colleagues and friends to provide me with information and advice. Bill Rowe and Mathew Roller patiently answered my questions about the Chinese and Roman worlds respectively. I have learned from Sanjay Subrahmanyam and Serge Grunzinski how to think globally, as much as about the individual histories of India, Iran and Spanish America. I owe a very special debt to the students of my class on empires and imperialism at the School for Advanced International Studies in Washington who provided me with information, questioned my more dubious assertions and, in their polyglot cosmopolitan enthusiasms, taught me much about the roots of restlessness. An earlier version of the text was read with great care by Toby Mundy at Weidenfeld & Nicolson and by Scott Moyers at Random House, and their careful, detailed comments have improved the final version immeasurably. I am grateful to them for their patience and perceptiveness. I am grateful, too, to Rebecca Wilson and Alice Hunt for their guidance in the final stages.

Giulia Sissa taught me about ancient Greece, and about life, and to her all of this is gratefully dedicated.

Paris, August 2000

Introduction

In 'The Story of the Warrior and the Captive', the Argentine writer Jorge Luis Borges tells two stories. In the first, a Lombard 'barbarian' named Droctulft reaches the gates of the Byzantine city of Ravenna, the last outpost of the crumbling empire of Constantine the Great. He has come there as a conqueror. Until that moment, which will change his life in ways over which he will have no further control, his only concern has been war and its spoils. His is a world of movement, of horses and tents, of transhumance and conflict. He knows nothing of cities, or of the arts or the sciences, or of the measurement of time. His world is his people. His loyalty, as Borges says, is to his chief, his tribe, 'not to the universe'. Space is infinite only because he knows nothing of its limits. He fights against men whose languages he does not understand and whose ways of life he cannot comprehend. He senses that these others, who live in cities, have goods that he desires and that his people cannot create for themselves.

On the day on which he enters the city he becomes another, a stranger to what he was. He becomes aware of desires he has never known before, is seized with wonder at the palaces and squares, the domes and cupolas, of the great city. This was what he had come to plunder. Overwhelmed by it all, he now realizes that he has no choice but to change allegiances and to fight in order to preserve what he had once thought only to destroy. By doing so, he acquires what he never knew he wanted: a place. There he will always be an outsider, a 'barbarian'. Because of that he will be compelled, as Borges says, to be little more than a child or a dog. But he and his descendants will have begun the long journey on the road towards the condition that Europeans have for centuries called 'civilization'.

Droctulft made one kind of journey. Borges' second story is about another. As a young woman, Borges' English grandmother was brought by her husband to the Pampas, the seemingly endless Argentine grasslands, staring at which, Charles Darwin once said, gave him 'horizontal vertigo'. There she met an English-woman, from Yorkshire, who as a child had been carried off in an Indian raid, had been raised as an Indian, and had married a chieftain to whom she had borne two sons. Borges' grandmother, shocked by what she could glimpse 'behind her story', the 'feasts of scorched meat or raw entrails ... the polygamy, the stench and the superstition', urged her to leave, to return to the world as she had once known it. But 'The woman answered that she was happy, and returned that night to the desert.'

Droctulft and the Indian captive crossed in opposite directions. This book is about the implications of those two stories, and the points at which they meet, cross and sometimes become confused one with the other. It is about what drives peoples into contact – and conflict – with one another. It is about restlessness. It is also, inevitably, about cruelty and anger, indif-ference and power, about loss and the passing of time. It is about empires and the peoples who have created them, and been created by them.

Empires, however we define the term, and wherever they occur, have always been way of imposing stability upon different groups who often have little love for one another. Most empires have offered their subject peoples a combination of opportunities and restraints. Many have chosen to accept the opportunities and put up with the restraints. Others, inevitably, have not. All, however, knew that what an empire of the size and power of Rome represented was what Droctulft had seen, in its final fading glory, at Ravenna. It was accumulated wealth, the comforts that a highly stratified, technologically advanced society can bring – at least for those who can afford them. It was – and, in the accounts from which Borges took his tale, this is what seems most to have persuaded Droctulft to devote himself to its preservation – the sheer sumptuousness of creativity: the paintings, the buildings, the garments of the peoples. It was also, although by the eighth century of the Christian era this was already a thing of the past, the possibility of security at least from external threat, of a calm and reflective life.

By contrast, the things Borges' grandmother could see in the life of the young English captive conjured up only images of a life of constant movement, a life lived in the open, a life without shape or ultimate purpose. For her, as for all Europeans, the only life in which it was possible to be fully human, to be, as she would have said, 'civilized', was one lived in cities. Our entire political and social vocabulary derives from this fact. 'Politics' and 'polity' have their root in the Greek term *polis*. Similarly 'civil', 'civility', 'civilization' all have their origins in the Latin word *civitas*. In time both words became abstract nouns translatable as the 'state', or the 'commonwealth'. But both had originally described the self-contained, urban spaces of the ancient world. Rome was the 'Eternal City', the 'Prince of Cities', which, in the words of the fourth-century poet Claudian, was the 'mother of arms, who casts empire [*imperium*] over all'.[1] The founding of empires has, therefore, always been closely associated with the creation of cities. Alexander the Great – whom we shall meet again – founded literally dozens in his name: in Egypt (the greatest of them, and the only one still to be called 'Alexandria'); at Herat in central Iran; at Arachosia (probably modern Kandahar); at Begram in the Hindu Kush; at Eschate (modern Leninabad). In one single year, 328 BC, he created six new cities north of the river Oxus. According to the Roman philosopher and historian Plutarch (although he was surely exaggerating), during the course of his reign Alexander established no less than seventy new settlements. Centuries later, when the Spanish conquistador Hernán Cortés marched through Mexico in 1519–20 he, too, founded cities as he went, first on the coast at Veracruz, then Cholula and Tlaxcala. Finally, after the great Aztec capital of Tenochtitlán had fallen in 1522, he rebuilt it and renamed it Mexico City.

Cities were, of course, by no means unique to Europe. Like much else that is defining of European culture, the walled, largely self-governing urban space had originated in Asia. But it is only with the rise of Athens after the sixth century BC that an association in the European political imagination began to form between an urban environment and a particular way of life. Man, said the Greek philosopher Aristotle, was *zoon politikon* – a term which means, quite literally, an animal 'made for life in the polis'. In the Greek world life in the *polis* was not merely the best attainable existence. It was the only life in

4

which it was possible for humanity to achieve the ends that nature, or the gods, had established for it. Little wonder then that for Aristotle there could be no life beyond the limits of the city but that of 'beasts and gods'. For centuries, those who chose, or were compelled, to leave their native cities were looked upon both as potentially degenerate and as potentially dangerous. Exile in the ancient world was a punishment comparable to death, and in Renaissance Europe it was often described, quite precisely, as a 'civil death'.

Those who have chosen to live beyond the limits of the city, the travellers and vagrants, even pilgrims, have in the course of European history been widely persecuted and abused. The most extreme case is that of Europe's Gypsies, whose history passes from initial astonishment and sympathy for what were believed to be the victims of the Ottoman conquest of the Byzantine empire, to suspicion and finally, in the gas chambers of Hitler's Reich, to attempted annihilation.

Yet, for all this distrust of journeying, this horror of the rootless and the homeless, most humans are, as St Francis once described them, *homines viatores*, perennial movers. When she met the young Englishwoman, Borges' grandmother was herself living on the frontier which, in nineteenth-century Argentina, was merely a step away from the condition of the Indians that so disgusted her. Most of us simply cannot avoid movement. Just as even the fiercest of endogamous societies must, on occasions, allow its members to 'marry out' if it is to survive, so all cultures, however concerned they might be with the virtues of immobility, have also to move if they are to progress. There have been few peoples for whom a state of permanent immobility is the norm. The happy Polynesians – the 'noble savages' – who figure so prominently in the eighteenth-century literary imagination of France, who went nowhere and who commanded all those Europeans who visited them to go home at once, could never, as the German philosopher Immanuel Kant said of them, 'give a satisfactory answer to the question of why they should exist at all'. Kant was being unduly harsh, not so much because the Tahitians had no desire to travel as because of his suspicion of what he took to be the description of a life of 'mere' enjoyment.[2] But he was right to see something inhuman in this idealization of Tahitian society.

Human history ends, as Kant insisted, as the history of settlement, of order, of peace and law. But it began in movement, in restlessness, in the quest for new resources, the search for more hospitable climates, and the insatiable desire for possession. These impulses drove the first humans out of Africa and across the world, and they continue to drive their descendants to this day. Probably all the cultures of all the races of the world have been the creations of prolonged periods of migration. Most of the stories we tell ourselves about our pasts, and many about our futures, are, therefore, stories of peregrination.

One such story, and it is typical of many early European accounts of the origins of humanity, is to be found in a curious collection of texts from the third century AD, known as the *Corpus Hermeticum*, supposedly the writings of the magus Hermes Trismegistus, whose wisdom was believed to predate even that of Moses. Here the Greek god Hermes is shown at work imprisoning the demiurges – the beings who had helped in the creation of the universe – in human bodies as a punishment for their attempt to rival the creativity of the gods. Even as he does so, the figure of Sarcasm (*Momos*) appears to congratulate him. 'It is a courageous thing you have done to have created man,' he mocks, 'this being with curious eyes and a bragging tongue ... For he will push his designing thoughts even to the limits of the earth. [These men] will extend their audacious busy hands even to the edge of the sea. They will cut down the forests, and will drive them [i.e. as ships] over the seas from bank to bank, all the way to those lands that are furthest away.'[3] As they travelled, these new and still more troublesome demiurges came together into families and then into tribes, all speaking separate languages and pursuing separate ways of life. This is the origin of peoples. Once divided, the stronger begin to seize possession of the weaker. This is the beginning of empire.

But what exactly is an empire? Macedonia, Rome, Byzantium, Ottoman Turkey, China, Peru, Mexico, the Soviet Union, the United States, even, by its enemies, the European Union, have all been described as 'empires'. We talk of 'informal' and 'economic' empires, of 'business' empires, even of the empire of the heart or reason's empire. 'Empire' has become as much a metaphor as the description of a particular kind of society. Today, the word is generally used as a term of abuse, although one that is also often tinged with nostalgia. 'Empire' suggests either the ruthless exploitation of largely defenceless, technologically unsophisticated peoples by the forces of technologically sophisticated ones – the kinds of empires carved out first in the Americas, then in Asia, and finally in Australia and the islands of the Pacific, by successive European powers. Or it conjures up images of the Third Reich or Stalinist Russia, where oppressor and oppressed come from much the same kind of cultures, and possess much the same kind of technologies. In both cases the 'empire' is represented as a mode of political oppression, a denial by one people of the rights – above all the right to self-determination – of countless others.

Empires, it is assumed, are in some sense artificial creations. They are created by conquest, and conquerors have always attempted to keep those they have conquered in subservience. This has been achieved by a mixture of simple force and some kind of ideology; in the case of the Roman empire this ideology was that of 'civilization', the lure of a more desirable, more comfortable and infinitely richer way of life. In the case of the Spanish, French and British empires, it was the same, but reinforced now by differing brands of Christianity. In the case of the Ottomans it was Islam, and in the case of the Soviet Union, Marxism. It is also assumed that virtually all of those who live under imperial rule would much rather not, and that sooner or later they will rise up and drive out their conquerors. Much of this, as we shall see, is undeniable, but by no means all of it. Empire has been a way of life for most of the peoples of the world, as either conqueror or conquered; and what we chose to call 'empires' have not only varied greatly from place to place and time to time, but have also marked the lives of those they involved in sometimes radically different ways.[4]

The modern term 'empire' and all its variants, 'emperor', 'imperialism', etc., derive, significantly, from the Latin word *imperium*, which in ancient Rome indicated supreme power involving both command in war and the magistrates' right to execute the law. The term has therefore linked the history of European imperialism very closely to the legacy of the Roman empire. Originally it meant little more than 'sovereignty', a sense which it retained until at least the eighteenth century. Ever since the days of the Roman republic, however, 'empire' has also been a word used to describe government over vast territories. When, for instance, in the early first century AD, the historian Tacitus spoke of the Roman world as an 'immense body of empire' he was alluding as much to its size as to its sovereignty, and ultimately it would be size which separated empires from mere kingdoms and principalities.[5] In 1914, the great Norwegian polar explorer Fridtjof Nansen calculated that the Russian empire had been expanding at an average daily rate of fifty-five square miles for over four centuries, or more than 20,000 square miles per year, an area roughly the size of modern Belgium. In terms of territory, the Russian empire was the largest the world has ever known, although most of it was unoccupied. But similar sorts of figures could be conjured up for most other imperial peoples. Under Philip II, the father of Alexander the Great, the Macedonian monarchy ceased at the Aegean and the Black Sea. By the time of Alexander's death in 323 BC, it reached from the Adriatic to the Indus, from the Punjab to the Sudan. In 1400, the empire of Timur – Christopher Marlowe's Tamburlaine – ran from the Black Sea to the gates of Kashgar. The Ottoman sultanate, which in the thirteenth century had been a small Anatolian province of *ghazi* ('holy') warriors sandwiched between the Byzantine empire and the Seljuk Turks, had by the beginning of the sixteenth century extended itself over more than 6,000 miles from Hungary to Central Asia. By the time the armies of Francisco Pizarro reached Peru in 1532, the domain of the Inca, which in the early fifteenth century had been limited to the region around Cuzco, stretched north through what are today Peru, Ecuador and

Colombia and south into Bolivia, northern Chile and north-west Argentina.

Because they have been large and relentlessly expansive, empires have also embraced peoples who have held a wide variety of different customs and beliefs, and often spoken an equally large number of different languages. It was in their sheer variety as much as their size that both their identity and their glory were to be found. The greatness of the Romans, said the second-century-BC Greek historian Polybius, lay in the fact that they now ruled over peoples of whom Alexander the Great had never even heard. Sixteen hundred years later, Spanish historians of the empire of Charles V would make much the same observation about their emperor.

Because of their size and sheer diversity, most empires have in time become cosmopolitan societies. In order to rule vast and widely separated domains, imperial governments have generally found themselves compelled to be broadly tolerant of diversity of culture and sometimes even of belief, so long as these posed no threat to their authority. In such extensive societies it was frequently a matter of indifference whether the supreme lord was a king in London or an emperor in Delhi. In many cases it might be preferable to be ruled by a distant sovereign than one close to hand. Better, said the Milanese in the sixteenth century, trapped between the contending powers of Spain and France, a king in Madrid than one in Paris. Madrid, at least, was further away.

But if they have generally tolerated diversity, empires have also inevitably transformed the peoples whom they have brought together. 'Empire,' said Charles Maurice de Talleyrand, Napoleon's foreign minister, in 1797, is 'the art of putting men in their place.' And putting men in their place inevitably resulted in prolonged and extensive migrations. Some of these were voluntary, the movement of the dispossessed, or, as happened in America and Asia, and later in Africa, of the marginalized in search of a better and richer life. Some, however, such as the Atlantic slave-trade – the greatest and most nefarious of them all – or the British transportation of indentured Indian servants in the 1840s to what Lord Salisbury called the 'warmer' British possessions, Mauritius, Trinidad, Fiji and Natal, were wholly involuntary.[6]

All the way from Europe to the Americas, these migrations have inevitably destroyed societies that were once flourishing. They have also brought into being entire societies that did not exist before. And in time these have created new peoples. The inhabitants of modern Greece and the Balkans are not what they were under Alexander, neither are the modern Italians Romans, nor the black populations of the Americas much like the West African peoples from whom they are descended. The majority of the inhabitants of Spanish America are neither fully European nor wholly Indian but, as the 'Liberator' Simón Bolívar said of them in 1810, 'a sort of middle species between the legitimate owners of this land and the Spanish usurpers'.

Empires have severely limited the freedoms of some peoples, but they have also given others opportunities they could not otherwise have imagined. As the 'father' of modern India, Jawaharlal Nehru, once observed, 'a foreign conquest, with all its evils, has one advantage: it widens the mental horizon of the people and compels them to look out of their shells. They realize that the world is much bigger and a more variegated place than they had imagined.'[7] In this way empires have been an inseparable part, real as well as metaphorical, of the development and spread of human knowledge. The 'through passage of the world', reflected Francis Bacon in 1620, by which he meant as much its occupation as its navigation, was clearly 'destined by divine providence' to be achieved in the same age as the 'advancement of learning'.[8]

Empires have, of course, also been responsible for a great deal of human suffering. They have been responsible, in the Americas and the Pacific, for the elimination of entire peoples, and have caused perhaps irreversible damage to vast areas of the surface of the planet. Now they are no more, at least in their traditional form. But they have, for centuries, comprised the history of the human race.

I   *The first world conqueror*

The story of the empires of the peoples of Europe begins in ancient Greece. For the Greeks, who devised the vocabularies with which we still think about how to live our lives, were also, as they described themselves, 'extreme travellers'. The Cyclopes, one of whom devoured members of Odysseus' crew, were the embodiment of barbarism because, among their other defects, they knew nothing of navigation and had never left their island home. Travel, as we know, broadens the mind. The first person to have made the connection between voyaging (*planê*) and wisdom (*sophia*) was supposedly Solon, who also gave the Athenians their laws and thus created the first true political society in European history.[1] Subsequent Greek history is filled with wanderers in search of knowledge. Sometime in the fifth century BC, Herodotus, the 'father of history', travelled well beyond the limits of his world, to Egypt and Libya, Babylon and the Phoenician city of Tyre, even to southern Russia, and reported extensively on what he found there. Pythagoras, the great sixth-century-BC mathematician, journeyed from his native Samos to Egypt and Crete before settling finally in Croton in southern Italy; and the earliest of the ancient geographers, Hecateus of Miletus, visited Egypt even before Herodotus.

The knowledge to be gained from travel was almost always, however, also a means to possession. The Greeks were not only great travellers, they were also great colonizers. Beginning in the eighth century BC when Corinth established a colony on what is today Corfu, the Greek city-states moved steadily across the entire Mediterranean until by 580 BC they had occupied, to some degree, all the most obviously desirable areas in the world then available to them.[2] Colonization and conquest on this scale required, obviously, skilled navigators and relatively large ships. Most of all, however, it required the evolution of a certain kind of warfare. Immanuel Kant believed that human conflict was nature's means of forcing primitive men to leave the settled, comfortable boundaries of their homes. There, like grazing cattle, they might be happy, but because they were not also anxious and active they could not be properly human. Kant credited nature with too much insight. But, in one way or another, war has contributed more than any other single factor to the steady distribution of peoples around the world.

Yet if all peoples engage in some kind of warfare, wars themselves are of many different kinds. The conflicts which took place between the tribal peoples of North and South America, parts of East Africa and Australia, and which still occur among the few remaining peoples of the world's rainforests, are often harsh, cruel and sudden; but they rarely do, or are intended to do, much lasting damage. Such struggles are, as one sympathetic Spanish observer in the sixteenth century described them, 'no more deadly than our jousting, or than many European children's games'.[3] They are fought for limited and often symbolic gains, and rarely aim at conquest or subjugation. They are not intended to change the world.

The kind of war of which Kant was thinking was something very different. It emerged out of the eastern Mediterranean and the Steppes in the late Bronze Age. It is the warfare celebrated in the *Iliad*, and it aimed at the total transformation of entire peoples or sometimes, as in the Trojan War, at their ultimate destruction. The Trojan War, not only the best-known but also one of the longest recorded wars in history, ushered in a new era in human conflict, at least in the Mediterranean. Agamemnon and his crew of semi-divine warriors had no objective beyond revenge for the insult inflicted upon the Spartan Menelaus by a Trojan prince. They were not conquerors, much less empire-builders. When they finally left after ten long years of unceasing conflict, Troy was no more. Their sole desire was to have done with the war and go home. But they left behind them a world in which conquest and subjugation had become possible. And they inspired at least one empire – possibly, by virtue of the story's constant retelling, the greatest of them all. Plutarch, who has left us so vivid a psychological portrait of Alexander the Great, tells us that his copies of the *Iliad* and the *Odyssey* never left his side.[4] He slept with them, and a dagger, under his pillow.

The Homeric poems are mythic celebrations of the emergence of a people. Similar stories have been told about other places and other peoples at other times. They serve many roles. But they all celebrate the moment when a group acquires the means to impose itself upon its world. In the Mediterranean world this moment was made possible by the discovery and invention of hard resistant metals, bronze and later iron, which could be sharpened and would remain sharp. As many contemporary observers pointed out, it was not their firearms – which often did more harm to their users than to their intended victims – nor even their horses which allowed the

Spanish to defeat the Aztecs and the Incas. It was rather their steel weapons, weapons that had not changed substantially for centuries. Against these, the brittle obsidian axes of the Aztecs, which shattered or blunted after the first blow, could make little impact.

Together with the new instruments of war, there emerged also a new kind of combat. The heroes of the *Iliad* still fought as individuals seeking individual gains and, in Achilles' case, pursuing private feuds onto the battlefield. But among the Greek ranks, who are of scant interest to Homer, there is evidence of cohesion, of organization, of a terrifying sense of purpose, a willingness to surrender the moment in order to win the day. All of this the earlier warriors hordes lacked, as did their American, African or Australian counterparts. The Aztecs could never understand the kind of war that was being made against them. Even though they had secured some kind of tributary authority over a vast area of Central Mexico, they were more concerned with acquiring sacrificial victims – the traditional objective of Mesoamerican warfare – than defending a civilization that was about to be extinguished.[5] This was to be the final cause of their downfall and, in general, the weakness of all those, in other parts of the world, who would over the centuries by swept aside by the technologies and the sheer relentlessness of the European powers.

The war machine, the capacity to transform a large body of men into a single instrument of destruction, was to prove decisive in what has come to be called the 'triumph of the West'.[6] The image of the Athenian army, whose soldiers held a spear in their right hands and in their left a shield with which they covered not themselves but their neighbours, has long been used as an image of Attic democracy. And so it probably is. It is also, however, an image of the people as an army. Each man shelters and is sheltered by his neighbour. The survival of one depends upon the survival of the whole. Cowardice or desertion could lead only to immediate destruction of the entire unit. The Greeks, and later the Romans, were good at this sort of thing. The Greek phalanx, particularly after the reforms of Philip II of Macedon in about 356 BC, was capable of organizing the resources of thousands of trained infantry, in conjunction with equally skilled cavalry regiments, into a solid compact fighting force more formidable than anything that could be pitched against them.

The person who benefited most from these new technologies of power, who used them to create what has since antiquity been looked upon as the first of the great European empires, was Alexander the Great.

During its relatively brief existence, from 336 until 323 BC, Alexander's empire was the most extensive the ancient world had ever seen. Although it did not last long, it transformed the world in ways that were to have immense consequences for the subsequent history of all the peoples of Europe. Alexander destroyed the great Achaemenid Persian empire which had been a constant threat to the cities of Greece since Xerxes' attacks on Athens in 480 BC. He united, if only briefly, vast regions of what we now call Europe and Asia. He also succeeded in uniting the quarrelsome independent Greek states. In doing so, however, he deprived them not only of their independence but also of their unique, democratic forms of government. Henceforth, until its resurgence in the late eighteenth century, the rule of the many would, ultimately, surrender to the rule of the one.

Alexander had been, if only briefly, the pupil of Aristotle who, with Plato, had created not only European philosophy but many of the natural sciences as well. In his *Politics* Aristotle had argued that in the ideal state a mixed constitution, one that combined democracy, aristocracy and monarchy, would be best. But he also knew that ideal states existed only in the imagination. In the real world he inhabited, a world dominated by the experience of civil war and inter-city conflict, monarchy was much to be preferred. This was one lesson from his old tutor which Alexander had taken to heart. The various leagues of the Greek city-states had ultimately proved to be ineffective against Persian aggression. As Cyrus the Great, the architect of the Achaemenid empire, is said to have remarked of the Spartans, 'I never yet feared men who have a place demarcated in their city in which to meet and deceive each other on oath!' In Persian eyes, talk, and the lies upon which the democratic assemblies of the people thrived, would always weaken the Greeks' powers of decision. Cyrus, of course, underestimated Sparta. But Greece was ill-equipped to defeat a consolidated monarchy. As early as the sixth century BC, the philosopher Thales of Miletus had suggested that the only way to resist the Persians was to transform the loose-knit alliances of the city-states into a true federal state with a council at Teos. No one, however, had paid any attention to him. The Greek states became progressively less able to resist outside aggression, so that by 346 the Athenian orator Isocrates was able to describe Thebes, Argos, Sparta and Athens – the once-great cities of the Greek world – as all equally 'reduced to a common level of disaster'. In the end it took a monarch to destroy the might of the Persian king of kings.

Alexander did not, however, create his vast empire entirely on his own. Much of what he achieved had already been prepared for him by his father Philip II (382–336 BC). It was he who had transformed Macedon from a kingdom divided by civil war and foreign intervention into the most powerful of the Greek states. It was he who had created the seemingly invincible Macedonian army which at Chaeronea in August 338 won a crushing victory over an alliance of southern Greek cities led by Athens and Thebes. Philip's forces on that occasion are said to have numbered 30,000 foot and 2000 horse, a staggering number at a time when the adult male population of Sparta has been estimated at less than one thousand. The battle of Chaeronea made Philip the effective master of the Greek world and Macedon an unchallenged superpower. Philip then turned his attention to the already weakened Persian empire. In 336 a Macedonian expeditionary force of 10,000 men began the subjugation of the coast of Asia Minor. Philip, however, never lived to complete his conquest. As with so many rulers in the ancient world, he fell victim to an assassin.

Two years later, Alexander, who had inherited both his father's throne and his ambition, crossed the Hellespont, determined to put an end to Persian power for ever. His army, the largest ever to leave Greek soil, numbered 43,000 foot, armed with fearsome pikes six metres long, and 5500 horse. The cities of the Achaemenid empire, Sardis, Ephesus, Miletus, Phaselis, Aspendus and the Phrygian city of Gordian, fell one after another. At Gordian, Alexander paused long enough to perform one of those symbolic acts the memory of which has survived long after his conquest. In the ancient palace of Phrygian kings he was shown the legendary wagon of Gordius, the mythical founder of the dynasty. The yoke of the wagon was fastened to its pole by an elaborate knot the ends of which were invisible. Legend had it that anyone who was able to untie the Gordian knot would become lord of Asia. Alexander did not bother trying to undo the knot; he simply took out his sword and cut it. For later historians this act became a sign of divine endorsement for the entire campaign, and 'cutting the Gordian knot' has remained a metaphor for decisive action, and a presage of empire, until this day.

In the early winter of 333 Alexander defeated the vast Persian army at Issus, which gave him control of what is now the Near East as far as the Euphrates. He then moved into Egypt and Mesopotamia and finally in the winter of 331–330 seized the Persian capital at Persepolis. Until this time Alexander had been relatively constrained in his handling of defeated populations. But his men were growing restless, eager to lay their hands on some of the booty they had been promised. Persepolis was turned over to the victorious army. The houses of the nobility were looted, the men slaughtered and the women enslaved. Some months later, after an orgiastic banquet, and urged on by the courtesan Thaïs (later to become the wife of Ptolemy), Alexander and his entourage burned down the great palace of the Persian king of kings. It was, or so the Greek historians claimed, the final act of revenge for Xerxes' despoliation of the Acropolis in Athens.

Alexander then marched eastwards to consolidate his hold over the empire. Moving in a great swathe through what is now eastern Iran and western Afghanistan he crossed the Hindu Kush and invaded Bactria in the spring of 329. Here, however, his empire finally reached its limit. In 326 his troops, soaked

and exhausted by monsoon rains and faced by an enemy equipped with elephant squadrons of legendary strength, refused to
cross the Beas river which separated them from the lands of the
Ganges. Like Achilles, his favourite Homeric hero, Alexander
retreated to his tent and for three days nursed his anger, waiting
for a change of heart. It did not come. Finally he made the
regular sacrifice for a river crossing and the omens proved,
conveniently, to be most inauspicious. Now that he could interpret his retreat as a concession not to his men but to the will of
the gods, he agreed to turn back.

Alexander returned to Persepolis and then moved to Babylon
where he began to prepare for the invasion of the Persian Gulf
and the Arabian littoral. For this he created a new army (one
less likely to challenge his ambitions) and a new navy. But
they were never put to the test. Towards the end of May 323
Alexander attended a banquet and, if the traditional accounts
are to believed, literally drank himself to death. The climax
came in an exchange of toasts in which he is said to have downed
twelve pints of undiluted wine in one steady draught. He
doubled up with a violent spasms and collapsed into a coma
from which his doctors were unable to revive him.[7]

This, briefly, is Alexander's story. In most senses it is exemplary. Like most empire-builders Alexander took over an earlier
and already weakened power. Although he moved large numbers
of Greek settlers into Persia, he did very little to alter the
administrative structure of the Persian empire. He ruled through
'satraps' – a Persian word meaning 'defenders of power' – as the
Persians themselves had done and, indeed, as most later empire-
builders, from the Romans to the British, were to do. In many
places, such as Sardes, the centre of Persian rule in Asia Minor,

he appointed his own men. In others he merely replaced local princes who had been loyal to the previous regime with ones of his own choosing.

Alexander's rule was always a personal one. At the centre of the empire was the figure and the legend of Alexander himself. He built up around him an elaborate court, something that had been largely absent from the traditional Greek *polis*. He invented a royal diadem, part Macedonian, part Persian in design, and even created a distinctive hairstyle for himself – the famous *anastole*, a quiff thrown back from a central parting. To ensure that all of this would survive him, he decreed that only one painter, one sculptor and one maker of medals – all men whom he could trust to produce the most flattering likenesses – were to be allowed to preserve his image.[8]

Like most rulers in the ancient world Alexander believed himself to be descended from semi-divine beings, from Andromache and Achilles on his mother's side and from Hercules on his father's. The final tribute that a man could pay to himself, however, was divinity itself. On a visit to the shrine of the god Ammon in the Libyan oasis of Siwah, Alexander told the chronicler Callisthenes that he had been greeted by the god as his son, and requested that after his death his body be taken to Siwah for burial. Ammon may have been Libyan by origin, but the Egyptians recognized in him the ram-god Amun and the Greeks, settled in nearby Cyrene, knew him as Zeus. It was characteristic of Alexander that he should have chosen as his divine parent not only the deity who had fathered Perseus and Hercules but also one who belonged to both the cultures, the East and the West, that he had hoped to unify.

An empire that was associated so clearly with the personal

authority and the carefully nurtured image of a single individual could not survive his death for long. Even in the final years of his life, Alexander was facing a mutiny of the Macedonian troops, a rising of the Greek settlers in Bactria, and imminent war in Greece itself. When he died his empire in effect died with him. He had appointed no heir and had no obvious successor. After a series of bloody civil wars the empire was divided up among his former generals. Even Macedon itself, weakened by Alexander's constant demand for manpower, was no longer able to dictate terms to the rest of the Greek world. In time the whole of Alexander's former domains would be overrun by another, greater imperial power: Rome.

For centuries, Alexander had been the archetypal empire-builder. 'The sole conqueror in the memory of mankind to have founded a universal empire,' enthused the Latin novelist Apuleius[9] – a model to be followed and an example to be surpassed. Julius Caesar tells how he wept when reading the history of Alexander, for 'Alexander had died at the age of thirty-two, king of so many peoples, while he himself had not achieved any brilliant success.' Some version of this story was repeated by both Pompey and Marc Antony (Pompey went so far as to copy Alexander's hairstyle, adopt the sobriquet 'the Great' and encourage his panegyrists to exaggerate his youth during his conquests of Judaea and Syria),[10] the emperor Trajan, Napoleon, and no doubt countless other would-be imperialists.[11] Nor was Alexander's image confined to the Western world. 'Sikander' became for generations of Persian monarchs a model of the world ruler, and in some accounts the precursor of the universal kingdom of Islam which would one day encompass the globe. 'My name is Shah Ismail,' wrote the founder of the Safavid dynasty in one of his self-aggrandizing poems, 'I am the living Khizr, and Jesus son of Mary, / I am the Alexander of my contemporaries.'

Alexander became 'the Great', however, not only because of his astonishing military successes. He became great for another more immediately modern reason. According to Plutarch, Aristotle had advised Alexander to treat only Greeks as human beings and to look upon all the other peoples he conquered as either animals or plants. This advice Alexander wisely ignored, for had he accepted his mentor's council he would have 'filled his kingdoms with exiles and clandestine rebellions'.[12] This anecdote is an allusion to the widespread Greek distinction between themselves and those whom they called 'barbarians'. The word 'barbarian' (*barbaros*) described all those who could not speak Greek and whose languages sounded, to Greek ears, merely like people stuttering 'bar bar'. Since only the Greeks had articulate speech only the Greeks were truly human. All the rest were, indeed, only animals or plants. For this reason, said Euripides (quoted approvingly by Aristotle) 'it is fit that the Greeks should rule over the barbarians'.[13] It had been this division of humankind and all that it implied which, in Kant's view, had been the cause of the ultimate collapse of Hellenic civilization. Alexander's vision of a universal empire was an explicit rejection of any such xenophobia. His ambition had been not merely to conquer or even to assimilate the mighty Persian empire, but to unite East and West, Asia and Europe, Hellene and barbarian. In this way he would be remembered not as a conqueror at all but, in Plutarch's words, 'as one sent by the gods to be the conciliator and arbitrator of the Universe'.[14] He had hoped that in his empire the old enmity between East and West – the origins of which are to be found in the myth of the Rape of Europa, an Asian princess abducted to Western shores, and in the story of the Trojan War, a struggle over a Western woman abducted to Eastern shores – would finally be brought to a close.

He did not, of course, succeed. But his image lived on after him on both sides of the Hellespont. In one Persian version of the Alexander legend, he is said to have erected a giant copper wall at the very edge of the world to protect the whole of 'civilization' from Gog and Magog, the twin giants which embody all that is untamed and inhuman.

Alexander's vision of empire, or at least the vision that later historians have attributed to him, had many of the properties which later empires would claim for themselves, from ancient Rome to the United States: the capacity to provide a living space for diverse peoples, to create peace and order in a world which would otherwise be at war with itself, and to defend a tenuous, hard-won and fragile civilization against all that might threaten it. The realities behind the legend were certainly very different. But that is unimportant; Alexander's greatness lies less in what he intended to achieve than in what he was believed to have achieved. It is for that reason that he has been looked upon by subsequent generations as the first world conqueror.

Alexander is a good starting point for our story for another reason. More than any other would-be world-ruler, his life became a tale of the elision of knowledge and understanding with power, of the merging of science and exploration with domination and settlement. It is doubtful if the real Alexander, despite his much publicized devotion to Homer, was overly concerned with learning, and despite his tutelage at the hands of Aristotle the science to which he could have been exposed was necessarily limited and in its infancy. Hostile later commentators such as the Greek comic dramatist Menander represented him as a drunkard, and the Roman philosopher Seneca called him 'swollen beyond the limits of human arrogance', unedifying, intemperate and wild.[15] But by the time Arrian in the second century AD sat down to write the history of his life, Alexander had already become a figure possessed not merely of the ability to conquer but also of an insatiable desire for knowledge. It was, or so legend had it, for Alexander that Aristotle had written not only the first treatise on politics but also one of the earliest studies of astronomy.

In the Middle Ages, this Alexander became a legendary figure whose desire to subjugate the entire world was matched only by his ambition to know all its secrets and visit all its parts. Stories were told of his quest for the hidden sources of the Nile, of his invention of a diving bell to reach the floor of the ocean, and of a great basket drawn by griffins in which he attempted to reach Heaven.[16] In the Persian, Indian and later Ottoman versions of his life he became a prophet, a seer, and – like Gilgamesh, the hero of a cycle of poems from Mesopotamia dating from the third millennium BC – a seeker after eternal life. In Walter of Châtillon's poem *Alexandreis*, which dates from the twelfth century, he is described as 'the prince who had called the earth too narrow and prepared armed throngs to lay open her secret parts', lines which run together in one erotic image both the conqueror's desire to possess and the scientist's desire to know. This Alexander, like the figure of Ulysses whom Dante meets in Hell (and who is given many of Alexander's attributes), tries to sail beyond the Pillars of Hercules and dreams of conquering the western sun.[17] The greatest empire-builder in the history of Europe thus becomes also its greatest explorer, traveller and seeker after truth.

2   *The empire of the Roman people*

In the end, Alexander himself might not have succeeded in holding together Europe and Asia. Their enmities survived him, and have lasted to this day, as the Ottoman Turks and then the Russians replaced the Persians, and as first the Romans and then the Christian Latin kingdoms of Europe replaced the Greeks. But something of Alexander's image of empire and his ambitions have remained: the wish to bring peace, stability, religious and cultural harmony, and ultimately to unite under one rule all the peoples of world.

Alexander created what has been looked upon since antiquity as the first European empire. Its successor in nearly every respect was Rome. Rome has consistently provided the inspiration, the imagery and the vocabulary for all the European empires from early modern Spain to late nineteenth-century Britain. All the former imperial capitals of Europe – London, Vienna, Berlin – are filled with grandiose architectural reminders of this indebtedness to Rome. Even the United States, which was created out of the dismemberment of one kind of empire and has throughout the course of its history done its best to avoid assuming the role of another, is ruled from a city that was built to replicate as far as possible parts of ancient Rome. No other modern nation is governed from a building called the Capitol.

Rome began sometime during the seventh century BC as a small city-state of farmers and tradesmen occupying a territory of a few square miles on the lower Tiber. Its original rulers had been kings, like those of the neighbouring peoples, the Sabines, the Etruscans, the Latins and the Umbrians. By the late sixth century, however, Rome had become a republic although, unlike the Greek city-states on which it was loosely modelled, it was in no sense a democracy.

Alexander's example, and that of the Achaemenid empire which he defeated, might seem to suggest that all truly successful empires have been monarchies. The early history of Rome, however, demonstrates that although most empires have in time succumbed to some kind of monarchical rule, as did Rome itself, there has never been any reason why a republic could not also be an empire. Republics, after all, are no more given to caring for the rights or the lives of others than are monarchies. Neither are republics any less expansive, or less concerned with glory, than monarchies. Those who are 'citizens' might enjoy more freedom and, in theory at least, have a greater say in the business of government than those who are mere 'subjects'. But those who live outside, who are neither fellow-citizens nor fellow-subjects, are quite as vulnerable to republicans as they are to monarchists.

Throughout European history expansion has generally been popular with the majority of the people, so long as it is going well and does not involve too onerous a tax burden. The empire of the Roman republic might have benefited most directly the patricians, the consuls and proconsuls who commanded the legions and whose power and wealth derived from their success in battle. But it had always been presented to the common people, the plebeians, as *their* empire, 'the empire of the people of Rome'. And, until the end, when the senate had long since ceased to wield political power, the legions of the empire still marched under the banner of the 'Senate and the People of Rome'. Scipio Africanus, a man who played an enduring role in much Roman history, was once accused by Naevius, the tribune of the senate, of accepting bribes from the Seleucid emperor Antiochus. It was a very serious charge. It was also an offence against Scipio's honour, a slur against his standing with the people. And it was to the people he turned. 'This,' he declared to the crowd which had gathered to hear him judged, 'is the anniversary of the great battle on African soil in which I defeated Hannibal, the Carthaginian, the most determined enemy of *your empire*.' Pointing at Naevius, he added, 'Let us not be ungrateful to the gods. Let us have done with that wretch and offer thanks to Jove.' He then walked to the Capitol. The crowd followed him and Naevius found himself alone. An invocation of the greatness of the empire had the power to make the people forget the petty misdemeanours of their rulers.[1]

The Romans, like the Macedonians before them, were highly skilled tacticians and military innovators. They were also thorough and ruthless. 'Virtue' – a word that derives from *vir*, the Latin word for 'man' – meant only courage in battle. This they possessed in abundance. By 272 BC they had already taken control of the Italian peninsula. They then moved overseas, first to Sicily and Carthage, a Phoenician colony which at the time occupied much of the hinterland of north and central Tunisia, and then into the eastern Mediterranean. By the first century BC most of what had survived of the empire of Alexander the Great had fallen into Roman hands. Roman armies put an end to the crumbling Macedonian monarchy at Pydna in 168 BC and destroyed Corinth in 146. The kingdoms of Macedonia, Asia and Syria now became Roman provinces. Egypt became a Roman protectorate, as did the vassal monarchies of the once vast Seleucid empire. The entire Mediterranean became a Roman lake: *mare nostrum*, 'our sea', as it came to be called. Most of what today is thought of as the Roman empire had been acquired under the republic. Britain, Dacia to the east of the Danube, Arabia, Mesopotamia and Armenia were taken by the emperors (most, with the exception of Britain, by Trajan between AD 101 and 117). But the full force of Roman expansion had stopped by the time Julius Caesar seized effective control of the senate in the first century BC. As the eighteenth-century English radical Richard Price sourly observed of his countrymen's self-serving idolization of the Roman republic, it had been 'nothing but a faction against the general liberties of the world'.[2]

The collapse of the republic and the creation of the principate were the outcome of what all empires have feared most: civil war. For if republics have been able to create empires, they have all sooner or later fallen prey to the ambitions of the strongest among them. This is what became of the Greek city-states, and it is what finally became of Rome when the empire had grown too big for the senate to able to control the army and the overweening ambitions of the mightiest of its generals. 'The empire of the Romans,' wrote the great eighteenth-century historian Edward Gibbon, 'filled the world, and when that empire fell into the hands of a single person, the world became a safe and dreary person for his enemies.'

The first of those men was Julius Caesar. Caesar had conquered Gaul in a spectacular if brutal campaign in 58 to 51 BC.

In 52 Pompey, who as sole consul was in effective control of the senate, fearful of Caesar's growing power and obvious autocratic ambitions, attempted to prevent him from returning to Rome as consul. Caesar's response was to invade Italy. Pompey had some initial success but was finally defeated near Pharsalus in Thessaly in 48. Caesar now proclaimed himself dictator (an office generally assumed only at moments of crisis and for a limited duration) and consul for life. He also adopted the style and dress of the old Roman kings (although he refused the title *rex*) and after much bullying succeeded in having himself declared a god. The republic had become in all but name a monarchy. On 15 March 44, he was stabbed to death on the steps of the senate, in what is probably one of the most celebrated assassinations in European history, by a motley group of 'republicans' and ex-Pompeians led by Brutus and Cassius, two of his former companions. Caesar's death did nothing to restore the republic as his assassins had hoped. Instead, it plunged the Roman world into a civil war which nearly destroyed the empire, something that no later Roman would ever forget.

Caesar's name has supplied the title for autocratic rulers of one kind or another until the twentieth century, the last being Tsar ('Caesar') Alexander of Russia. In fact, despite his openly despotic behaviour he did little to change the republican constitution of Rome beyond grafting his divine and hereditary rule onto it. It was his successor Octavian who in 27 BC had the title Augustus ('revered one') conferred upon himself, who was the first to adopt the term Emperor (*Imperator*) as a title, and who was the ideological and institutional founder of what is now called the principate, the period in the history of the empire when it was in effect ruled by one man. It was Augustus who succeeded in bringing the civil war to an end, brought peace to the empire and established a centralized system of government. He reined in the power of local aristocrats, deprived the senate and the people of most of their authority, and reformed and hugely extended the rule of law.[3]

Augustus also radically overhauled the tax system, on which his ability to pay his troops depended. Previously, cash flows to the treasury had been erratic and uncertain. Now the whole Roman world was enrolled and a census was held of every potential contributor. One of the unintended consequences of this new fiscal order was the journey of an obscure Judaean carpenter named Joseph and his pregnant wife to be registered at the town of Bethlehem. As Christian historians would repeat over and over, it was no accident of history that Augustus' new order should have come into being at the same moment as the birth of the man whose teaching would usher in another and, in their eyes, final, God-ordained, world order. God had sent Augustus to unite the world and, in doing so, to prepare the way for the coming of Christ.

Augustus also presided over the Golden Age of Latin literature, the age of the epic poet Virgil, whose *Aeneid*, a celebration of the origins of Rome, became for the Roman people something similar to what the *Iliad* and the *Odyssey* had been for the Greeks. It was the age, too, of Ovid (although Augustus banished him to Tomis on the Black Sea, probably because of his part in some scandal involving the imperial house), whose writings have had more impact on later European literature than perhaps any other classical author, as well as of the poets Horace, Tibullus and Propertius, and the historian Livy. In their different ways all of these writers celebrated the greatness, past, present and to come, of the new Roman order. Augustus thus became a hero who over the centuries would be venerated by pagan and Christian alike; and, like Caesar and the title of Emperor, the name of Augustus was also adopted by later princes with aspirations to empire. 'Most invincible Caesar and August Emperor ...' began one version of the roll-call of titles of the Holy Roman Emperor Charles V.

To its citizens, Rome offered some measure of protection, a way of life that, for better or for worse, we have come to call 'civilized', and membership of the greatest state the Western world had ever known. To the patrician classes it offered, too, the prospect of wealth and, more importantly, glory. Glory is the desire for the esteem and admiration of others. In the ancient world, and indeed in most worlds until perhaps very recently, the most obvious and in some cases the only field in which it could easily be won was the field of battle. The orator, jurist and philosopher Marcus Tullius Cicero (106–43 BC) even looked upon what he described as 'fighting for empire and seeking glory' as a particular kind of warfare. It was, he said, one that was 'waged less bitterly' than war for 'defence or restitution' since what was at stake here was not who would survive but who would rule.[4] A man might be praised or admired, or loved, for being a just and benign ruler, but glory was an altogether noisier, flashier and ultimately more deadly affair. The people, wrote the sixteenth-century Italian political philosopher Giovanni Botero, reflecting on the lessons to be learned from Rome's history, will always prefer a strong, irascible and triumphant ruler to a wise and prudent one, just as they 'prefer a tumbling torrent to a calm river'.[5]

Glory-seeking strategists carried the Roman empire, just as they had the Macedonian monarchy. Empire was about the rewards to be had from war, and as it grew the Roman empire increasingly became less a people with a standing army than a population in arms, a military culture which embraced the entire free male population. By the time imperial rule had been fully established under Augustus, what the Romans referred to as the *domi*, that which pertains to the home, or what today we would 'civil society', had been virtually subsumed into the military, the *militae*. Towards the end, Roman society became a world in which scribes were soldiers, bishops were soldiers, local governors were soldiers, and, of course, the emperor was a soldier. Ultimately this was to become not only the source of Rome's greatness, but also, as Edward Gibbon recognized, the cause of its downfall. Later imperial cultures from sixteenth-century Spain to twenty-first-century America, with their far greater social complexity, would learn to distinguish more clearly between civil and military power and to ensure the subservience of the latter to the former. Yet the office of the president of the United States still combines supreme, if also highly restricted, command over the military as well as the civil sphere, as the French monarchy did in its time and in theory at least the British monarch (who biannually dispenses honours in the name of the now vanished British empire) does to this day.

Rome's greatness was not, however, built on military might alone. The more extended the empire and the greater the distance, both geographically and politically, between the centre and the periphery, the more difficult the task of governance becomes. Even modern societies, with all the immense power available to the state, can only be ruled for prolonged periods of time with the consent of their members – as numerous auto-crats, both ancient and modern, have discovered to their cost. 'It is on opinion only that government is founded,' wrote the philosopher David Hume in the eighteenth century. And what is true of all governments is especially so of those that seek to unite a diversity of peoples with a variety of expectations, customs, beliefs, and loyalties.

If the empire was to outlast its founder and be proof against intruders, it had to have something to offer its conquered peoples, something that would persuade them that their way of life under the conqueror would be ultimately better than that which they had enjoyed before. It was not only Roman roads and Roman architecture, or even the much spoken of but not always so obvious *pax Romana*, which persuaded non-Roman patricians from North Africa to Scotland to identify themselves with the empire. It was the lure of luxury, opulence and the trappings of power. It had been precisely his encounter with the splendours of the doomed city of Ravenna, the glittering gilded domes, the opulent buildings with their arched and pillared porticoes, the symmetry and, even at this time of siege, the orderliness of its streets, the elaborate dress of its inhabitants, in particular the women with their stacked hair and tottering shoes – it had been this prospect of a life far richer than any the wandering Lombard warrior had experienced elsewhere that persuaded Droctulft that this was not something he could help to destroy.

The Roman empire thus constituted not only a state but a way of living, what Cicero identified as 'our wise grasp of a single truth'.[6] And it was embodied in that all-precious commodity, citizenship. To be a citizen, a *civis*, meant to be able to say, in that celebrated phrase, 'I am a Roman citizen' – *civis Romanus sum* – not a Gaul or a Spaniard or an Egyptian, but a Roman. It meant to belong to what was called the *civitas*, the Roman civil community, and the word from which the more ambiguous modern term 'civilization' derives. Above all, it meant, in a sense that the word has retained to this day, to live in a society which, for all its great injustices (by modern standards), was looked upon as the embodiment of the rule of law. To be a Roman citizen meant to acquire a legal identity and a place in a system of understanding and controlling human behaviour which was intended to extend over the entire planet.

Roman law became the law of the whole of Europe, and despite having been extensively modified by the legal customs of the Germanic tribes which overran the empire in the fifth century, it has remained the basis of most of our understanding of what law is until this day. It was the Romans' great intellectual achievement, as moral philosophy and the natural sciences had been that of the Greeks. For Roman jurists the law was the supreme expression of human rationality. 'However we may define man,' wrote Cicero, 'a single definition will apply to all ... For those creatures who have received the gift of reason from Nature have also received right reason, and therefore they have also received the gift of law ... And if they have received law they have received justice. Now all men have received reason; therefore all men have received justice.'[7]

The history of Roman law begins, in effect, with the Twelve Tables, said to have been composed between 451 and 450 BC. The effect of these was to ensure that henceforth all customary law would be given a legislative basis and enacted by statute. Later Roman jurists attempted to gather all these enactments together in series of codes, of which the most enduring was compiled under the Eastern emperor Justinian in the fifth century AD. Justinian's codification is divided into four books, running to over a million words: the *Codex*, the *Digest*, the *Pandect* and the *Institutes*. Like most legislators, Justinian hoped that his definition of the law would prove to be so authoritative that there would be no further need for lawyers to interpret it. He turned out, of course, to be wrong. His codification was only the beginning of a vast proliferation of later commentaries and interpretations which, from the eleventh century onwards, became the basis for all legal education and administration throughout Europe.

Roman law was predominantly civil law, which is to say that it was concerned with the laws governing the peoples of Rome and, as Rome spread, of the empire as a whole. But the Romans also created a legal category called the 'law of nations'. In practical terms this was that part of the Roman civil law that was open to Roman citizens and foreigners alike. In a wider sense, however, it was taken to be what the second-century jurist Gaius called 'the law observed by all nations'. This concept was to have a prolonged and powerful impact on all subsequent European legal thinking. As the European powers reached outwards into other areas of the globe, many of which the Romans had never imagined, it became the basis for what is now called 'public international law', and it still governs all the actions, in theory if not consistently in practice, of the 'international community'.

Roman law also introduced into Europe the crucial idea that warfare itself had to be regulated, and above all that wars could not be fought simply for personal gain. 'The imperial majesty,'

Justinian began his *Institutes*, 'should be armed with laws as well as glorified with arms.'[8] The Greeks, and their antagonists, had been largely unconcerned with the justice of war. When Alexander invaded the Persian empire he did so initially, he claimed, to avenge the wrongs committed by the Persians against the Greeks. But the territories he seized and attempted to Hellenize were what was called 'spear-won'. The conqueror's right to possession lay merely in his success in battle. The Romans, however, introduced a complex distinction, which still governs the conduct of most modern conflicts, between 'just' and 'unjust' wars.[9] In general, the Roman jurists looked upon war as a means of last resort, the objective of which must always be to acquire not cultural and religious transformation, much less territory, but peace and justice. Human beings, Cicero insisted, used language to resolve their differences and resorted to violence only when language had failed.[10] This was one of the things which distinguished them from mere brutes. A just war could only be waged defensively and in pursuit of compensation for some alleged act of aggression against either the Romans or their allies. 'The best state,' according to Cicero, 'never undertakes war except to keep faith or in defence of its safety.'[11] Most Romans, however, fully recognized that Rome, like the United States and the Soviet Union in the 1950s and 1960s, frequently acquired clients with the sole purpose of 'defending' them against enemies, real or imaginary, whose territories they wished to acquire. Neither did the doctrine of the just war prevent Roman warfare from being in reality spectacularly brutal. When the Romans sacked a city, observed Polybius, they were so ferocious that they even killed all the animals.

Ultimately, Roman law was intended not merely to create political and social order, but also to confer an ethical purpose upon the entire community. Under the late republic, and then more forcibly under the principate, the legal formulation of *imperium* merged with the Stoic ideal of a single universal human race, in Cicero's phrase 'a single joint community of gods and men'.[12] To be a member of the community meant to acquire an identity more enduring, more compelling than anything that the membership of a village or a tribe could confer. In the real world of ancient Rome, Astérix and his friends would have been a quaint anomaly with very little motive for continuing to resist the lure of Roman civilization. (True, the Isaurians, *montagnard* warriors from the Taurus, proved to be so indomitable that they were given their own frontier, yet even they, at the end of the fifth century, placed their own candidate, Zeno, on the imperial throne in Constantinople.) As James Wilson observed in 1790, as he mused upon the possible future of the United States as the new Rome in the West, 'It might be said, not that the Romans extended themselves over the whole globe, but that the inhabitants of the globe poured themselves upon the Romans.' This, he concluded, was clearly 'the most secure method of enlarging an empire'.[13]

Nearly three centuries earlier, an admiring Niccolò Machiavelli had observed that Rome had 'ruined her neighbours' and created a world empire in the process precisely by 'freely admitting strangers to her privileges and honours'. Compare, he went on, Rome with Sparta. Lycurgus, the legendary father of the Spartan republic, because he 'believed that nothing would more readily destroy its laws, did everything to prevent strangers from coming into the city'. As a consequence Sparta had slowly stagnated until it was forcibly incorporated into the Roman province of Achaea.[14]

Rome, by contrast, had flourished. By the time Augustus came to power, it had become in effect a huge cosmopolitan state. For its most skilful and fortunate subjects the empire was a vast resource, often more enriching than the narrow limits of the original communities from which they came. Peoples from all over the empire could be found in almost every Roman province. Even the emperors themselves, after the second and third centuries AD, were sometimes neither Roman nor even Italian, at least by birth: Septimus Severus was born in North Africa; Trajan, who took the empire to its furthermost limits, in Spain; and Diocletian in Dalmatia. In this way, Roman imperialism came to be seen not as a form of oppression, as the seizure by one people of the lands, the goods and the persons of others, but as a form of beneficent rule which involved not conquest but patronage, and the first purpose of which was the improvement of the lives of others. As Cicero also said of the imperial republic he served, 'We could more truly have been titled a protectorate [*patrocinium*] than an empire of the world.'[15]

When in AD 212 the emperor Caracalla granted citizenship to all the free inhabitants of the empire a common bond was created, at least in theory, which extended the Roman *civitas* to all the many peoples of which the empire was composed. 'Those within the Roman world,' declared the edict of Caracalla, 'have become Roman citizens.' From there it was but a brief step to declaring that Rome was the 'common homeland' of the entire world, and an even shorter step to declaring that those who were not citizens and showed no desire to become citizens should, if only in their own long-term interests, be obliged to do so. As Cicero had pointed out, even Africans, Spaniards and Gauls, 'savage and barbarous nations', were entitled to just government. If their own rulers were unable to provide it then the Romans would be happy to do so for them.

Like Alexander before them, the Roman rulers created an ideology which aimed at world domination. There were to be no limits to the rule of Rome – which is why, the historian Livy tells us, Terminus, the god of boundaries, had refused to be present at the birth of the city. Already by 75 BC coins were being struck with images of a sceptre, a globe, a wreath and a rudder, symbols of Rome's power over all the lands and oceans of the world. By the time Augustus came to power 'the World' – the *orbis terrarum* – and the empire had come to be identified as one. 'We look neither to this corner nor to that,' wrote the first-century playwright and philosopher Seneca, 'but measure the boundaries of our nation by the sun.'[16] When a century later the emperor Antoninus Pius took the title 'Lord of all the World' – *dominus totius orbis* – he was merely making explicit what all the Roman emperors had always assumed.

The Roman claim to rule the universe was not unique. Most rulers of very large areas of the world have aimed at one time or another at what they understood to be world domination. The Mughal emperors of northern India styled themselves 'Lords of the Universe'. The rulers of Vijayanagara, the 'City of Victory' on the Tungabhadra river in southern India, claimed 'to rule the vast world under a single umbrella'.[17] The Chinese emperor, the Huang Di, was the supreme lord of all humankind, for even if the Chinese knew full well that he did not literally rule over the entire world, all that he did was believed to affect even those who were not, or not yet, his subjects. The idea of Roman citizenship, however, expressed more than the exercise of simple power. It was about creating a world which would outlive even the empire itself. Even as Britain became independent, Gaul fell to usurpers, the Goths took possession of the Eternal City and the emperors in Ravenna (the city which would become a nemesis for Droctulft) began issuing laws to safeguard the Holy Roman and Catholic Church, the poet Claudian could still offer to the Teutonic vice-regent of the emperor Honorius (that 'pale flower of the women's quarters') lines in praise of universal citizenship: 'She [Rome] alone who has received the conquered into her bosom, and like a mother not an empress, protected the human race with a common name, summoning those whom she has defeated to share her citizenship.'[18]

Such sentiments would remain an aspiration of all later Western empires. As one British political philosopher expressed it in 1923, 'the thought on which the best of the Romans fed was a thought of a World-State, the universal law of nature, the brotherhood and the equality of men.'[19] This was meant to be as much a description of the British empire, at a time when it was still a going concern, as it was of the Romans. And some conception of universal citizenship has sustained every cry for justice, sincere or mendacious, that has ever been made in the name of 'humanity', 'mankind' or, more recently, that shifting and amorphous body, 'the international community'.

Until the late eighteenth century, however, 'the world' over which in their various ways its would-be rulers claimed sovereignty was an immense, uncertain place. In Cicero's *Scipio's*

Dream, which became one of the most popular accounts of the frightening infinitude of space, the Roman general Scipio Aemilianus has a dream in which he finds himself talking to his deceased adoptive grandfather, Scipio Africanus. Africanus takes him on a tour of the heavens, from where he is able to gaze down upon the earth.

> You see that the earth is inhabited in only a few portions, and those very small, while vast deserts lie between them ... You see that the inhabitants are so widely separated that there can be no communication whatever among the different areas; and that some of the inhabitants live in parts of the earth that are oblique, transverse and sometimes directly opposite your own, from such you can expect nothing surely that is glory. Examine this northern zone which you inhabit and you will see what a small portion of it belongs to you Romans. You cannot fail to see what a narrow territory it is over which your glory is so eager to spread.

In reality, the younger Scipio (as his adoptive grandfather is also made to predict) would go on to destroy Carthage in 146 BC, thus bringing the third Punic War to a victorious conclusion, and to take Numantia in northern Spain. But Scipio Africanus' vision of a vast, unknowable and ultimately unpossessable globe would remain to haunt the imagination not only of the Romans but of most subsequent would-be empire-builders in Europe. 'Empire', as Cicero knew, is about glory. And, as Africanus makes clear, if you cannot aspire to hold all of the world, it would be better to give up hope of any of it. Better to think about the pleasures of the afterlife or the things of the spirit which alone are of lasting value. For even, says Africanus, if what we achieve in our own lifetimes is glorious, 'even if future generations should wish to hand down to those yet unborn the eulogies of every one of us' – even then the disasters which overrun the world would prevent anyone 'from gaining a glory which would be long-enduring, much less eternal'.[20]

Cicero attributed these sentiments to one of the greatest of Roman generals, the man who, if Livy is to be believed, declared that 'The empire of the Roman people shall be extended to the furthest ends of the earth.'[21] Scipio Africanus may have been permitted to see how small his own triumphs had been when viewed from the heavens, and he may have come to the conclusion that his achievements, and those of all the other glory-seekers who have plagued the world, were ultimately illusory, grains of chaff in the wind. Cicero himself could certainly think that way. But Africanus' grandson was destined to go on in the same way, as was Rome itself, until it finally fell to other peoples with imperial ambitions.

For all Cicero's scepticism about the capacity of the Romans to occupy anything more than a very small portion of 'the world', the Roman empire was, before the arrival of the British in the nineteenth century, the most extensive in terms of inhabitable lands and population that the world had ever known. (The Russians, and before them the Mongols, ruled over more territory but most of it was unoccupied, and, prior to the development of modern technologies, largely unoccupiable.) At its height in the second century AD the Roman empire covered an area from the Atlas Mountains to Scotland and the Indus valley to the Atlantic, a territory of approximately five million square miles and a population which has been estimated at about fifty-five million. By one account, the process of expansion had only stopped when the Romans believed that they had reached the furthermost limits of what the Greeks called the *oikoumene*, the inhabitable world.[22] More prosaically, they stopped expanding when they reached the real limits of their capabilities, checked by the Parthians in the east and the vastness of the Atlantic Ocean in the west. By then, however, the empire had already become too large to be managed from a single centre, too diverse politically and culturally to sustain its claim to being a single state under a single rule of law.

In the end Rome fell prey to the limitlessness of its own ambitions. As the empire grew and the diversity of the peoples it included increased, so its sheer heterogeneity became more difficult to handle. Like all extensive empires it eventually reached a stage where it was no longer able to keep ahead of the competition and to satisfy its subject peoples.[23] Having reached a point of equilibrium in the second century, it began slowly but inexorably to be hollowed out from within as long-quiescent subject peoples revolted and once-loyal subjects seized the opportunity to carve out independent states for themselves. A similar fate befell the state of Vijayanagara in southern India, and the Muslim empires of the Ottomans, the Safavids and the Mughals. It is what became of Spain and Britain and, in its own way, the Soviet Union.

The dangers of overextension had been there since before the time of Augustus although no one had paid them much attention. Livy, writing in the early days of the principate, tells how, when Scipio Africanus took his army into Asia in 190 BC, he was met by Heraclides of Byzantium, ambassador of the Seleucid emperor Antiochus. Heraclides warned him to 'let the Romans limit their empire to Europe, that even this was very large; that it was easier to gain it part by part than to hold the whole'.[24] Scipio was unimpressed: 'What seemed to the ambassador great incentives for conducting peace,' commented Livy, 'seemed unimportant to the Romans.' Scipio marched on to begin what would be the final annexation of the empire of Alexander the Great. But Heraclides' words would return again and again to haunt not only later generations of Romans but most subsequent empire-builders.

By the end of the second century AD, the empire, as Heraclides predicted, had become impossible to hold together. Already, by 200, a serious trade recession had hit the Mediterranean. In the middle years of the century the Roman legions had suffered terrible defeats at the hands of Persians, Goths, and other Germanic tribes, and civil war had brought the imperial government to the verge of disintegration.[25] In a last attempt to keep it intact, the emperor Diocletian divided the empire into a Western and an Eastern half. The division was carried still further by his successor Constantine the Great, who in 324 created on the site of Byzantium on the shores of the Bosphorus a 'New Rome' for the Eastern empire and called it Constantinople, Greek for 'Constantine's city'.

In 312, at the battle of the Mulvian Bridge, Constantine had defeated his rival Maxentius for control of the entire empire. His victory, or so he later claimed, had come after he had seen in the sky a cross with the words 'Be victorious in this'. After his triumph, which later historians inevitably attributed to divine intervention, Constantine converted to Christianity, made it the official religion of the empire, and began the slow process of transforming a polytheistic pagan society into a monotheistic Christian one.[26] Henceforth the Roman empire, and with it the whole of what had now become Europe, acquired two separate identities: a Latin Western part, and a progressively Hellenized East which has come to be called the Byzantine empire. The latter remained until its end in 1453 the empire of the Romans, although by the fifth century it had become a Greek-speaking, wholly Hellenized culture. Roman culture under both the republic and the empire had always been heavily indebted to that of Greece. Men like Cicero, if never quite bilingual, had had Greek tutors and derived all of their philosophical training from Greek texts. Greek art, Greek architecture, Greek modes of dress and Greek ceremonial all left their mark on the Roman world. After the division of the empire Romans not only spoke two different languages, they adopted two distinct forms of Christianity: Greek Orthodoxy in the East and Catholicism in the West. In time these differences would deepen until finally any dialogue between the *basileus* in the East and the emperor in the West became impossible.

Byzantium outlived Rome. By the early years of the fifth century the empire in the West had been overrun by waves of Germanic tribes. In August 410, the traditional date for the formal end of the Roman empire in the West, the Eternal City was sacked and pillaged for three days by the armies of the Visigothic ruler Alaric. What remained of Rome revived briefly, but when in 476 the German Odoacer deposed the emperor Romulus Augustulus, the Western empire was finally extinguished.[27]

Byzantium, however, remained firmly in control of most of the East for another 500 years. In the eleventh century, however, Seljuk Turks seized Byzantine Armenia. In 1204 Constantinople itself fell to the marauding soldiery of the Fourth Crusade who held it until 1261. But it was the Ottoman Turks who were to carry out the final destruction of the Christian East. Beginning in the thirteenth century they moved steadily and inexorably westwards until in 1453, after a prolonged siege, Constantinople fell to the armies of Sultan Mehmet II, 'The Conqueror'. Thereafter it would become Istanbul and be rebuilt as the capital of another great power, the only Muslim empire the Christian world was ever prepared to accept as such. With the demise of the last Byzantine ruler, there would be 'two suns' shining upon the globe, two rulers competing for universal supremacy, a Christian emperor in the West and a Muslim sultan in the East.

3 *Universal empire*

The modern European world remains the heir to both of the civilizations of the ancient world. But with the final collapse of the Byzantine empire Greek culture was submerged for nearly 400 years. European society, despite its continuing indebtedness to Greek science and philosophy, became predominantly a Latin one on which the customs and languages of the Germanic invaders left deep and enduring marks. The former Roman *civitas* was transformed into a succession of fiefdoms, principalities, duchies, city-states and bishoprics. In time, all that remained of the status of the ancient Roman *imperium* belonged to the pope. The pope was the titular head of a secular state which was limited to southern and central Italy. But he was also the leader of a religious community which had always claimed that one day it would cover the entire globe – and this, as we shall see, was to have some far-reaching implications for subsequent relationships between the European imperial powers.

In 800 Pope Leo III, in the name of the people and city of Rome, conferred upon Charles I, the king of the Lombards and the Franks, who was subsequently known as Charlemagne (742–814), the title of Emperor. Between 771 and 778, Charlemagne had made himself sole ruler of the once-divided Frankish peoples, conquered the Lombard kingdom, and subdued and

Christianized the tribes of what is today Lower Saxony and Westphalia. He was a very long way from restoring the former Roman *imperium*, even within the traditional frontiers of Europe. But he had done more than any previous ruler. The new emperor was, as all his predecessors since Constantine had been, the defender of the church. He was the 'second sword' – the pope still wielded the first – of all Christendom. In 1157, in recognition of this role, Frederick I added the word Sanctus to his title and the empire thus became not merely Roman but also Holy.

Charlemagne's success in reuniting at least some of the many peoples which the dissolution of the Roman world had scattered into different communities did not, however, last for long. By 924 the Carolingian empire had been dissolved in Italy, and both France and Germany were in the process of becoming separate kingdoms. For Rome's true successor in the West was not to be yet another empire but instead a number of different kingdoms. By the mid-twelfth century each of the kings of Europe was claiming to be an emperor in his own kingdom, and what remained of the empire itself was gradually confined to the Germanic kingdoms. There it would remain, as Voltaire sarcastically remarked, 'neither Holy nor Roman nor an empire', for another 700 years until it was brought to an end by Napoleon in August 1806.

For most of the empire's long history, the Holy Roman emperors were princes who used their status to maintain an uneasy peace between the various political groups – free and imperial towns, landgraves and dukes, princes and prince-bishops, and the footloose Free Imperial Knights – which ruled over the German lands. (On the eve of the Reformation there were about 300 such political powers which were of real significance, and a host more which were not but believed themselves to be.) The emperor was, in that time-hallowed Latin phrase, *primus inter pares* – 'first amongst equals'. He was also, after the Frankish custom, not an hereditary but an elected ruler. By the fifteenth century, however, the imperial crown had become effectively hereditary within the Austrian Habsburg family, and with their ever-increasing power some of the real independence of the German princes began steadily to be eroded.

The ruler who did most to reassert the power of the empire and briefly transformed it from a merely German affair back into a true *imperium* was Charles V (1500–58). Charles had inherited from his grandfather Maximilian I most of what is now central and eastern Europe, and the Duchy of Burgundy which then included modern Holland and Belgium. He had inherited from his maternal grandparents, Ferdinand of Aragon and Isabella of Castile, the kingdoms of Spain, Castile and Aragon, and the Aragonese empire in Italy and the eastern Mediterranean. More significantly for the future of all the European states, he had also acquired a vast and as yet largely unexplored territory in the Western hemisphere, then known simply as the Indies.

When Charles of Burgundy, as he then was, set sail from the port of Flushing in Zeeland in September 1517 to claim the thrones of Castile and Aragon, the ship that carried him had painted on its sails an emblem depicting the Pillars of Hercules encircled with a banner nearing the legend *Plus Oultre*, 'further beyond'. The Pillars of Hercules was the name given to Mount Hacho and the Rock of Gibraltar, on the African and European sides of the Straits of Gibraltar. Legend had it that they had been set down to mark the limits of the known world and inscribed upon them had been the words *ne plus ultra*, 'no further beyond'. Beyond, for the ancients who knew nothing of oceanic navigation, lay only what the Arabs would later call the Green Sea of Darkness, which swallowed every vessel that dared to venture into it. Charles's removal of the word 'no' was an assertion made in the future tense. It was both a declaration that his empire had already passed the limits of that of Augustus, whose name he would later assume, and a statement about the further possibilities that were open to him.

According to the mythic genealogy which the eulogists of the house of Habsburg had provided for him, Charles had inherited his empire from Aeneas, Augustus and Constantine the Great, via Charlemagne.[1] It was an unbroken line which reached all the way back to the fall of Troy. The history of Rome, wrote the sixteenth-century Spanish imperial historian Pedro de Mexia, was the history of an empire which in 'longevity, size and power' was the greatest of all empires because it had begun 'a little less than 2300 years ago and is still alive today'.[2] Charles would complete the task which his ancestor, whose name he bore, had begun and reunite the whole of Europe under a single ruler. Moreover, the emblem of the Pillars proclaimed, he would go further than Caesar and Augustus. He would literally go forward and conquer the entire world. He himself, it must be said, claimed never to have harboured any such ambitions. In 1535, as suspicion of his intentions mounted, particularly in France, he went so far as to declare publicly before Pope Pius III that he had no aspirations whatsoever for universal empire. Not many, however, perhaps least of all the pope, ever wary of the objectives of the second sword of Christendom, believed him.

Charles' empire was not a single *imperium* but a vast,

sprawling, cosmopolitan conglomerate ruled over by an emperor who had no established capital, travelled ceaselessly to be with his loyal subjects, and tried to maintain the illusion, in the words of one seventeenth-century Milanese, that the ruler who held all these disparate realms together 'was only the king of each one of them'. Charles' empire resembled a modern multinational corporation more than a state. Although it was governed in accordance with an overarching legal principle, the imperial public law (*ius publicum*), it had no common legal system and no single administrative structure. It did not even have a single language. There is a woodcut by Albrecht Altdorfer which shows Maximilian I quelling a mutiny among his polyglot troops by addressing each one in his own tongue. Charles himself was said to have spoken Spanish to God, French to his mistress and German to his horse. Under the aegis of the emperor all his subjects supposedly enjoyed the same status whether they were Spanish, Walloons, Flemings, Neapolitans or even American Indians. God, wrote the sixteenth-century Italian poet Ludovico Ariosto, had willed it that 'under this emperor there should be only one flock and only one pastor', an inescapable allusion to St John's Gospel. For this reason making war on the Indians, declared the Spanish theologian Francisco de Vitoria in 1534, was making war not 'against strangers' but against vassals of the emperor 'as if they were natives of Seville'. Milanese, Florentines and Genoese settled in Spanish Naples and prospered there, acquiring Neapolitan lands and Neapolitan titles. Germans ran the printing presses of Seville, and Spaniards settled in the Netherlands (before the Dutch threw them out).

Charles' cosmopolitanism and claims to universalism were matched only by the rulers of the remainder of what had once been the ancient Hellenic and Roman worlds: the Ottoman empire (the Habsburg empire's immediate rival) and, further to the east the Safavid and Mughal empires. These were, if anything, even more porous than their Christian counterpart. The intelligentsia and guardians of the faith of the Muslim world shared a common body of texts: the Qur'an, the *Hadith* or traditions of the prophet, and the vast body of Arabic writings on philosophy and science which had been responsible for the diffusion of much Greek science, including most of Aristotle, into the Western world. Arabic and Persian were *linguae francae*, understood in educated circles at least from Budapest to Chittagong. Gujarati Hindus, Syrian Muslims, Jews, Armenians, and Christians from south and central Europe operated trading routes which supplied Persian and Arab horses to the armies of all three empires, Mocha coffee to Delhi and Belgrade, and Persian silk to India and Istanbul.[3] Arching over this international community and economy was the law of Islam which, like the *pax Romana*, offered considerable benefits to those who were prepared to accept the limitations it inevitably imposed.

All of these states saw themselves as heirs to the ancient empires which had preceded them. But the Habsburg empire was unlike both its Muslim rivals and its Roman and Greek predecessors in one crucial respect. All previous European and Asian empires – from those of the Medes and Achaemenids in Iran and the Ch'in in China, Vijayanagara in southern India, the empires of Alexander the Great, Genghis Khan, Tamburlaine, Caesar and Augustus, right up to the empire of Charles' paternal grandfather Maximilian – had been linked to large, well-trained and highly mobile land forces. They comprised territorial land-masses embracing myriad peoples and reaching over thousands of miles, but they were unbroken by large expanses of ocean. Charles' empire was also still land-based. It included most of central and eastern Europe, the Spanish kingdoms of Castile and Aragon, a large portion of southern Italy, the Duchy of Milan, and what are now Holland and Belgium. The greater part of it, however, at least as far as territory was concerned, lay overseas in America. And from the late fifteenth century on, the direction of European expansion would be increasingly maritime.

4   *Conquering the ocean*

In *Scipio's Dream* Cicero had created a vision of the real world, or at least of the world as Cicero thought it might be. Just how large that world was and just how many peoples it might contain was, of course, unknown. It was and would remain, until at least the late eighteenth century for most Europeans and well beyond for many others, a place of vertiginous geographical uncertainty. The Romans, the Mughals or the Chinese, even the Spanish and the Ottomans, all had very different visions of the planet from one another and from the one we have today. Maps were crude, inaccurate and impressionistic. Even within Europe itself the size and topography of individual states was often wildly imprecise. Alessandro Farnese, the commander of Philip II's armies fighting the rebellious Dutch in 1585, appears to have believed that Holland was an island; and when the first truly accurate survey was made of the kingdom of France, Louis XIV complained that his cartographers had robbed him of several hundred square miles of territory.

Yet, if the limits of Europe itself were unclear, those of Africa, Asia and America were frequently only mythical. For most ancient geographers the globe had contained a single landmass divided into three linked continents: Europe, Asia and Africa. Herodotus grumbled that he could not see 'why three names, and women's names at that, should have been given to a tract which is in reality one'.) Later, Asia was divided into three: China, Japan and what were generally called 'the Indies', the lands east of the Indus, the traditional limit of the Hellenistic world. The whole of this landmass was believed to be encircled by a massive river consisting roughly of what we know as the Atlantic and Pacific Oceans. It was called by the Greeks *Okeanos*, and by later Europeans the Ocean Sea.

In the early fifteenth century, however, this vision of the world began to change. In 1434 a small fleet of lateen-rigged vessels known as caravels, barely more than fishing boats, slipped out of the Tagus estuary bound for the unknown waters of West Africa. It successfully passed Cape Bojador which jutted far out into the Atlantic from the Western Sahara and was believed by many to mark the limit of the navigable ocean. The fleet made landfall just south of the cape and then turned for home. The expedition achieved little else but it had demonstrated that it was possible to sail down the west coast of Africa and, more importantly, to return.

The early Portuguese voyages to Africa were sponsored by Prince Henry, called 'the Navigator' by later generations of admiring English sailors. In the early fifteenth century Portugal was one of the poorest nations in Europe. Denied access to the reserves of silver and gold it required, and with severely limited trading capacities, its only hope of improving its condition was to exploit its long Atlantic coastline and considerable maritime experience. Henry hoped to find a direct route to the gold which was mined somewhere in the interior of Africa and then transported overland across the Sahara by Arab middlemen to Europe. He also hoped to discover new grounds for his crusading ambitions, which had been largely frustrated on the shores of North

Africa some years before, and to make contact with the legendary Prester John. This fantastical Christian ruler of an empire of vast wealth (a confused memory of the Coptic kingdom of Ethiopia) would, so Henry hoped, make common cause with the Portuguese against the forces of Islam and help them to regain the kingdom of Jerusalem. Prince Henry found none of the things he had hoped for. The gold stayed shut up in the interior of Africa. Prester John remained confined to the realms of myth. The only crusading ventures, shameful struggles between mounted Portuguese knights and unarmed fishermen on the coasts of Mauritania, rapidly came to an end when the Portuguese moved south and the peoples of Senegal and Senegambia turned poisoned arrows upon their assailants and tsetse flies destroyed their horses. In 1448 Henry forbade any further attempt at armed conflict except in self-defence. It is often forgotten that in the first encounter between a European colonizing power and an African people the Europeans were soundly defeated.[1]

Later voyages, however, aimed at securing direct access to the silks, spices, precious woods and other luxury commodities of the East and, with more enduring and sinister consequences, to opening up the trade in African slaves. Henry died in 1460. But his initiative changed the economies of Europe, the relations of Europeans with the peoples of the world beyond, and the nature of European imperial ambitions. At first the voyages had been modest. Even in 1497, by which time the Portuguese had established a secure base in West Africa, the fleet with which on 22 November Vasco da Gama rounded the Cape of Good Hope and sailed into the Indian Ocean consisted of only four small ships. They carried a startlingly inappropriate collection of trading goods: hawks' bells, brass chamberpots, and the brass bracelets which later became the currency of the African slave trade. It was a tawdry collection of junk with which to do business with the highly sophisticated merchants of the fabled Orient. When da Gama returned to Lisbon in April 1499 and laid out before King Manuel II the precious goods he had brought back with him, the king is said to have thought for a while and then remarked that 'it would seem that it is not we who have discovered them, but they who have discovered us.'

Despite these beginnings, by the seventeenth century the Portuguese empire reached all the way from West Africa to India and southern China, and the overladen carracks of the *Carrera da India* annually carried immense fortunes back to Europe.[2] Some idea of the profits to be made from the trade in spices and silks with Asia can be had from the voyage led by Fernão de Magalhães (known to the English as Magellan), a Portuguese in the service of the Spanish crown, to find a route south to the so-called Spice Islands (the Moluccas). Magellan set sail from Sanlúcar de Barrameda on 20 September 1519 with five ships. The voyage, which led to the first circumnavigation of the globe, lasted for three years. One by one the ships foundered or sank and Magellan himself died in a skirmish on Mactan Island in the Philippines. In the end only one vessel, the *Victoria*, remained. On 8 September 1522 she sailed into Seville, leaking and with only seventeen Europeans and four Indians on board. But the spices she carried in her holds were enough to cover the costs of the entire voyage, with the loss of four ships, and still make a profit.

The Portuguese navigators had sailed into waters which many had believed to be unnavigable. They had travelled down the coast of Africa, rounded the Cape of Good Hope and reached India. More importantly, they had done all this and returned. The impact they have had on the subsequent history of the world has been enormous. But their voyage was neither so dramatic nor, arguably, so far-reaching as that undertaken in 1492 by an obscure but insistent Genoese who was convinced that the world was roughly half the size it was and that what were known as the Lands of the Great Khan – China and South-East Asia – could therefore be reached by sailing west. When on 12 October 1492 Columbus landed on a still unidentified island in the Caribbean which its inhabitants called Guarahani, he changed the European perception of the planet for ever. He did so, however, entirely unintentionally and against his own judgement. He insisted until his dying day that what he had encountered out there in the Atlantic was not a new world but merely the easternmost rim of Asia. He was not at all interested in new worlds. In his geographical understanding, the vast Ocean Sea was dotted with islands of no great wealth or significance. What Columbus had promised his sponsors, Ferdinand and Isabel, the monarchs of the united kingdoms of Castile and Aragon, was direct access by sea to the wealth of the Orient. The last thing they wanted was an unknown land peopled by naked 'savages' who had no spices or silks to offer and precious little gold or silver.

By the time Columbus returned from his third voyage in 1498, however, it had become obvious to all in Europe that America was no mere island but a continent which had been wholly unknown to antiquity (although maps were still being produced in the 1510s which eliminated the Pacific and declared Cuba to be a part of Asia). Columbus himself remained a stubbornly medieval figure who preferred to believe that the vast quantities of fresh water flowing from the Orinoco into the Gulf of Paria in modern Venezuela came from the earthly paradise rather than any new world. He was buried in Franciscan habit and left what little money remained to him at his death to sponsor a crusade.[3] But for later generations he became, like Galileo, with whom he was often compared, a hero of the new science who in defiance of the wisdom of the day had shattered all conceptions of what was known about the globe and, more importantly, what could be known. Here was a man who had demonstrated that the moderns could indeed surpass the wisdom of the ancients. Little wonder that for later generations the 'discovery' of America, along with Vasco da Gama's voyage around the Cape of Good Hope to India, came to be seen as the beginnings of the modern world.

The discovery of the existence of America, a hitherto unknown landmass of immense size and complexity, not only upset all previous notions of geography but led many to wonder if other undiscovered continents might lie to the south in the fabled Antipodes. According to St Augustine, it was absurd to suppose that men might live there because they would have to do so hanging upside down. Augustine had not supposed that the world was flat – almost no one did that. But neither had he fully grasped the significance of the sphericity of the earth. By the early sixteenth century, however, all Europeans had come to suppose that, excluding some of the deserts and the furthermost northern reaches (which were recognized as being too cold for habitation by most humans), all the world was at least potentially inhabitable. A new continent called by the cartographers 'the unknown southern land' – *Terra australis incognita* – was projected into the South Pacific. When in 1642 the Dutchman Abel Tasman landed on what is now Tasmania and the south island of New Zealand, the possibility that there existed inhabitable land in that shadowy region became a certainty – although it would take more than another century, until Captain Cook's second voyage of 1772–5, before anyone was to realize the full extent of what in 1817 was baptized by Governor Macquarie as Australia.

Charles V and his heirs, Philips II, III and IV, laid claim to all of this even though they had very little notion of what it contained. When Columbus returned in 1493 the Spanish crown immediately petitioned the papacy for title to what he had 'discovered'. This was not an unusual move. Not only did the papacy at this time act as an arbiter in international disputes, it was believed by some (although by no means all) to exercise by divine decree authority over the lands not just of Christian but also of non-Christian rulers. In 1455 Pope Nicolas V had licensed King Afonso V of Portugal to 'reduce to perpetual slavery' all the inhabitants of Africa, 'and all southern coasts until their end', as the 'enemies of Christ'. And Castile was not to be outdone. In 1493 Pope Alexander VI duly issued a series of decrees (known as bulls) which gave Ferdinand and Isabella control over all those lands 'you have discovered or are about to discover'. The peoples who inhabited these places, although the pope insisted that they should be well treated and led as gently as possible into the Christian fold, had no identity but a negative one. They were not Christians and had not yet fallen under the authority of a Christian ruler. The pope, as the American lawyer James Otis observed in 1764 with the withering sarcasm of a devout Calvinist, had thus with a single flourish of his pen 'granted away the kingdoms of the earth with as little ceremony as a man would leave a sheepcote'.

A year later, still under the watchful eye of the papacy, Spain and Portugal signed a treaty in the Spanish town of Tordesillas which for the first (and the last) time in human history divided the entire world into two areas of jurisdiction. The Tordesillas Line, as it came to be called, was drawn along longitude 46° 30' W, calculated at 370 leagues west of the Cape Verde Islands. (Before the invention of stable marine chronometers in the seventeenth century, lines of longitude were only ever approximate, and in the eighteenth century this led to bitter border disputes between Spain and Portugal in South America.) The western half went to Castile which believed that it now controlled an unhindered route to the Orient. The eastern half went to Portugal, intent mainly on keeping its Castilian rivals out of the South Atlantic, which thereby came into possession of Brazil. But the agreement failed to say anything about what happened where East met West on the far side of the world, or who would be entitled to what portions of the fabled southern continent should one prove to exist. The treaty and the Alexandrine bulls were regarded with predictable contempt by the other European powers. Yet, despite their obvious flimsiness as documents in international law, the Spanish crown continued to insist on what one British official in 1749 described as 'their whimsical notion of exclusive right in those seas' until the final demise of the empire at the end of the eighteenth century.

In 1494 neither the Spanish nor the Portuguese had any but the vaguest of notions of what the vast tracts of ocean to which they had laid claim might contain. By the time Ferdinand's grandson, the future Charles V, set out to claim his inheritance, however, it was becoming obvious that the Indies were more than a cluster of islands inhabited by simple Stone Age cultures. The fantasy of lands filled with gold which the Portuguese had pursued along the shores of Africa, and which was to cost Sir Walter Raleigh his head, was now being relocated to America. With the conquest of Mexico in the 1520s and that of Peru a decade later, the fantasy was suddenly and dramatically transformed into reality. On this occasion, wryly commented the eighteenth-century philosopher and economist Adam Smith, Fortune had done what Fortune rarely ever does and 'favoured its devotees' with 'something not very unlike that profusion of precious metals which they sought for'. From the 1530s, when the massively rich silver mines of Mexico and Peru were discovered, until well into the eighteenth century, American silver poured unceasingly eastwards, first into the coffers of the Spanish crown and then outwards through German, Dutch and Italian bankers until it reached every part of the continent.

The 'discovery' of America meant more, however, than access to huge deposits of precious metals. The voyages of Columbus and Vasco da Gama were, said Adam Smith, 'the most important events recorded in the history of mankind', not because they had provided Europe with gold and silver, but because they had made her peoples vastly more mobile than they had ever been before.[4] They had brought them closer to the great civilizations of the Indian Ocean and into ultimately tragic contact with entire races of whose very existence they had previously known nothing. By the time Smith published *The Wealth of Nations* in 1776 the two Iberian empires had truly encompassed the globe. They had come closer to creating a single world economy than ever before. They had distributed populations across the continents and circulated new diseases, new foodstuffs, and new drugs all the way from Seville to Manila. And all of this they had done by exploiting the waters and winds of the world.

The Europeans were, of course, not alone in their use of the sea. The Arabs had extensive seaborne trading networks in the waters around the Arabian peninsula. Long before the Europeans reached them, the Polynesians had crossed vast expanses of ocean, sailing their double-hulled canoes against the wind, to colonize areas thousands of miles from their homelands, and had drawn maps to prove it – maps which astonished Captain Cook when he was shown them. Between 1405 and 1433 a Chinese admiral, Zheng He, had made seven voyages in giant, 400-foot-long, nine-masted junks called *bao chuan* or 'treasure ships', through the China Seas and the Indian Ocean from Taiwan to the Persian Gulf and down the east coast of Africa as far as Malindi and Mombassa. Zheng's mission was trade and most of his ships were laden with merchandise. But the fleet was also accompanied by supply ships, water tankers, transport for horses, warships and numerous lighter boats, with crews amounting to more than 28,000 sailors and soldiers. It was a small population under sail, the largest fleet the world had then seen, dwarfing the 100-foot vessels with which Vasco da Gama entered the same waters over half a century later.

But the Arab traders confined themselves largely to their own coastal waters, and the Polynesians never left the Pacific. After Zheng's last voyage the Chinese decided to cease all long-distance overseas trade. Why they did so no one really knows. In 1477, when a later attempt was made to revive overseas trading, the vice-president of the Ministry of War, Liu Daxia, confiscated

Zheng He's documents from the archives and either hid or burned them. They were, he said, 'deceitful exaggerations of bizarre things, far removed from the testimony of people's eyes and ears' and all that the ships had brought home had been 'betel, bamboo staves, grape wine, pomegranates, ostrich eggs and such like odd things'. China had turned its back upon any further expansion of the empire, on overseas trade and, so far as was possible, on any further contact with outsiders. It was a decision which, in the longer run, was to prove calamitous. By the mid-seventeenth century the Europeans had effective mastery of the Atlantic and were the most powerful trading presence in the Indian Ocean. By the end of the eighteenth century they had taken over most of the Pacific. When at last in 1860 the war junks of the Dragon Throne, technically unchanged since the days of Zheng, confronted the iron-clad, steam-driven gunboats of the British intruders the entire fleet was reduced to matchwood. All the English suffered was the death of one sailor, struck by a stray cannonball.

Navigation changed dramatically the future relationships between the peoples of the world. It not only brought Europeans into ever closer contact with increasingly larger areas of the globe but allowed them to transport large numbers of individuals from one part of the planet to another. Migrations, which before the creation of ocean-going sailing ships had been predominantly overland and slow and irreversible, became rapid and potentially reversible. True, the colonies of the ancient world had also depended upon the ship; and Viking seafarers had reached as far as the shores of North America, and some seem to have returned to tell the tale. But these journeys had all been dependent upon tiny, oared vessels capable of covering relatively small stretches of water. The great flotillas which would cross and recross the Atlantic and the Pacific became in the space of a very few years capable of carrying the equivalent of an entire population.

When in 1519 Charles set out for his coronation as the official heir of Augustus, he was already in name at least master of a vast new continent, and his apologists and historians were busy making good his claim in the name of the universality of the Roman *imperium* to be lord of the still vaster regions that lay beyond. Without the ship none of this would have been imaginable. Charles had had his emblem put on a sail and it was the sail which would carry it to the ends, or at least very nearly the ends, of the earth. As a result, his empire was to be the first in human history on which, in Ariosto's words, 'the sun never set'.

5   *Spreading the word*

The empire of Charles V was not only Roman, it was also Holy. Throughout his life Charles saw himself as the defender of Christendom against all its enemies, both external and internal. And his heirs, down to the final disintegration of the Spanish empire at the end of the eighteenth century, would remain loyal to this image. In this, too, Charles was conscious of his place as the successor to Augustus and Constantine, for Roman imperialism had also marched under the banner of religious devotion. This was focused on the emperor's own person; and all the pagan emperors had themselves deified so that their *imperium* became not merely a mundane right to rule, as it had been for the senate, but a quasi-mystic power reserved to them alone. Aurelian, in the third century AD, in emulation of Alexander, brought back to Rome the Persian worship of the unconquered sun; and his successor Diocletian came to regard himself as Jovius, the earthly representation of Jupiter. After Constantine's conversion to Christianity the practice ceased, but all Roman emperors and most Christian monarchs after them believed that the authority they possessed had been granted to them by God – until the French Revolution swept the whole notion of the divinity of kings away for ever.

For the Romans, the divinity of the emperor was indissolubly linked to the grandeur of the homeland, the *patria*, and love of the *patria* had always been an expression of individual piety among the Roman people. The Latin word *pietas*, however, meant something rather different to a pagan Roman than its modern, Christianized counterpart does. Piety, like virtue, described qualities associated ultimately with warfare: devotion, loyalty and trust, adherence to the laws of the community, and the willingness to sacrifice one's life for the common good. The truly pious man was inevitably also a warrior. 'A man outstanding in arms and piety' is how the poet Virgil introduces Aeneas, the founder of Rome, in the *Aeneid*. It was this piety which in the view of St Augustine had led God to entrust the Romans with the task of uniting the world prior to the coming of Christ. Universal empire had been their reward, he believed, for 'the virtues by which they pursued the hard road which brought them at last to such glory ... They disregarded private wealth for the sake of the common wealth. They stood firm against avarice, gave advice to their country with an unshakeable mind and were not guilty of any crime against the laws, nor of any unlawful desire.'[1]

It is not a very convincing account of the historical Roman empire, but it captures the ambiguities which followed the attempt to turn Roman martial virtues into the rather more gentle Christian ones. Piety became submissiveness before God. Virtue, which for the Romans had meant only the qualities of manliness, came to be associated with an ethic of renunciation.

Under its Christian rulers Rome would become the place where the universalizing message of Christ would find its ultimate if also unintended political expression. Christ himself might have wished the things of Caesar to remain Caesar's and, more importantly, those of God to remain for ever and only God's. But under Peter's successors in the see of Rome the borders between church and state, although hotly contested, became increasingly blurred. After Constantine's conversion Christianity, which had begun by turning its back upon empire, became and in the West was to remain empire's most valuable ally. The divinity which hedged the pagan emperors was transferred to the Christian. 'The emperor,' wrote the second-century theologian Tertullian, father of the church and scourge of deviants of any kind, 'is established in dignity by God, and [the Christian] must honour him and wish for his preservation.' Now that they could no longer claim to be divinities in their own right, the Christian Roman emperors took upon themselves the role of defenders of the church. Even after the disappearance of the empire and the rise of the new nation-states the kings of Europe acquired semi-sacred titles: 'Most Christian king' was bestowed upon Francis I of France, 'Most Catholic Monarchs' on Ferdinand and Isabella of Spain, and 'Defender of the Faith', somewhat ironically in the light of subsequent developments, on Henry VIII of England.

Christianity was also a truly universalizing creed. The 'new man', St Paul informed the Colossians, 'is being renewed unto knowledge after the image of him that created him, where there cannot be Greek or Jew, circumcision and uncircumcision, barbarian, Scythian, bondman, freeman: but Christ is all and in all'.[2] This new Christian world order, the origins of which could not now be separated from those of the Roman empire, would, as Tertullian had also said, endure as long as 'this earthly world'. It thus came to imagine itself not only as the common *patria* of humankind, but as a spiritual, cultural and moral order with no natural frontiers. From this the Christian Roman emperors took upon themselves a duty not only to uphold and protect Christendom, but also to extend the knowledge of Christ to those non-Christians who because of their ignorance had been denied historical access to the 'congregation of the faithful'.

Thenceforth, Christianity accompanied the expanding European empires almost until their final demise in the middle of the twentieth century. Where the conquerors and the settlers and traders went the missionaries followed hard behind. Priests and friars travelled on all the Portuguese voyages and accompanied all the conquering Spanish armies. For a brief period in the early sixteenth century the Spanish Caribbean was even administered by the Hieronymite order. Calvinist ministers travelled into Dutch Asia and Africa. French Huguenot pastors occupied a short-lived settlement in Brazil in the sixteenth century where one of them, Jean de Lery, wrote one of the earliest and most sympathetic accounts of a 'primitive' people ever written by a European.[3] Anglican clergymen, and even a few women, followed the flag into India and then into Uganda and Nyasaland and what became Rhodesia. Some of them did so in order to provide legitimacy to barely legitimate enterprises. Many, however, went in the hope that the journey on which they had embarked would be a stage in the final triumph of Christ over the whole world. In the Americas the fact that Hernán Cortés' conquest of Mexico had roughly coincided with Luther's rebellion was taken as a sign that God had given to the church territories in the new hemisphere to compensate for those it had lost in the old. Such millenarianism is possibly a feature of all early empires. It provided an ideology and a goal but it also offered a prediction, a certainty which could help to uplift those who felt, as many did, that sometimes things were not going quite as they had expected.

In its transition from world-renouncing sect to state religion, Christianity had become something none of its founders could ever have imagined, or wanted. The Christian church, unlike Islam, is based on layer upon layer of highly sophisticated – not to say sophistical – interpretation of its founders' words, filtered through Greek philosophy and Roman jurisprudence. In the process those words have become obscured, darkened, sometimes wilfully distorted. As a consequence the Church militant has, at least since the Middle Ages, been the constant companion of the Church pastoral. Yet Christianity itself has not always been the entirely pliant handmaiden of empire. Christ's message, with its insistence on the priority of the spiritual over the temporal, was there to be read by those who could do so. The religious orders in particular were inclined, to the displeasure not only of their secular overlords but sometimes also of their own superiors, to insist that it should be taken seriously and literally – that 'love thy neighbour as thyself' should be a real deterrent against pillage and the unwarranted expropriation of the goods of others, even when, as was generally the case, those others were not Christians.

Most of the missionaries lived in an uneasy alliance with the soldiers, adventurers, merchants, royal officials and lawyers who made up the advance forces of most colonizing voyages. The friar who protested to that archetypal conquistador Francisco Pizarro that he was not doing enough to convert the Incas to Christianity before slaughtering them received the tart reply: 'I have not come for that. I have come to take their gold away from them.' He was not alone. Jesuit and Dominican missionaries, Anglican chaplains and Huguenot pastors similarly protested against the excesses of the settlers from Brazil to

Timor. Most of them went unheard. But by no means all. One who started a debate over the rights of conquerors which was to echo down the centuries was an otherwise obscure Spanish Dominican named Antonio de Montesinos.

On the Sunday before Christmas 1511, the small and motley Spanish population of the island of Hispaniola filed into the main church of the town, then barely more than a village, of Santo Domingo. It was hot and humid and the church was a small rudimentary structure of adobe bricks under an agave roof. Diego Colón, Columbus' brother and the governor of the island, was there with all the other king's men. Most of those who made up the congregation were 'holders' (*encomenderos*) of Indians, as they were called. *Encomenderos* were entitled to exploit the labour of the Indians, although not to take their lands, and in exchange they were supposed to look after their spiritual welfare and even to pay them a small wage. Most, however, did none of this. They had crossed the ocean in the belief that they could become in this new world what they could never have been in the old, and they resented the crown's refusal to allow them simply to enslave the Indians and appropriate their lands. That morning, they had all come to the church because they had been told that the sermon would contain a special message for them. One of them, who left an impassioned and detailed account of all that followed, was a lay-priest called Bartolomé de Las Casas. When Las Casas entered the church that day he was a holder of Indians like all the rest, a little kinder perhaps than most but largely untroubled by the misery he saw about him. He would leave a changed man, the man who would become the 'Defender and Apostle to the Indians', the perpetual moral scourge of the Spanish settler community and a hero for anticolonialists from that day to this.

The dignitaries of the island had also come to hear Montesinos because he was known as a 'great lover of the rigours of religion', a very devout and fiery preacher, 'very chloeric in his words'. The sermon they got was certainly choleric. But it was no ordinary exhortation of the kind to which they were accustomed. Montesinos mounted the crude wooden pulpit. Having begun with a few obvious and unthreatening things about Advent, he launched 'with pugnacious and terrible words' into an attack on the conscience of the Spaniards which he likened to a 'sterile desert'. They were words, Las Casas later remembered, which 'made the Spaniards' flesh creep as if they already stood before divine judgement'. Montesinos thundered at them, demanding to know by what right they treated 'these innocent people', the Indians, 'with such cruelty and tyranny', by what authority they had 'made such detestable wars against peoples who were living pacifically and gently on their own lands'. Montesinos' ringing questions culminated in three which were to become the rallying cry of the struggle against colonial rulers in the Spanish-speaking world and far beyond. 'Are these not men?' he asked. 'Do they not have rational souls? Are you not obliged to love them as yourselves?'[4]

Las Casas listened appalled. From that moment, which he thought of as his 'conversion', right until the end of his very long life (he lived to be ninety-two years old), he dedicated himself to a single objective: that of demonstrating first to his king, then to the royal administration – the Council of the Indies – and finally to the world at large that the American Indians were human beings and had a right to be treated as what they were in law, true subjects of the Castilian crown. Las Casas wrote a great deal: histories, political and theological treatises, ethnographies, and innumerable pamphlets. He also did a great deal. In 1543 he was made bishop of Chiapus in southern Mexico, a region which from his day to this has been a predominantly Indian area and has always refused to accept quietly the rule of usurpers, be they Spanish conquistadors or modern Mexican *politicos*. Twice between 1545 and 1560, once in Cumaná on the Venezuelan coast and then in the optimistically named Verapaz ('True Peace') in what is now Honduras, he attempted to establish communities of the kind the missionaries believed they might have been able to create if the Spanish colonists had not got there first: settlements of priests and honest farmers. Both projects, however, turned out to be based upon a tragic illusion. No one leaves his home for an uncertain life in remote lands except in the hope of being able to better himself. The 'honest farmers' recruited for Las Casas' experiments had a rather more conventional view of what improvement meant than he did. Even before they had reached America they were boasting of how they would be wearing swords in the new world and that they had gone there to command not to obey.

Las Casas' main objectives were intellectual. He was an agitator, a rhetorician, and a pamphleteer. He fought the royal administration unremittingly, until finally in 1542 he persuaded the crown to introduce a body of legislation, the New Laws, which attempted to curb the worst excesses of the settlers and to return to the Indians at least some of their rights. These proved to be unworkable, almost provoked a settler revolt and were repealed a few years later, but they did demonstrate that rulers could be swayed by the sheer force of moral and religious indignation. Today Las Casas is probably best remembered for two things. The first is a brief and gory chronicle of all the horrors perpetrated against the Indians from the occupation of Hispaniola to Pizarro's conquest of the Inca kingdom of Peru, called succinctly *A Short Account of the Destruction of the Indies.*[5] This became a bestseller in a number of European languages. It was the book which launched the 'Black Legend' against Spain, the often distorted record of Spanish atrocities which was to darken every attempt to exonerate or even to describe Spanish imperial ventures from the sixteenth to the eighteenth centuries. The second was his role in a debate with a humanist historian' and translator of Aristotle named Juan Ginés de Sepúlveda, on the rationality of the American Indians.[6]

In 1544 Sepúlveda had written a dialogue in Latin justifying the 'wars' waged against the Indians by the Spaniards. A large part of his argument hinged on the image of the Indians as subhuman creatures, filthy, ignorant, 'like pigs with their eyes fixed always on the ground', lascivious and idolatrous, given to unnatural practices such as incest, cannibalism and human sacrifice. 'Homunculi', he called them, in whom 'hardly a vestige of humanity remains'. Sepúlveda's work circulated widely in manuscript and unsurprisingly met with the approval of the settler community in Mexico which sent its author a gift of 200 pesos' worth of jewels and clothing, no small sum, to 'encourage him in the future'. When, as part of the complex business of sixteenth-century censorship, the work was submitted to the theology faculty of the University of Salamanca for approval, the theologians turned it down on the grounds that its doctrines were not 'sound' and that it was likely to cause a 'scandal'. Sepúlveda was furious. He was the official royal historian and one of the king's chaplains. He had produced a ringing defence of imperial policy and practice. To reject him in this humiliating fashion was little short of treason. Behind the decisions of the university professors he thought he saw, probably correctly, the intrigues of Las Casas. In 1549 he wrote to the future Philip II, then regent of Castile, demanding a public hearing, a debate in which his views could be made public before the Council of the Indies. This would surely vindicate all he had said.

Sepúlveda got what he had asked for. The 'debate' – although the two men seem never to have met face to face – was staged in Valladolid in 1550–51, in the presence of a number of judges appointed by both sides. Las Casas spoke for five days without ceasing from a text which he had written with 'so much sweat and sleepless nights'. He challenged not only what Sepúlveda had said but all that had ever been written against the Indians until he was asked by the Dominican Domingo de Soto, who was presiding over the whole affair, to limit himself to the arguments he was trying to refute. Some days later Sepúlveda replied to this tirade with twelve objections, to which Las Casas in turn replied with twelve replies. And so it might have gone on if Soto had not put an end to a debate which, as he said, had 'now grown as long and prolix as the years of this matter'.

The outcome was inconclusive. One of judges, Melchor Cano, left before the end and was still being asked for his judgement seven years later; and Soto himself, although he was generally unsympathetic to most forms of empire, abstained. Sepúlveda's little book was not published until the nineteenth century so in some sense Las Casas and the theologians of Salamanca could be said to have won. This is certainly how the whole event was later understood. When in 1763 Boswell asked Doctor Johnson what he thought of the Spanish empire, Johnson replied, 'I love the university of Salamanca, for when the Spaniards were in doubt as to the lawfulness of their conquering America, the university of Salamanca gave it as their opinion that it was not lawful.'[7]

Johnson had not got it quite right. But for him and for many of those who, as he did, cordially detested most forms of colonialism, the debate had become symbolic of the power of moral outrage to halt, or at least slow down, the process of empire. It has been seen, too, as evidence of the other side of European imperialism, the self-scrutinizing, even self-hating fear that in the end all this might have done far greater damage than it had ever done good – far greater damage, furthermore, not only to the benighted peoples of the worlds beyond Europe but also to the Europeans themselves. Las Casas had expressed this in eschatological, apocalyptic, prophetic terms, warning Spaniards that if they did not soon mend their ways God would destroy them as he had done once before, by sending the Muslims to conquer them in 711. Later writers, such as the French philosopher Montesquieu, reflecting on the Spanish case in the eighteenth century, and the liberal political theorist Alexis de Tocqueville, commenting on French Algeria in the nineteenth, would warn other generations of unrepentant imperialists that no one can afford for long to practise atrocities and tyrannies overseas without the evil that they do seeping back to contaminate the homeland.

To later generations Las Casas became a symbol of the fight

against the injustices of colonialism. In 1810, Simón Bolívar, 'The Liberator' of South America, described him as, 'that friend of humanity who with such fervour and determination denounced to his government and his contemporaries the most horrific acts of that sanguineous frenzy'. Even in Spain itself, despite murmurings of protest from the Catholic reactionaries of the late nineteenth century, he has been hailed as the 'authentic expression of the true Spanish conscience', in an attempt to explain away the destruction of the Amerindian peoples as a passing aberration in the nation's history. For many, in Spain and beyond, his presence has seemed somehow to redeem the inescapable complicity of all Europe in the Spanish conquests. The Abbé Guillaume Raynal, author together with the philosopher and man-of-letters Denis Diderot, of the *Philosophical and Political History of the Two Indies* of 1780, the fiercest and most widely read condemnation of European colonialism written during the Enlightenment, looked forward to a more generous age when 'these unfortunate lands which have been destroyed will be repopulated and acquire laws, customs, justice and liberty'. He imagined a statue, 'In which you will be shown standing between the American and the Spaniard, holding out your breast to the dagger of the latter to save the life of the former. And on the base such words as these should be inscribed: IN A CENTURY OF FEROCITY, LAS CASAS, WHO YOU SEE BEFORE YOU, WAS A BENEVOLENT MAN.'[8] Today, throughout the Americas there are many such statues. In Latin America Las Casas' presence remains a powerful one. He has been represented as a kind of Catholic Marxist *avant la lettre* and is looked upon as the founding father of liberation theology, the semi-heterodox movement within the Latin American church which has tried to direct the attention of the clergy once again to the suffering of the poor and the oppressed.

But for all the passion of his rhetoric, Las Casas was no modern critic of colonialism. He was firmly committed to the view that the Americas were the legitimate property of the crown of Spain. He even went so far as to say so in his will. He never doubted the superiority of European civilization, never doubted that without Christ the inhabitants of the Americas would have been doomed to eternal damnation, never doubted that it was only with the coming of Columbus that 'these numberless peoples who had laid in oblivion throughout so many centuries' had finally entered history. Las Casas' reading of history both legitimated the Spanish occupation of the Americas in the name of the church and ultimately made the Europeans the paternal instructors of all those who would later come to be called the 'backward' races of the world. What it did not do was to sanction the indiscriminate exploitation of these races, nor did it deprive them of their humanity or their rights. As Las Casas insisted time and again, although God's deliverance of the Americas to the Castilian crown had granted it incontestable political rights, it had imposed upon it a severe moral duty which, at least during his lifetime, it had done very little to fulfil.

6   *The decline of the Iberian world*

Las Casas' protests against the cruelty of the Spanish settlers had been made not only when Spain was the most powerful state in Europe but when its ruler, Charles V, could reasonably claim to be the heir to Augustus, the bringer of order and peace to the entire world. In 1555–6, exhausted by his struggles to keep his scattered domains together and to contain the menace of Protestantism, Charles abdicated in favour of his son Philip and retired to the remote Spanish monastery of Juste. There he spent the remainder of his days eating gargantuan meals and playing with ingenious clockwork toys. In the complex process of succession Philip lost the Austrian homelands, Germany and Bohemia, together with the imperial title, to his uncle Ferdinand. But in 1580 he acquired through the uncertainties of dynastic succession the kingdom of Portugal and with it the now sprawling Portuguese overseas empire. This vast conglomerate, the Catholic Monarchy as it came to be known, lasted until 1640 and it spanned the entire globe.

Only parts of Asia, China and India now lay seemingly beyond Philip's reach. In 1565, Spanish forces seized what were called in his honour the Philippines, and there, close to the Asian mainland, fantastical plots began to be hatched for the invasion of China. In 1584, the bishop of Malacca, João Ribeiro Gaio, came up with a scheme for a joint Spanish and Portuguese attack on the Chinese mainland by way of Sumatra, Patani and Thailand. Two years later a 'general assembly of the Spanish inhabitants of the Philippines' led by the bishop and the governor drew up a petition urging the king to prepare for the conquest of China and entrusted a Jesuit, Alonso Sánchez, to carry it in person to the king. Nothing came of this. The great Italian Jesuit sinologist Matteo Ricci, who had adopted Chinese dress and been accepted into the Chinese intelligentsia, poured scorn on the project. He knew that China was endless and alien, that no European monarch, however great, could sustain the allegiance of such distant and complex peoples, that his armies would lose themselves in the inner wastes of the empire and starve to death.[1] Neither was Philip himself, despite his occasional messianic claims to universal empire, able to contemplate any further expansion. For all his conviction that he was doing God's work in the world, he was not a Holy Roman emperor and most of his efforts and most of his wealth went not into conquering and converting all that remained of the world but into sustaining what he had inherited, a monarchy which slowly but inexorably was beginning to unravel.

What contemporaries called 'the decline of Spain' had, however, already begun by the mid-sixteenth century.[2] In 1568 the Netherlands, the heart of the old Duchy of Burgundy where Charles V had been born, rose in revolt. A long and bitter war ensued which gradually drew in most of the states of Europe, squandered massive resources and millions of lives and, in its final stages, spread across half the globe. It lasted, on and off, for eighty years until in 1648 the Spanish were finally driven to acknowledge the existence of the new state. Already in 1579 the United Netherlands (modern Holland) as it was known, had become first in practice and then in law a republic. For the first time in European history, a rebellious vassal state had succeeded in acquiring self-determination. The new republic now stood poised to become an imperial power in its own right.

Spain was financially and morally bankrupted by what the Dutch call the Eighty Years War (and the Spanish the Revolt of the Netherlands). Burdened with the need to hold together diverse, over-extended states, Philip II and his successors Philip III and IV had been overly concerned with the short-term gains of war and insufficiently mindful of the long-term economic needs of the various peoples of which their monarchy was composed. Spain, and Castile in particular, had been hit by the runaway inflation that had followed the importation of astonishing quantities of silver and gold from America. No one at the time really understood the mechanisms of inflation or had very much idea about how economics in general worked. In a world without monetary policies, economic crises were all too often attributed to God's disfavour. Neither did anyone have any clear idea about the relationship between wealth and scarcity, and precious metals tended to be treated as fetishes rather than as means of exchange. Columbus had been so certain of the inherent power of gold that he had once declared it could make a man 'jump into heaven'. As Adam Smith pointed out later, Spain's problems could all be attributed to the failure to understand that the increase in the production of bullion could only ever lead to its devaluation. 'The same passion,' he wrote, 'which has suggested to many people the absurd idea of the philosopher's stone, has suggested to others the equally absurd one of immense rich mines of gold and silver. They did not consider that the value of those metals has, in all ages and nations, arisen chiefly from their scarcity.'[3]

Because of its rulers' obsession with the illusory wealth to be found in precious metals, Spain had also failed to develop the potential of its overseas possessions for trade and agriculture. Many of the more far-sighted conquistadors, Hernán Cortés among them, had been eager to stress the potentially disastrous consequences of the grab-and-run mentality that had marked the early conquests. Few wanted to see a repetition of the virtual devastation of the population of the Antilles, which followed on the Spanish conquest. Yet despite moderate reforms, the maintenance of the supply of gold and silver continued to be the crown's principal economic concern. Even in the 1770s and 1780s, when a concerted effort was made to modernize the empire according to free-trade principles, the final objective was the reinvigoration of the production of the silver mines. Time and again the Spanish crown was forced to default on its loans. The economy slid into stagnation. What resources there were went increasingly into protecting Spanish and Portuguese overseas possessions and shipping from attack by the new contenders for control of the world's oceans, the English, the French and, as they broke free of their Spanish masters, the Dutch.

Even by the late sixteenth century, the Dutch had begun an onslaught on the Portuguese possessions in Asia, which were far more vulnerable than the Spanish colonies in America. By the mid-seventeenth century they had taken Cochin, Malacca, Sumatra, Java, Borneo, the Celebes, the Moluccas, the western end of New Guinea, Formosa and, most importantly, Indonesia. When in 1658 they finally managed to seize Ceylon all that remained of the Portuguese empire in the East Indies was Goa in southern India and Macao. Portugal held on to Brazil until 1822, despite Dutch and French incursions, and her settlements in West Africa until the mid-twentieth century, but the empire that Prince Henry had set in motion in 1434 had relinquished most of its wealth and all its power by the end of the seventeenth century.[4]

Slowly Spain also began to lose its grip on its overseas empire. By the mid-seventeenth century much of the trade between the colonies was being carried in foreign ships, largely to the benefit of foreign merchants. By the 1680s, the French had moved south from Canada to found New Orleans, French and English buccaneers had sacked Panama, Cartagena and Veracruz; and Spain's naval power had fallen so low that during the War of the Spanish Succession (1702–13) French warships were used to escort the treasure fleets home from New Spain. The war followed the death in 1700 of the last of the Habsburg kings, Charles II, known as the 'bewitched', a man who was probably impotent, certainly feeble-minded, and whose reign had been, in the words of the Venetian ambassador, 'an uninterrupted series of disasters'. When the war ended, a branch of the French Bourbon family had gained control of the Spanish throne which they have retained, with interruptions, to this day. In the process Spain lost all her remaining European possessions and the empire was reduced, in effect, to the Americas and the Philippines. These would remain, although increasingly independent and reliant upon foreign trade, for another century.

By the beginning of the nineteenth century, however, the Spanish colonists, as the English had done before them, began to resent the autocratic presence of a remote and declining European power with which few of them could now identify.

Between 1808 and 1826 in a series of bloody wars the Kingdoms of the Indies, as they had been called, were finally extinguished. In their place there arose a number of competing, mutually hostile and internally unstable republics, which have remained divided and unsettled to this day. Finally in 1898, the United States occupied and 'liberated' the Philippines, and drove the Spanish out of Cuba and Puerto Rico. The sun had now set on an empire which, at its height, had covered more than half the globe.

7   *Empires of liberty, empires of trade*

Within less than a century Europeans had taken possession of much of America and had established enduring footholds in Asia and Africa. This rapid overseas expansion had been made possible by social and economic changes in the emerging European nation-states, the development of new navigational techniques, and the evolution of ships that could sail rapidly and effectively against the wind. They had taken place, too, against the background of one of the most enduring social transformations in the history of the continent of Europe itself. On 18 April 1521, an otherwise obscure Augustinian monk named Martin Luther appeared before Charles V at the imperial diet at the city of Worms to answer charges of heterodoxy. Luther's rebellion against the Catholic church might have passed largely unperceived. There had, after all, been many protests against the corruptions of the clergy as well as theological objections, like Luther's, to the notion that the church might have some say in who gained God's favour and who did not. But the German princes and free cities chose to make use of this somewhat dyspeptic monk to mount a resistance to Charles V's increasing attempt to transform the Holy Roman empire from a loose federation of independent states into a true empire.

Their quarrel with the emperor broadened into prolonged confessional conflict. Since it was always hard to distinguish religion from politics, this rapidly developed into ideological warfare. It was the first time that the peoples of Europe had confronted one another not over dynastic claims or rights of succession, but over differences in belief. From the War of the League of Schmalkalden (an alliance of Protestant princes and cities) in 1546–7 until the Treaty of Westphalia in 1648, which finally brought to an end the Thirty Years War, one or another region of Europe was convulsed by the most bloody and ferocious civil and ideological struggle in its history prior to the outbreak of the Second World War.

The Treaty of Westphalia changed all this – or at least so it seemed to contemporaries. It was the first truly modern treaty. (Most previous ones had been little more than agreements to cease hostilities.) It created what has come to be called the Europe of Nations. It established, if only in a shadowy way, the conception of an international community and it ratified the existence of two new states, both republics: the United Netherlands and the Swiss Confederation. By the terms of the agreement, to which all the major powers of Europe were party, it would no longer be possible for nations to fight among themselves over how to interpret God's intentions for humankind. Now it would be the ruler of each state who would decide what brand of Christianity was followed in his realm. The papacy, which had acted, if often fitfully and ineffectually, as an arbiter in international disputes, would henceforth be relegated to the sidelines, its power limited to the realm of the sacred and no longer universal or very powerful even there.

By the time the treaty was signed, the map of Europe had undergone a transformation. Where once there had been religious unity across most of the continent, a confessional curtain had been lowered which separated a largely Protestant north from a largely Catholic south. This divide was not merely religious. It was also cultural, political and economic. By the middle of the seventeenth century new ideas in the arts and the sciences were moving steadily northwards. The imperial powers of the Iberian peninsula, although still among the richest in Europe, were clearly in decline. Their old enemies, France, England and the Netherlands, were in the ascendant. London and Amsterdam replaced Lisbon and Madrid. A pattern had been set which would last until the twentieth century.

In the process of transformation the old European visions of universal empire had faded away. Among other things, the Reformation had been a struggle against a new kind of imperialism in Europe. It is not surprising that the new Protestant nations which it finally created should have evolved their own notions of what empire could and should be. No one nation in Europe could aspire to dominate even a substantial part of the continent. Nor could any one claim to be entitled to conquer the world, although they might attempt to gain some other kind of control over it.

The balance had shifted in other ways, too. The lure of the Spanish empire had lain initially in the vast quantities of gold and silver it had been able to extract from the Americas. At first, the French and the English had merely set out to do the same. The French navigator Jacques Cartier embarked on his first expedition to what is now Canada in 1534, just as Columbus had before him, with the aim of 'discovering certain islands and lands where it is said that a great quantity of gold and other rich things might be discovered'. Like Columbus, he had returned with tales of a mysterious land of untold wealth.

But all he had to show for it were some samples of ore which on examination turned out to be not gold and silver but iron pyrites and quartz.[1] Similarly, the expeditions that Martin Frobisher led to Newfoundland in 1576, 1577 and 1578 had all gone in search of precious metals. They, too, had returned empty-handed. All Frobisher had been able to bring back were two 'Eskimos' from Baffin Island who, he explained, were, in the absence of anything more serviceable, 'tokens from thence of his being there'. They only lived for a year, exhibits for the amusement of the aristocracy, who watched them hunting the royal swans on the Thames from a skin-covered boat. They were nothing more than curiosities, part of the contemporary passion for exotica, the living equivalent of the unicorn horns and pickled mermaids to be found in the cabinets of curios which adorned many noblemen's homes.[2]

By the beginning of the seventeenth century it had become evident to all the new would-be imperial powers that the future lay not in the vain pursuit of further Aztec and Inca empires or the fantastical El Dorado – the elusive land of gold, the failure to find which had in 1618 cost Sir Walter Raleigh his head. It lay instead in trade, that new 'golden ball', as the Scot Andrew Fletcher of Saltoun called it in 1704, 'for which all nations of the world are contending'. And the only way to secure this golden ball was through mastery of the world's oceans. In the end even Raleigh, England's only would-be conquistador, came to see this. 'Whosoever commands the Sea,' he reflected, 'commands the trade, whosoever commands the trade of the world, commands the riches of the world and consequently the world itself.'[3]

The new discoveries made it obvious to all that domination of the lands and peoples of the world was beyond the reach of even the most powerful European nation. Control of the seas, however, clearly was not. A new form of universalism took hold. The empires of the largely Protestant and increasingly capitalist north would, like their predecessors, encircle the globe. But unlike their predecessors, they would all be, nominally at least, trading empires, largely eschewing colonization and conquest except as a means of last resort. They were to be built upon wealth, not military might. This involved what, by the mid-eighteenth century, was to become a massive shift in sensibilities. The rise in Britain and France of a new merchant class, educated, generally enlightened and with very little stake in the older military aristocracies, led to a powerful celebration of the civilizing and humanizing power of commerce. For commerce involved not merely the exchange of goods. It also demanded contact between peoples and with that, or so it was hoped, greater understanding and tolerance among them. 'Everything in the universe,' wrote the Marquis de Mirabeau in 1758, 'is commerce because by commerce one must understand all the natural and indispensable relationships of the entire species, which are, and will always be those between one man and another, between one family, one society, one nation and another.'

Many were also convinced that commerce was the only means to put an end to international conflict, for there was a widespread conviction that, in Diderot's words, 'A war among commercial nations is a fire that destroys them all.' Like the not dissimilar modern belief that democracies never go to war with one another, this proved in time to be an illusion since commerce could, and generally did, become as much a source of conflict as of peace. But the association of commerce with both peace and liberty survived even the great trade wars of the late eighteenth and early nineteenth centuries. 'War then comes before commerce,' as the French liberal Benjamin Constant expressed it in 1813, after witnessing the collapse of the Napoleonic empire; 'the former is all savage impulse, the latter civilized calculation.'[4]

Paradoxically perhaps, the earliest European overseas empire to be almost wholly concerned with trade rather than conquest was the Portuguese. As we have seen, the first Portuguese attempts at settlement and conquest in Africa had been thwarted by the skill of the Africans, the climate and disease. In the end, the Portuguese had been compelled to confine their settlements to coastal enclaves leased to them by local rulers. These, which they called *feitorias* or factories, a term which the British would later adopt, were established throughout Africa, India and Asia: on the island of San Jorge da Mina, at Arguin, Mozambique and Melindi, in Hormuz in the Persian Gulf, Goa and Cochin in India, and Malacca and Macao in China. They were self-governing, independent communities which, although fortified and garrisoned, existed with the consent and in most cases the active participation of the local populations. The propagandists of the Portuguese empire, in particular the epic poet Luís de Camões, were inclined to describe trade as a kind of conquest. They insisted in their legal wrangles with the Dutch that they had 'discovered' both Africa and India; and ever since the mid-fifteenth century Portuguese kings had styled themselves Lords of India and Lords of Guinea. In fact, though, the only true colony the Portuguese established anywhere was in Brazil.

Britain and Holland were the European powers that truly made commerce the ideological basis of far-reaching imperial claims. Each recognized its similarity to the other. (England had, after all, played an important role in securing Dutch independence from Spain.) They also accused one another of exploiting commerce to achieve the kind of world dominance which had for so long eluded the Spanish. The Dutch, declared the English poet Robert Wild in 1673, 'Though to grasp a power as great as old Rome / Striving to carry all commerce away / And make the universe their only prey'. When a Dutchman in a tavern asked why the English called him a 'butterbox', he was told it was because 'you are so apt to spread everywhere, and for your sauciness must be melted down'.[5] To which the Dutch could have replied that they had not driven the Spanish out of the Netherlands and pursued the Portuguese to Java and beyond only to find the British trying to take their place.

Trade, as both peoples understood it, was not merely a different means of pursuing similar universal objectives to the older imperial orders. It was an entirely different way of perceiving both what an empire was and what it might become. Trade represented a different way of construing the relationships between imperialists and aboriginal peoples, and a new approach to building colonial settlements. Whereas Alexander the Great, the Romans and all their would-be heirs had sought the possession of lands and the subjugation of peoples, the maritime empires had no concern for either land or subjugation. 'The Sea,' declared Andrew Fletcher in 1698, 'is the only Empire which can naturally belong to us. Conquest is not our Interest.'[6]

These seaborne empires were also built upon the conviction, which survives in one form or another to this day, that successful commerce and capital accumulation can only take place in free societies. In their own eyes, the British and the Dutch lived under free constitutional governments, unlike the priest-ridden subjects of the Catholic Monarchy. Their empires would encircle the entire globe as surely as those of their rivals, but they would avoid all the horrors – the unrestrained destruction of indigenous peoples, depopulation, and massive inflation – which had afflicted their Iberian rivals. They would bring the maximum benefit to the metropolis at the minimum cost to all those involved, Europeans and non-Europeans, colonizers and colonized alike. Their role would not be to exploit the resources of the defenceless peoples of the non-European world but to help them overcome paganism and primitive modes of production as well, of course, as the tyranny of other Europeans. The American Indians, declared the sixteenth-century historian and geographer Richard Hakluyt, were a people 'crying out to us ... to come and help'. (This sentiment was even incorporated in 1629 into the seal of the Massachusetts Bay Company, on which an Indian is depicted saying 'Come Over and Help Us'.)[7] Little wonder that when in the 1690s the Scots attempted to found a settlement on the Isthmus of Darien, 'peaceably ... without either Fraud or Force', they fully expected the Indians to welcome them as liberators from the 'hellish servitude and oppression' they had suffered at the hands of the Spanish. To Indian eyes, however, one heavily-armed white interloper was much like another and they fled, leaving the Spanish to finish with the Scots.[8]

England's great rival for empire in the Americas, and, to a lesser degree, India, however, was not Spain or Portugal but France. The French and the English engaged in a prolonged and heated territorial dispute from the very early seventeenth century. In 1609, when only a handful of settlers were clinging to the malarial swamps of the St James River, the first royal charter for the Virginia Company solemnly laid claim to all of America north of the border with what is now New Mexico and all the islands 'thereunto adjacent or within one hundred miles of the coast thereof'. The French retaliated in 1627 when they had just 107 settlers in Canada, situated in the regions of Acadia and the St Lawrence and completely isolated from one another, by asserting their rights over a territory reaching from Florida to the Arctic Circle, nearly all of which was uncharted. These disputes led to intermittent warfare between the two powers, in which the Indians skilfully played one side off against the other so as to preserve their own autonomy, a strategy which Peter Wraxall, secretary for Indian affairs in New York in the mid-eighteenth century, called 'the Modern Indian Politics'.[9]

Before the mid-eighteenth century these clashes had been sporadic and indecisive. In 1756, however, the two nations went to war as a consequence of a dispute involving the attempt by the Austrian Habsburgs to seize the Duchy of Silesia. The Seven Years War (or the French and Indian War), as it came to be called, was the first prolonged conflict between two European imperial powers which was fought extensively in their overseas territories. In 1763, by which time it had become obvious that France had nothing further to gain by continuing the struggle, the two sides signed the Treaty of Paris. This gave Britain all of North American east of the Mississippi, including Spanish Florida, as well as Senegal and French India, the capital of which, Pondichery, had been captured in 1761. The end of the Seven Years War left Britain indisputably the most powerful of the European maritime powers. It also left the crown with a crippling debt. For the next twelve years the government attempted to make up some of its financial losses by taxing the American colonists. This, and the crown's refusal to allow the colonies direct representation in parliament, precipitated the crisis which led ultimately to the American War of Independence.

In 1775, the British government prepared to fight a long and bitter war of attrition in its American colonies. It was, in the view of many, including the Irish orator and political philosopher Edmund Burke and the philosopher and economist Adam Smith, a doomed enterprise. The distance alone meant that any such struggle could only result in a British defeat, if not in the short then certainly in the long run. 'The Ocean remains,' Burke told the House of Commons on the outbreak of the war, 'you cannot pump it dry; and as long as it continues in its present bed, so long all the causes which weaken authority by distance will continue.'[10] It would be far better, suggested Adam Smith the following year, to let the American colonists go their own way in peace. They would make firmer friends and more valuable trading partners than they had ever made subjects.[11] The government of George III, of course, paid no heed since, as Smith himself sadly acknowledged, what was at stake in the war was not merely economic benefit. It was also honour. Had Britain surrendered America without a struggle, her empire would have been 'so much curtailed, [that] her power and dignity would be supposed to be proportionately diminished'. It would take a war – a civil war as it has sometimes been described – lasting eight bitter years to make her finally relinquish her hold over the colonies.

For men like Burke and Smith, the War of Independence made it obvious that the patterns of colonization that had evolved over the centuries since Columbus' first voyage had been a disaster. In the first instance, conquest and settlement created dependent communities which demanded massive and constant assistance from the metropolis if they were to survive. Later, when these had become strong (and potentially profitable), they obstinately insisted on going their own way like troublesome children grown to adulthood. Their inhabitants inevitably became new and different peoples. Edmund Burke could see this even before the English Americans had become simply Americans. 'The object,' he wrote of America, 'is wholly new in the world. It is singular ... nothing in history is parallel to it. All the reasoning about it, that are likely to be solid, must be drawn from its actual circumstances.'[12] Something similar was said by Simón Bolívar in 1810 about the peoples of his future, all-too brief state of Gran Colombia. Something like it was also voiced much later, perhaps in a more muted way, by New Zealanders, Australians and Afrikaners.

For the British, the American War and the loss of the Thirteen Colonies marked a watershed between what have come to be called the first and the second British empires. The focus of the latter would be in Asia, Africa and, later, the Pacific. It was an empire which set out to be all that the older empires had not been: commercial, benevolent, and liberal. As the British were proud of saying, even before the American revolution, Britain's empire was one of liberty. Not liberty, or at least not complete liberty, for its subject peoples, but liberty for its settler populations and, above all, liberty from the kind of crushing power which the creation of large empires so often placed in the hands of the military. Building such an empire was not, however, to be an easy task. 'There is not,' Edmund Burke had warned the House of Commons in 1766, any 'more difficult subject for the understanding of men than to govern a Large Empire upon a plan of Liberty.'

Burke, and many of the more perceptive thinkers in the troubled years of the American War of Independence, struggled hard to replace the vision of the British empire as a new Augustan Rome with Cicero's image of a 'commonwealth of all the world'. In 1775 the English radical John Cartwright came up with a plan to transform the empire into a 'Grand League of Confederacy'. This would have granted independence to all but a few of the strategic colonies – Newfoundland, Gibraltar, Minorca – and incorporated them within a kind of harmonious alliance in which, as he put it, 'this enlightened, this Christian kingdom' would go on to 'extend the influence of her religion and laws, not the limits of her empire' over the rest of the globe.[13] It was a vision rather than a proposal because, as Cartwright knew, no state, let alone a powerful centralist monarchy, has ever been known to relinquish what it has to the interests of some possible future, however attractive. But it captured an acceptable image of empire, one which in a not dissimilar form would reappear nearly two hundred years later as the Commonwealth, even if today that has become little more than a desperate attempt to preserve a vanished past.

In keeping with their image of themselves as nations of enlightened merchant adventurers rather than conquistadors, the first English and Dutch settlements in Asia were not colonies as they had been in America but factories similar to the Portuguese. The Dutch and English factories in Amboina, Surat, Madras, Calcutta and Bombay were all acquired by treaty and rapidly became international entrepôts, mixed communities of European and Asian merchants. Even if they had wanted to pursue more aggressive policies, neither power was in a position to do so. Although by 1658 the Dutch had ousted the Portuguese, neither they nor the English were any match for the forces of the Mughal empire. The brief skirmish between the East India Company and the Mughal armies in 1688–9 only resulted in the closure of the factory at Surat and the blockade of Bombay.

However, as the East India Company grew in strength so, too, did the temptation to use its power to control as well as to trade. In the early decades of the eighteenth century the Asian world had begun slowly but inexorably to change. The Muslim empires – Safavid, Ottoman and Mughal – which even at the middle of the century still nominally controlled between them all the lands from Algeria to the borders of Burma, were everywhere in retreat or decline. By 1765 the British were dominant in Bengal, the Deccan and Arcot. Gradually the East India Company became the true ruler of large areas of India although it remained until its dissolution by the crown in 1858 a vassal state, in name at least, of the Mughal emperor in Delhi.[14]

By the time Benjamin Disraeli had Queen Victoria declared 'Empress of India' in 1878, India and large areas of Africa had become in effect conquest states. Despite what might seem to be a reversion to earlier methods of conquest and settlement, British India differed in many crucial respects from British America – and from the European colonies which were to emerge in southern Africa in the nineteenth century. India, and Asia generally, was always a place of passage, not of settlement. It was governed by the British in British interests. But it was manned and at the lower levels administered largely by Indians. As the Persian chronicler Ghulam Husain Khan had noticed by the late eighteenth century, the English had 'a custom of coming for a number of years, and then of going away to pay a visit to their native land, without any one of them showing an inclination to fix himself in this land'.[15] The American colonists, by contrast, had gone with every intention of 'fixing' themselves in the land. They had gone to create in what they took to be a natural wilderness the worlds that they had lost in Europe or from which their social position had excluded them. Those who went to India did so only in order to return home richer than they had left. No sense of being a distinct people ever emerged among the Europeans in India. There was never a creole population or very much of the interracial breeding which transformed the population of many of the former Spanish-American colonies into truly multiethnic communities. The Anglo-Indians are still entitled to separate representation in the Indian parliament, but this remains a courtesy to the departed regime and reflects neither their numbers nor their political importance.

The absence of a dominant settler population and the fact that the British in India ruled through, and nominally on behalf of, the Mughal Emperor did not, however, prevent the agents of the Company from attempting to replicate all the worst excesses, real and imaginary, of the Spaniards in America. 'Turn your eyes to India,' wrote the English radical Richard Price in 1776. 'There more has been done than is now attempted in America. There Englishmen, actuated by the love of plunder and the spirit of conquest, have depopulated whole kingdoms and ruined millions of innocent peoples by the most infamous oppression and rapacity. The justice of the nation has slept over these enormities. Will the justice of heaven sleep? Are we not now execrated on both sides of the globe?'[16]

At the centre of this image was the figure of Warren Hastings, governor-general of Bengal from 1772 to 1785. Hastings had amassed a personal fortune, it was said, at the Company's expense and had extorted funds by force from the rulers of Benares and Avadh. 'There would seem,' remarked one of the judges at the trial for his impeachment in 1788, 'no species of peculation from which the Honourable Governor-General has thought it reasonable to abstain.' He had also, on his own admission, ruled Bengal as an 'Oriental despot'. Hastings was finally acquitted in 1795, but his trail was a great theatrical event in which were played out all the passions and anxieties that by the late eighteenth century had come to torment most European imperial states. It was stage-managed in large measure by Edmund Burke.

Burke was a great conservative and passionate denouncer of all modes of political passion. But he shared with such radicals as Price, whom he otherwise loathed, a hatred of any kind of behaviour he saw as tyrannical. The East India Company had, he claimed, become 'one of the most corrupt and destructive tyrannies that probably ever existed'.[17] Under Hastings' governorship it had perpetrated 'cruelties unheard-of, and devastations almost without name'. It had abused its power to further its own ends and, worse, it had trampled on those of its Indian subjects to whom, in Burke's conception of liberty, it owed a duty of benevolence every bit as great as to any of its European agents. To argue, as Hastings had done, that to win respect in Asia one had to rule as an Asian was to threaten all the principles, political and moral, on which the British constitution rested. It was to let 'barbarism' in. It was that most unforgivable of colonial crimes, to 'go native'.

Hastings' views horrified Burke for much the same reason as the presence of the Yorkshirewoman turned Indian would later horrify Borges' grandmother. For Burke knew, as did she, how delicate the tissue of 'civilization' and 'liberty' was, and how very easy it was to slip through it and then on down the human scale into the disordered worlds that lay only a very short distance below. Empire had given the Europeans enormous responsibilities towards the poor benighted 'savages'. It had hugely enhanced their sense of their superior grasp of what it was to be fully human. But it had also brought them face to face with both the realities and the temptations of barbarism. Burke and the enlightened rationalists of his day understood all human history to be a perpetual cycle in which barbarism gave way to civilization, only to be replaced once more by barbarism as civilization decayed, became weak, corrupt, and overrun by that most feared of eighteenth-century ills, 'luxury'. In 1776, at the precise moment when the British empire was first beginning to disintegrate, Edward Gibbon argued that in the enlightened century in which he lived the cycle appeared to have come to an end. The constant threat of a return to barbarism was, he believed, no more. But those like Burke who had heard of what had gone on beyond Europe knew otherwise.

What was on trial between 1788 and 1795 was therefore not only Warren Hastings, it was a way of governing, a way of conceiving of empire itself. Burke and the other mangers of Hastings' trial clearly harboured a deep and dispassionate concern for the well-being of the Indian subjects of the Company. They were quite sincere in their horror at what they had heard of its treatment of those who, after all, were not only free subjects but belonged to a civilization which, in some vaguely conceived sense, they recognized to be as ancient and once as great as their own. The trial was, unsurprisingly, never a popular one. Yet Burke pursued Hastings in the face of fierce opposition from those whom he once described in a letter as the 'white-men' – perhaps the first time a European has employed such an epithet for his own people.

Burke's dogged pursuit of Hastings was driven, however, by another more urgent concern. Like Las Casas before him, he realized that nothing could be practised with impunity in some distant outpost without it having consequences for the metropolis. What applied to Spain might equally apply to Britain. An Englishman could not, as Hastings had done, be an Asian despot in India without sooner or later becoming a despot also in England. To deny liberty and the right of freedom from cruelty and oppression to others could only come to undermine one's own right to such things. An empire was a whole and could only be governed as a whole. 'In order to prove that the Americans have no right to their liberties,' Burke had written of the American War, 'we are every day endeavouring to subvert the maxims which preserve the whole Spirit of our own.' The same was now true of the rights of the Indians. 'I am certain,' he wrote, 'that every means effectual to preserve India from oppression is a guard to preserve the British Constitution from its worst corruption.'[18] Empire was not the means to personal aggrandizement Hastings had made of it. It was a sacred trust 'given by an incomprehensible dispensation of Divine providence into our hands'. To abuse it might not call down the wrath of God on the head of King George – Burke shared none of Las Casas' faith in divine retribution – but it did threaten the collapse of what Burke thought of as 'the civilization of Europe'.[19]

Burke's warning, however, fell on deaf ears. The history of the British domination of India perhaps demonstrated that the lure of conquest and possession was inescapable. Britain, which had begun by condemning the Spanish and by insisting that theirs was to be an empire of trade governed in the name of liberty, had ended by becoming one of the most aggressive and rapacious of imperial powers. Yet the vision of empire as the expansion of civilization, as the benevolent rule of the more gifted and more able, as a duty as well as a right, survived the trial of Warren Hastings. By the early nineteenth century what Napoleon would call the 'civilizing mission' of the European powers came to be looked upon as an integral part of the culture of Europe. It was, after all, the one aspect of the Roman world which the modern imperialist could adopt with pride. Later, as we shall see, it became tinged with a racism which had been virtually absent from the ancient world, and in so doing it sowed the seeds of the end not only of the European overseas empires but of empire itself.

8 *Slavery*

The British concern to build an 'empire of liberty' for its subject peoples failed in the long run to suppress entirely the desire for the acquisition of territory. For much of its existence it also turned its face away from the dark stain that had spread across all European overseas empires: slavery.

All empires in history prior to the beginning of the nineteenth century have been slave-owning societies. Slaves were everywhere the silent and silenced masses, the peoples with whose labour Athenian democracy and Roman republicanism had been created. In antiquity 'the people' meant only the citizenry, and that excluded all slaves, as well as all women and children. The Greeks, wrote Herodotus, in what has subsequently become a commonplace, were the most free of peoples because they alone were subject not to the will of an individual but only to the law. For Herodotus the vast slave populations on which the city-states of Greece were built simply did not exist. The same was true for every Greek or Roman citizen. Occasionally, but only occasionally, slaves surface briefly in the literature to remind us that beneath this rich and varied culture there were other peoples, other races who had made all this possible.

In antiquity slaves had come from all over the Greek and Roman worlds, from Syria, Egypt, Judaea, Dacia, Moesia, Germany, Gaul and Britain. They had performed many tasks.

Some had even occupied positions of considerable responsibility and relatively high social standing, which is probably why Odysseus believed that it was generally better in the world he knew to be a slave than a free labourer. The Romans had employed Greek slaves as tutors and household administrators. Athens in the fourth century BC was policed by a body of 300 Scythian archers who were slaves. Cicero's confidential secretary, who invented a form of shorthand which was named after him, was a slave called Tiro.[1] The Muslim world relied heavily on slave armies known as mamlûks, and in Egypt and Syria in the thirteenth century they succeeded in taking control of the state itself.

With the collapse of the Roman empire, however, this diversity rapidly vanished in the West. The Germanic peoples who overran the empire belonged to fragmentary societies with only limited engineering capabilities. Tribal in organization and nomadic or pastoral in origin, they were in no position either to acquire or to control the vast slave populations which had sustained the extensive building programmes, civic projects and complex urban lifestyles of those they had vanquished. In medieval Europe slaves were employed predominantly as agricultural labourers and supplemented a largely peasant workforce. In the end even field slavery was driven out by the spread of feudalism, the expansion of an agrarian economy and new agricultural technologies. Indentured peasants were easier to control than slaves and generally more productive. Slaves still continued to act as domestic servants; but within Europe at least, by the end of the Middle Ages the institution had ceased to fulfil any significant economic function.

Modern slavery was in many ways a new beginning and quite

unlike its ancient and medieval predecessors. It began on the morning of 8 August 1444 when the first cargo of 235 Africans, taken from what is now Senegal, was put ashore at the Portuguese port of Lagos. A rudimentary slave market was improvised on the docks and the confused and cowed Africans, reeling from weeks confined in the insalubrious holds of the tiny ships on which they had come, were herded into groups by age, sex and the state of their health. 'What heart could be so hard,' wrote the chronicler Gomes Eannes de Zurara who recorded the event,

> as not to be pierced with piteous feeling to see that company? Some held their heads low, their faces bathed in tears as they looked at each other; some groaned very piteously looking towards the heavens fixedly and crying out loud, as if they were calling on the father of the universe to help them. To increase their anguish still more, those who were in charge of the divisions then arrived and began to separate them one from another so that they formed five equal lots. This made it necessary to separate sons from their fathers and wives from their husbands, and brother from brother ... And as soon as the children who had been assigned to one group saw their parents in another they jumped up and ran towards them; mothers clasped their children in their arms and lay face downwards on the ground, accepting wounds with contempt for the suffering of their flesh rather than let their children be torn from them.

One person, it seems, who remained entirely unmoved was Prince Henry 'the Navigator' who had sponsored the voyage. He rode, according to Zurara, 'on a powerful horse accompanied by his people'. He extracted, as was his due, the royal fifth of all the sales – forty-six slaves in all – and then rode away. The traffic in 'Black Gold' had begun.[2]

The slaves sold that day would have found their way into private households in Portugal or on to private estates. But those who were to follow them in their hundreds of thousands were shipped not to Europe but across the Atlantic to the American colonies. Modern slavery was the creation of a new form of empire-building. It was developed to supply the manpower for a particular socio-economic unit – the sugar plantation – which had been unknown in the old world.[3] It was sugar which was responsible for the massive growth in the slave trade, between the fifteenth and eighteenth centuries, and it was the value of sugar to the economies of the slaving nations which made the abolition of slavery at the end of the eighteenth century such a protracted and uncertain business. As Daniel Defoe put it in 1713, 'No African Trade, no Negroes, No Negroes, No Sugar; no Sugar no Islands, no Islands no Continent, no Continent no Trade; that is to say farewell to your American Trade, your West Indian Trade.'

In its scale and its long-term consequences for population distribution – not to mention its sheer barbarity – it surpassed anything that had previously taken place. After the failure of the initial slave raids in Senegal and Senegambia, the Portuguese purchased their slaves from Africa and Arab middlemen. (Prince Henry justified this on the grounds that by buying slaves from Muslims he was turning their greed against them, and ultimately depriving them of vital manpower. Buy enough slaves, he argued, and the way would soon be open for a new Portuguese crusade against the African Infidel.) The slave trade had been endemic within Africa for centuries – a fact upon which its supporters tirelessly insisted. But the Europeans hugely increased the demand and by so doing encouraged African slavers to devastate whole areas and effectively exterminate entire peoples in the African hinterland. Europe, as the Marquis de Condorcet protested in 1781, 'is thus guilty not only of the crime of making slaves of men, but, on top of that, of all the slaughter committed in Africa in order to prepare for that crime'.[4]

The European demand for slaves transformed what had been a local commercial practice into the greatest forced migration in human history. Between 1492 and 1820 five or six times as many Africans went to America as did white Europeans. Modern slavery shattered entire cultures within Africa and built new ones on the far side of the Atlantic. It contributed to the creation of interracial communities, of Europeans and Africans, Africans and Native Americans, Asians and Africans, and it fragmented and dissipated communities which once were, or believed themselves to be, solidly endogamous. It also provided vast fortunes for those who lived by it and turned otherwise small, unremarkable seaports – Liverpool and Nantes, Bristol and Newport – into thriving, wealthy and sometimes sophisticated metropolises. It transformed small African communities such as Dahomey into powerful states. It made Brazil, the Caribbean and southern North America into multiracial societies in which Africans soon outnumbered the dwindling indigenous inhabitants or replaced them altogether.

Modern slavery was new, too, in its reliance upon a massive transatlantic trade. Trading in slaves had been a feature of both antiquity and the Middle Ages, and it had formed an important part of the Scandinavian economy between the eighth and eleventh centuries. But all of this was on a relatively small scale in comparison with the massive exportation of human merchandise that took place between the late sixteenth and early nineteenth centuries. Few had died in the ancient world as a consequence of the trade; countless millions perished during the infamous 'middle passage' between Africa and the Americas.[5]

Modern slavery also required a new conception of the relationship between slave and master. In antiquity slavery had been accepted as part of the order of the world. Some, such as Aristotle and Cicero, had tried to theorize the master-slave relationship as one between two types of persons: those who were naturally wise and masterful, and those who were naturally servile. But even Aristotle had been unable to distinguish clearly between the two. Natural slaves should, he argued, be everywhere robust, and natural rulers everywhere delicate and refined, 'making the one strong for servile labour, the other upright and although useless for service, useful for the political life in the arts of both peace and war'. Yet he was forced to concede that 'the opposite frequently happens – that some have the souls and others the bodies of freemen'.[6] Nature, it would seem, is not always able to fulfil her own intentions. The idea, however, had a rich afterlife. It was much used by the Spanish in America, and employed in a slightly modified, more emphatically biological form in the nineteenth century by both the British in Australia and the French in Africa.[7]

In practice, however, one became a slave in antiquity as a 'punishment' for having fought on the losing side in a war. (Unwanted children who had been exposed by their parents could also be enslaved, although this does not seem to have happened very often.) Those who were defeated in battle were generally slain, those who were not were 'saved', the price of their salvation being enslavement. As late as 1804, one of opponents of the abolitionists, William Devyanes, a former Chairman of the East India Company, following the same general logic, proposed that the slave trade could be defended on the grounds that 'if the slave merchants did not purchase from him and others, their prisoners taken in war would be killed'.

The triumph of Christianity made very little difference to this view. Both the Old Testament and the Qur'an accepted that it was legitimate to enslave individuals, and indeed entire populations, in the pursuit of supposedly just wars, and there is nothing in the gospels to contradict this. The church did attempt to restrict the degree to which Christians might themselves be enslaved by other Christians, but was prepared to countenance the enslavement of Christians by non-Christians. (Martin Luther even warned Christian slaves against 'stealing themselves' away from their Muslim masters.)

The vast majority of modern slaves, and all those employed on the plantations in America, were Africans who had clearly not been acquired in a 'just' war. How then could such enslavement possibly be legitimate? Some early attempts were made by the Portuguese, the Spanish and the French to argue that the African internal warfare of which they were the beneficiaries, and which they had, if not created, certainly greatly exacerbated, had itself been 'just'. When in 1546 the Spanish theologian Francisco de Vitoria, who was otherwise so severe in his criticism of the Spanish occupation of America, was asked about the moral validity of the Portuguese claim to have purchased slaves who had been taken in a 'just' African war, he replied that it was not up to the slavers to discover 'the justice of wars between barbarians'. All they needed was the assurance of the traders that the human merchandise they were buying had been legitimately acquired, 'and they may be bought without a qualm'.[8] Needless to say, when they were called upon to do so the African slavers were all too happy to provide such assurances, although they must have found the European need for them deeply puzzling.

Few, however, found such arguments very convincing. Between 1684 and 1686 the Holy Office (the papal Inquisition) received a number of petitions, mostly from a Portuguese mulatto named Lourenço da Silva, denouncing such self-serving justifications of the trade. Da Silva's initiative received considerable support from the Capuchin order whose missionary efforts in the Congo had been constantly thwarted by the slave-traders. In 1686 the Holy Office actually went so far as to condemn the slave trade (although not slavery as such). Since it took no action against the slavers themselves, the injunction was wholly ignored. But it did give some moral weight to the opponents of the trade; and some of Da Silva's arguments, in particular that free peoples of colour should be treated just as free whites, may have inspired the French *Code noir* of 1688. This remained in force in the French overseas possessions until the revolution and, although on most issues it followed the Roman law on slavery, it did guarantee at least in theory a greater measure of independence to slaves than existed in any of the other European colonies.

As protests against slavery and the slave trade in particular mounted, it became increasingly difficult to find any sustainable argument for its existence. Neither the just war thesis nor any kind of racism could finally stand up to close examination. The conviction that the slave was some kind of lesser being ran counter to the very nature of the master-slave relationship, which demanded of slaves a far higher degree of comprehension and rational calculation than were possessed by the domestic animals after which, in a sustained attempt to deny the obvious fact of their humanity, their masters frequently named them: Jumper, Juno, Fido, and so on. Slaves could, after all, breed with their masters – a persistent fear in slave-holding societies. They could converse with their masters; they could even, as Benjamin Franklin observed, unlike sheep, rise in revolt against their masters.

For a convinced Christian, there was always the claim that although the slave might be constituted like any other human being, Africans knew nothing of Christianity before they were enslaved. Slavery, therefore, had saved them from eternal damnation. No matter how appalling the slaves' condition might be – and many claimed to believe that it was in fact no worse than that of day-labourers in Europe – it was far better for their minds and their souls to be enslaved among civilized beings than free among their own savage kind. What was a little suffering and privation in this world in comparison with hell-fire in the next? Zurara might have been somewhat disingenuous when he claimed that Prince Henry's 'entire riches' lay not in the forty-six slaves he had taken in August 1444 but in the certainty 'of the salvation of those souls which had before been lost', but he was in effect stating what in the following centuries was to become a commonplace. The philosopher John Locke, who passionately denounced slavery as 'so vile and miserable an estate of Man, and so directly opposed to the Generous Temper and Spirit of our Nation' that ' 'tis hardly to be conceived that an *Englishman* much less a *Gentleman* would plead for it', nevertheless held shares in the Royal Africa Company, the main business of which was the slave trade, and defended slavery for Africans on the ground that it rescued them from the worse fate of barbarism and eternal damnation. Even the seventeenth-century Jesuit Antonio de Vieira, who was one of the very few to speak openly against all forms of slavery, transformed the sufferings of the Indians in Brazil into a vocation which had 'illuminated' them and for which they would receive 'eternal inheritance as a reward'. 'Oh what a change of fortune,' he told them, 'will be yours at that time, and what astonishment and confusion for those who have so little humanity today!'

What is missing from Zurara's account and even from Vieira's indignation, what is missing from nearly all the pleas for the abolition of slavery before the middle of the eighteenth century, is the awareness that suffering is a human universal. Because the curious creatures Zurara had seen on the docks at Lagos could suffer as he could they must indeed be human, and their humanity necessarily imposed an obligation to alleviate it. There are, after all, many better ways of becoming Christian.

The slave's right to freedom of choice, even the right to select his or her own forms of indebtedness – which most clearly distinguished the slave from the European day-labourer – was a mode, as Diderot phrased it, of 'an enjoyment in one's own mind' to which all human beings are entitled. The slave, denied this feature of what it is to be a person, was thus reduced to a level lower even than that of the dogs which the Spaniards had brought with them to America. For the dog is only an auto-maton, whereas the slave still retains some grasp on what nothing can deprive him of, his consciousness. He or she alone *knows* that he or she is a slave. Only the slave among living beings has been denied all cause for hope, all expectation of what Diderot called 'those happy times, those centuries of Enlightenment and of prosperity' which might one day allow even the most miserable labourer to recover his identity to the full.

In the end, it was humanitarian arguments such as these which brought the whole business to an end – that and the fact that by the mid-eighteenth century the slave trade had begun to be far less profitable than it had once been.[9] Yet even the abolitionists, while they loathed both the trade and the institution, still clung firmly to a belief in the civilizing potential of European culture. William Wilberforce, the most outspoken, dogged and successful of them, remained convinced that emancipating the Africans might ultimately be less important than bringing 'the reign of light and truth and happiness among them', by which he meant primarily Christianity and British 'laws, institutions and manners'.

The abolitionists recognized that as humans the Africans had an absolute right to freedom, but this did not make them the equal of the Europeans, nor did it exempt them from certain kinds of tutelage. Claims for the inferiority of the African and the consequent rights of the European to long-term tutelage remained a significant ideological prop for the European overseas empires in the nineteenth century. They had, and in some areas continue to have, a determining impact on the modern relationship between the developed and developing worlds.

Slavery of any formal kind – for there are many informal kinds still in existence – came to an end in the territories of the European overseas empires during the first decades of the nineteenth century. The first European state to outlaw the slave trade was Denmark in 1792. British involvement in the trade ended in 1805–7 and by 1824 slaving had become a capital offence. The African reaction to all this was, predictably, one of bewilderment. Why, the King of the Ashanti asked a British official in 1820, had his people sudden stopped buying slaves when the Muslims continued to do so? Were not their Gods the same and if the Qur'an did not forbid slavery why was it that the Bible had suddenly begun to do so? He received no answer.

Together with the attempts to outlaw the trade, the Western powers had also made a number of sporadic attempts to return some of the victims of the trade if not exactly to their homes then at least to Africa. In 1792 a settlement duly named Freetown had been created on the Sierra Leone peninsula in West Africa by a group of British philanthropists to provide a new home for escaped or liberated slaves. After 1808 Freetown became in effect a British colony and its harbour provided the base for the British warships which patrolled the West African coast in search of slave-traders. During the next sixty years the original population of Freetown was increased by some 60,000 men, women and children who had been freed from captured slave ships.[10] Similar settlements, although far smaller and less successful, were established by the French at Libreville on the estuary of the Gabon in 1839–48, and by private American initiatives on the Grain Coast (modern Liberia) in 1821.

By the end of 1870 the trade worldwide was effectively at an end. (The last verified landing was in Cuba in January of that year.) Slavery, however, survived in Brazil until 1888, and it was not until 1890 that the General Act of Brussels committed the European colonial powers in Africa to stamp it out in their territories. In doing so they transformed the abolition of an institution which had for so long been the mainstay of their overseas empires into a part of their own 'civilizing mission'.[11]

Slavery was officially at an end. A painful period in human history, which had lasted for millennia, had been, or so it seemed, extinguished. In 1890 the Brazilian abolitionist Rui Barbosa ordered all the papers in the Ministry of the Treasury relating to slavery to be publicly burned. Among those who turned out to watch this conflagration was a worker in the customhouse, who claimed to be 108 years old. He had come, he said, to witness for himself the 'complete destruction' of the documents which contained the history of the 'martyrdom' of his race.[12] He could never perhaps have imagined that his race was also about to enter upon another kind of martyrdom, one which would not only lead to other kinds of divisions and conflicts in almost all the societies which had once benefited from the African slave trade, but which would also lead to seemingly endemic civil war within Africa itself.

9   *The final frontier*

The fight against slavery began in the middle years of the eighteenth century as Britain was in the process of losing one empire and acquiring another. It began, too, at the same time as a quite different development in the long history of the relationship between peoples. By this period most of the earth's surface had been explored, charted and in some cases colonized by Europeans. Most parts, that is, except one: the Pacific. The Pacific had, of course, been crossed and recrossed many times since the circumnavigation by the fleet which set out in 1519 under the command of Magellan. But for Europeans it remained a largely uncharted mystery, the imprecise location of 'the unknown southern land', the very existence of which comprised (along with the Northwest Passage) the last remaining geographical myth. In the eighteenth century the Pacific became the final frontier.

The fantasies that since antiquity had plagued or delighted the European imagination had been moving steadily further and further away from Europe itself. The marvels and monsters with which the ancients had populated the globe but which had failed to turn up in Europe, Africa or 'Ethiopia' were later found in 'India' or, after 1492, in America. In 1512 Juan Ponce de León went to Florida in search of the fountain of eternal youth, and Francisco de Orellana was so convincing in his description of the Amazons that he had seen there that their name, not his, was given to the great river that he was the first to navigate.

The horizon of these possibilities began to recede, however, with the advance of modern science which made increasingly improbable such curiosities as men with their faces in the middle of their chests or with one large foot which they raised over their heads at noon to protect themselves from the sun. By the time first the British, then the French and Spanish, began to explore the South Pacific no one believed any longer in such things. They did, however, still believe in something else perhaps no less chimerical. They believed that somewhere in the world there existed lands where nature provided all that humankind required, and where peoples lived wholly virtuous lives free from the terrible constraints of civilization. This vision, part fantasy and part ethnographic curiosity, was loosely based upon impressionistic travellers' tales. It was a transposed version of the dream of the earthly paradise or what in antiquity were called the Islands of the Blest. Alexander had visited it, in myth if not in reality, and it had been glimpsed briefly by eager European readers in Amerigo Vespucci's account of America – until that was shown to be a forgery. Thomas More's *Utopia* (1516), which claims to be an account by one of Vespucci's sailors, is in part at least a satire on the possibility that any such place could exist in reality.

In 1766 a French nobleman, mathematician and explorer named Antoine de Bougainville left Nantes on the frigate *La Boudeuse* with instructions to observe the transit of Venus (a means of measuring the distance of the earth from the sun) – a somewhat ironic commission in the circumstances – and if possible to complete a circumnavigation of the globe. The following year he joined up with *L'Étoile* off the Malvinas/ Falklands and headed out into the Pacific. On the morning of 4 April 1768 he landed on an island where, he later declared, 'one might think oneself in the Elysian Fields'. It had a perfect climate (untroubled, he noticed immediately, by the fearsome insects which infest most tropical paradises), an abundance of food which required no cultivation, and was inhabited by a people who seemed to have no social organization, possessed only a rudimentary religion, and lived together as one large family. Not only were they happy and peaceful, they were also beautiful, more beautiful than anything to be seen in Europe. 'The men are six feet or more,' he wrote, 'and better proportioned and better made than any I have ever encountered; no painter could find a finer model for a Hercules or a Mars.' All of them, even the aged, had 'the most beautiful teeth in the world' – no small virtue in the eighteenth century when few people over the age of thirty could count many of their own. (The botanist Sir Joseph Banks, who visited the island the following year, noted in much the same tone of surprise that their breath was 'entirely free from any disagreeable smell'.)

But it was the women who really caught Bougainville's attention and that of his crew. They were beautiful, unadorned and entirely natural. The contours of their bodies in particular had, as he observed, 'not been disfigured by fifty years of torture', a reference to the constraining corsets into which most women in Europe were strapped. Above all, 'their sole passion is love ... sweet indolence and the concern to please is their most serious occupation'. Jealousy was apparently unknown among them, and 'all are encouraged to follow the inclinations of their hearts or the law of their senses, and are publicly applauded for doing so. The air they breathe, their songs, their dances, which are almost always accompanied with lascivious gestures, all speak at every moment of the pleasures of love.' 'These people,' Bougainville concluded, 'live only in the tranquillity and the pleasure of the senses.' Because of this he called the place 'The New Cythera', after the island in the Peloponnese on which Venus had been born. We, of course, know it as Tahiti.[1]

In 1771 Bougainville published an account of his voyage, the *Voyage autour du monde*, which became a bestseller. This, and a letter by the surgeon of *La Boudeuse*, Philibert Commerson, which had appeared in the *Mercure de France* the year before, established Tahiti as an exotic – and erotic – paradise. Thereafter it became the final resting place of the myth of the 'noble savage'. For Bougainville, and later for Diderot who wrote a review of the *Voyage autour du monde* and a famous (and fictional) supplement to it, the Tahitians seemed as no other 'primitive' people had before to provide proof that somewhere in the world it was possible to live wholly fulfilled lives beyond the reach of religious dogma, laws or social conventions. In Bougainville's account Tahiti was a place without warfare or hardships. It was a place in which humankind's better instincts had not, as Diderot expressed it, been smothered by those of the 'artificial man' which European civilization had created in their stead.

Most of this, as Bougainville himself later came to recognize, was either misleading or simply false. The Tahitians were by no means unwarlike, nor did they lack either social laws or deeply-held religious beliefs. The dedication of the women to 'sweet indolence and the concern to please' was real enough, but it derived from a set of social practices and expectations no less rigid than those that in France compelled women to behave in quite other ways. Yet for all that, the Tahitians were undeniably untainted by contact with Europeans, came closer to meeting European aesthetic expectations than most other 'primitive' peoples and were certainly far more exotic than anything that had been seen since Columbus made his first landfall in 1492.

Bougainville made Tahiti famous throughout Europe. In the years that followed his voyage, British and French ships would sail across the entire length and breadth of the Pacific Ocean until virtually every island had been mapped and in most cases formally, if only fleetingly, 'possessed' by one or another of the European powers. The most celebrated of these voyages were those made under the patronage of the Royal Society by Captain James Cook between 1768 and 1778. Like Bougainville, Cook had gone to the Pacific to observe the transit of Venus and, while doing so to observe, map and record. Like Bougainville, too, though more restrained in his enthusiasms, he saw the Polynesians as living lives very close to those which all humankind must have lived before being transformed by 'civilization'. The Pacific Ocean thus became a kind of living anthropological laboratory, 'a fit soil', as John Douglas described it in the preface he wrote for the official account of Captain Cook's third voyage, 'from whence a careful observer could collect facts for forming a judgement, how far human nature will be apt to degenerate, and in what respects it can ever be able to excel'. What he termed the *novelties* of the Society or Sandwich Islands' were a record of the whole of humankind in its infancy.[2]

Bougainville and Cook enjoyed cordial, even amicable, relationships with these samples of early humankind, in so far, that is, as they were able to control their crews – not an easy task, as both men noted, with a gang of sex-starved males confronted with hordes of women whose sole passion was 'love ... sweet indolence and the concern to please'. But as with all such contacts, relationships soon became strained as more and more navigators visited the islands. The much publicized death of Cook himself in Hawaii on his third voyage in 1778, of Marion de Fresne in New Zealand in 1772, and the slaughter of twelve of the companions of the French navigator La Pérouse on Samoa, darkened the vision of the noble, gentle savage. 'No person,' wrote La Pérouse on his return, 'can imagine the Indians of the South Seas to be in a savage state. On the contrary they must have made very great progress in civilization, and I believe them to be as corrupt as the circumstances they are placed in will allow them to be.'

Yet for all that, Bougainville's elegiac and Cook's somewhat more matter-of-fact descriptions of their encounters with the Tahitians created an enduring image of the Pacific as a place where it was possible to act out all the European fantasies of sexual freedom and complete liberty from social constraint. It was an image that was still powerful enough over a hundred years later to persuade the painter Paul Gauguin to abandon home, family and a secure job for a life in the South Seas. There he found, alas, a very different Tahiti, riven by European disease, its tranquillity turned to despair by Christian missionaries.

The Pacific islands were not, however, merely the rococo pleasure grounds that Bougainville's and Commerson's descriptions had made of them. They were also revictualling places for European merchant ships and potential stages on the route to the fabled southern continent, should it exist. Both France and

Britain, watched anxiously by Spain which still looked upon the Pacific as its own special sphere of influence, had vague but quite evident designs on the potential riches of the southern ocean. Since the end of the Seven Years War the French, in particular the circles around the influential duc de Choiseul and the Ministère de la Marine et Colonies, had begun to think about the possibility of a French overseas empire in the Pacific.

For some optimistic spirits in France, the Pacific seemed to hold out the promise of a new kind of imperialism, one which would truly benefit equally the colonizer and the colonized. As early as 1756, even before the loss of Canada, the influential polymath Charles de Brosses had set out a project for a new kind of settlement in the Pacific which would, he hoped, compensate for what the Europeans had done to the Americas. 'Imagine,' he wrote,

> a future which is not at all like that which Christopher Columbus secured for our neighbours ... For we would avoid the two vices from which the Spaniards then suffered, avarice and cruelty. The former emptied their own country in pursuit of an illusory fortune, something which should never have been attempted. The latter, whose causes were national pride and superstition, has all but destroyed the human race in America. They massacred disdainfully, and as if they were base and alien beasts, millions of Indians whom they could have made into men.

No longer, insisted De Brosses, could the Europeans aspire to 'establishing imaginary kingdoms beyond the equator'. Like the empire which Burke had hoped to see in India, De Brosses' enlightened French presence in the Pacific would combine trade with education. It would purchase from the 'savages' the hardwoods and pearls which the Europeans required and in time, through the benign influence of commerce, the Polynesians would come to see 'the advantages of human and social laws'. The model for all future French empires, concluded De Brosses, should be not the Spaniards or the Romans but the Phoenicians. For the Phoenicians, as a peaceful trading people, had created not dependencies or colonies but new nations, and 'what greater objective could a sovereign have' than that?[3]

This vision was shared by many later French writers, by Diderot and the Abbé Guillaume Raynal in particular. But despite the enthusiasm which greeted the Pacific voyages, it was to remain only a vision. In the sands of Tahiti, Bougainville had planted a wooden plaque, together with a bottle containing the names of all the officers on his three ships, which declared this and all Polynesia to be French territory. (Two years earlier, however, the English navigator Samuel Wallis had visited the island and renamed it, rather more prosaically, 'King George's Island'.) No attempt was ever made to make good this claim. After the creation of the French republic in 1792 the revolutionary government turned its back on any future colonizing ventures – until, that is, the creation of the Napoleonic empire. When Tahiti was finally established as a French colony in 1880 after having been devastated by Protestant missionaries, European traders and beachcombers for nearly a century, the vision of enlightened co-operation between over-civilized Europeans and simple 'noble savages' in which, as Diderot had hoped, each might learn from the other, had been entirely forgotten.

Like Bougainville, Cook was also involved in plans for some future occupation of the Pacific. James Douglas, Earl of Morton and President of the Royal Society, provided him with a set of 'Hints' as to how he was to conduct his voyage. These warned him in the strongest terms against doing anything that would cause harm to the natives, and roundly condemned any form of colonization. He was cautioned, 'To have it still in view that shedding the blood of these people is a crime of the highest nature. They are human creatures, the work of the same omnipotent Author, equally under His care with the most polished European; perhaps being less offensive more entitled to His favour. They are the natural, and in the strict sense of the word, the legal possessors of the several Regions they inhabit.'[4] Cook also carried with him, however, a set of 'Instructions' marked 'Secret' and given to him by the Admiralty. These were rather less interested in science and rather more in the possibilities of future imperial expansion. Cook was similarly advised against any conflict but he was also told to 'take possession of Convenient Situations in the Country in the name of the King of Great Britain' and to 'take Possession for his Majesty by setting up Proper Marks and inscriptions, as first discoverers and possessors'.

Yet for all this it would be a mistake to see any of these early expeditions as merely covert colonizing operations. For one thing neither Bougainville's nor Cook's ships had been designed for such purposes. All were shallow-draught vessels, lightly armed and built for working close inshore. Then there is a wholly different sensibility in Bougainville's and Cook's accounts of their encounters with the Polynesians from that found in any of the travel narratives that preceded them. Both men talk of the Polynesians with wonder and sometimes incredulity, but also with respect and even at times with a kind of baffled affection. Nowhere is settlement ever seriously envisaged, even in Cook's supposedly nefarious secret instructions, except with the express 'Consent of the Natives' and even then only 'if you find the Country uninhabited'. Cook himself refused to do even this. In the journal of his final voyage he remarked that the Tahitians had shown him 'with what facility a settlement might be made at Otaheite, which grateful as I am for their repeated good offers, I hope will never happen'.[5] Bougainville and Cook carried back to Europe a greater knowledge of the extent and nature of the South Pacific. They returned with data, calculations and charts. They came carrying specimens of minerals and plants. Both also returned with people, living human specimens of the diversity of humankind.

When Bougainville arrived in Paris in May 1769, he was accompanied by a Tahitian he called Aotourou. Aotourou had joined the French fleet of his own free will in order to accompany it home and to see the wonders that France had to offer. (Since he assumed, not unreasonably, that France was a nearby island he can have had no idea of the length or the kind of journey on which he had embarked.) In Paris, he became something of a celebrity. He was welcomed into the circle of the duchesse de Choiseul, taken to the Opéra and the zoo, paraded in the Tuileries and introduced to various salons where he met some of the leading scientists and philosophers of the day. Among others, he was scrutinized by the natural historian Buffon; the explorer of the Amazon, Charles de la Condamine, who later wrote an account of his visit; Diderot, who in a fiction entitled *Supplément au voyage de Bougainville* transformed him into a harsh critic of the irrationality of Christian moral laws; the philosophers Helvétius and Holbach. He was examined by a celebrated French phonetician to discover why his language sounded the way it did and why he had failed to learn French. He may even have been presented to the king. His one defect, it seems (apart from his failure to master French), was his ugliness. Bougainville recorded with irritation that the *beau monde* of Paris persisted in asking why, 'from an island where the men are generally so beautiful I should have chosen someone so ugly'. To which Bougainville replied that 'I repeat once and for all that I did not choose him, he chose me.' Bougainville also insisted that Aotourou made up in intelligence for what he lacked in looks – although since he was never able to master French and there is no suggestion that Bougainville ever learnt a word of Tahitian, how the two men communicated is unclear.

Aotourou was a specimen, but he was treated as a human being, a curious and puzzling human being perhaps, an object of scientific inquiry, but a human being nonetheless. No attempt was even made to convert him to Christianity. Finally he was sent home (at the by now bankrupt Bougainville's own expense), carrying gifts from the king and the duc de Choiseul, but he died of measles en route in November 1771. Three years later, when he returned from his second voyage, Captain Cook also brought back a native, this time from Huahine in the Sandwich Islands (now Hawaii). Although Cook seems to have had a low opinion of his intellect, based largely on his failure to be impressed by the splendours of London, Mai, or Omai as he came to be called, was undoubtedly handsome. He, too, became a celebrity. He had his portrait painted by Reynolds, in which he appears dressed in a belted version of a toga and in the traditional pose of the Roman orator, and by William Parry. He proved to be a great favourite at court and became the subject of several popular plays.

Omai returned home on board the *Resolution* on Cook's third and last voyage in 1776. Like Aotourou, he was given a number of what might seem to be inappropriate gifts: a sword presented to him by Joseph Banks who had had himself painted with Omai, and a suit of armour from Lord Sandwich which had been made specially by the armourers of the Tower of London.[6] These and a number of other more useful items Cook hoped 'would be the means of rising him into consequence, and of making him respected, and even courted by the first persons throughout the extent of the Society Islands'. On finally reaching Huahine on 13 October 1777, Omai was set up in a new house negotiated for him by Cook and given a number of European weapons (about which Cook had some misgivings) together with a horse and mare, a goat 'big with kid', a boar and two sows 'of the English breed', and a number of European plants. Omai took his leave of Cook on the deck of the *Resolution* and wept all the way to the shore. As Cook put out to sea he wrote in his journal that, 'It was no small satisfaction to reflect, that we had brought him safe back to the very spot from which he was taken. And yet such is the strange nature of human affairs, that it is probable that we left him in a less desirable situation than he was in before his connection with us.' What became of him after that we do not know since, as Cook somewhat wistfully concluded, that was a matter for 'the future navigators of this ocean; with whom it cannot be a principal object of curiosity to trace the future fortunes of our traveller'.

Cook had brought Omai back home. He had also brought with him, in addition to the animals he had given to Omai, some horses, goats and cows with which he hoped the islanders might be able to improve what he (unlike Bougainville) saw as their restricted and impoverished diet. It was, as he conceived it, an act of simple magnanimity – evidence, as had been the repatriation of Omai, of the Europeans' goodwill. 'The trouble and vexation that attended bringing this living cargo thus far,' he recorded, 'is hardly to be conceived. But the satisfaction of mind that I felt in having been so fortunate as to fulfil his Majesty's humane design in sending such valuable animals to supply the wants of two worthy nations, sufficiently recompensed me for the many anxious hours I had passed.'[7] We are a long way from Columbus, on the island he called Hispaniola, trading pieces of glass and 'other trinkets of little worth' for gold and silver ornaments.

Contact between the Europeans and these 'two worthy nations' was, nonetheless, not entirely disinterested. The offspring of Cook's cattle would serve later generations of European sailors well. Cook's reticence to settle would not be followed by later, less considerate generations. Soon the missionaries and the merchants arrived, and after them came the colonizers, first British, then French and finally, with the annexation of Hawaii in 1893, American.

During the late eighteenth century an astonishing number of voyages of exploration left from various parts of Europe, few if any of which had obvious colonizing intentions. Charles de la Condamine travelled down the Amazon in 1743 and 1744 in a voyage which was a joint French–Spanish venture. The Portuguese Xavier Ribeiro de Sampaio left the following year for the Rio Negro. Nicolas le Caille went to observe the transit of

Mercury from the Cape of Good Hope in 1751. La Pérouse followed Bougainville into the Pacific in 1785. In 1789, Alejandro Malaspina set out to chart all the possessions claimed by the Spanish crown, 'in the wake of Messes Cook and La Pérouse', and to prove to the world at large that Spain was every bit as enlightened a nation as France and Britain.

All these expeditions carried botanists, engineers, hydrographers, physicists, physicians, astronomers and painters, but very few soldiers and no missionaries. Even the names of their ships were intended to reflect their purpose: *Discovery*, *Resolution*, *Adventure* and *Endeavour*; *Géographie* and *Naturaliste*; *L'Astrolabe* and *La Boussole* (compass). They were something new in the history of empires and the peoples who created them. They represented the point at which the pursuit of power and the pursuit of knowledge met. 'Abstract science, Gentlemen,' La Roncière la Noury, President of the Paris Geographical Society, told its members in 1874, 'is not sufficient to serve humanity. Science is not truly fruitful unless it is the instrument of progress and production.'

Some of these scientific ventures, such as the expedition in 1735–6 under Louis Godin to test Newton's hypothesis about the shape of the globe, were devoid of any secondary purposes; some, in the manner of the Pacific voyages, had mixed objectives. Others, like the great ordnance survey carried out by the British in India between 1765 and 1843, served quite specific political ends. All were intended to enhance the reputation of the nation both at home and abroad. When Bougainville's account of his journey appeared in 1771, Johann Reinhold Forster (who later accompanied Cook to the Pacific) rapidly made a translation of it because, he said, 'Every true patriot would wish that the East India Company would imitate the French' and 'despatch men properly acquainted with mathematics, natural history [and] physic' to discover 'new branches of trade and commerce'.

Competition between the European powers had acquired an extra and, with the rapid spread of industrialization, potentially more sinister dimension. Science became a recognized source of power and a terrain on which the European powers fought one another for pre-eminence. It might be fanciful to see this as similar to the space-race between the world's most recent empires, the United States and the Soviet Union, in the mid-twentieth century – fanciful, but not entirely wrong. As with the space-race, military advantage, or in the case of the Pacific the possibility of colonization, was a secondary consideration. What mattered most was national prestige. The disinterested pursuit of science was transformed into a new kind of ideology, and the scientist became a new kind of hero.

After Cook was killed in Hawaii in 1779 he became not merely yet another casualty of the dangerous business of seafaring but a martyr to science and a new vision of empire. All of the many tributes paid to him, which were published in French and Italian as well as English, contrasted his deeds with those of the older heroes of empire: Alexander, Scipio, Cortés and Pizarro. They had only conquered men and destroyed peoples in doing so. Cook, enthused the Italian Michelangelo Gianetti in a eulogy published by the Royal Academy of Florence in 1785, had cleared the seas of terror and embraced rather than slaughtered those whom he had encountered in the Pacific. In doing so, he had carried the banner of 'an Enlightened Monarch and Enlightened Society' around the earth. Philip James de Loutherbourg's engraving of 1794, *The Apotheosis of Captain James Cook*, shows him being transported aloft by the figures of Britannia and Universal Fame. In keeping with ancient Greek practice, he is a hero who has been transformed into a god. Nothing could capture so neatly the alliance of science and empire, which had first been dreamt up by the mythologizers of Alexander the Great and would endure until the end of empire itself.[8]

10 *Empire, race and nation*

Cook's triumph, as his panegyrists made plain, had been the triumph not only of science but also of the British nation. The imperialism which he represented was the creation of a new mode of identity and political creed, one that has done more than any other to shape the world since the early nineteenth century: nationalism. Nationalism is the idea that peoples have separate, distinct and indissoluble features, that they are united by a common language and culture, and live under a single and indigenous ruler. When it first emerged at the end of the eighteenth century, this creed made the older empires of the world look like doomed attempts to prevent the evolution of national, and natural, human features.

The German philosopher Johann Gottfried von Herder (1744–1803), who is often somewhat unjustly identified as the father of German and hence most European nationalism, argued that 'Nature has separated nations, not only by woods and mountains, seas and deserts, rivers and climates, but most particularly by languages, inclinations and characters, that the work of subjugating despotism might be rendered more difficult, that all the four quarters of the globe might not be crammed into the belly of a wooden horse.'[1] The use of force and economic interest might have temporarily 'glued together' the world's empires into 'fragile machines of state' but underneath this apparatus they were all, he insisted, 'destitute of internal unification and sympathy of parts'. For Herder the concepts of a people – a *Volk* – and an empire were simply incompatible. Sooner or later all the world's empires – those 'Trojan Horses' as he called them, which conspired against the natural plurality of the human race – were destined to collapse back into their constituent parts. The colonists and settlers would either be driven out or would in time become absorbed by the indigenous peoples. In this way 'does not Nature revenge every insult offered her?'[2]

But the European empires proved to be far more adaptable and a good deal more amorphous than Herder had allowed for. Far from disappearing with the rise of the nation, all the great empires of the nineteenth century, the French and the British in particular, were created in its shadow. Since antiquity empire has been one way of uniting a people. It had after all, as Aristotle observed, been the people of Athens, the *demos*, and not the better sort, the *aristoi*, who had been responsible for the growth of the Athenian empire. And as we have already seen, in his struggle with the tribune Naevius, Scipio Africanus was able to appeal to the Roman people in the name of 'their' empire. Profitable adventures beyond the boundaries of the homeland have always been a way for rulers to give their subjects what Machiavelli shrewdly called 'great expectation of themselves' – one way of making them forget if only briefly their present divisions and miseries. Only as long as Rome was expanding, as Machiavelli also observed, had she been free from corruption. When she stopped, her peoples fell to squabbling among themselves and instantly lost the martial spirit which had held the state together.

Similar uses of the images of empire and the greatness it

evoked were made by later generations of Europeans. Nowhere is this more striking, and nowhere perhaps has it had more lasting consequences, than in France. In the immediate aftermath of the revolution, when France was surrounded on all sides by enemies and internally disunited, 'The Empire' or 'Our Empire' came to denote the personality of the entire French nation. It stood very much as it had once done throughout Europe for the unification of disparate local groups into a single whole. An empire was understood to be not the rule of a single individual but a federation entered into voluntarily. 'Emperor,' declared one enthusiast in the 1790s, 'means he who rules over a free people.' The title King by contrast, as the Romans had known, meant only 'tyrant'.[3] 'We are always hearing about the great empire of the whole nation,' mocked the French liberal Benjamin Constant in 1815, 'abstract notions which have no reality. The great empire is nothing independently of its provinces. The whole nation is nothing separated from the parts that compose it.'

Constant, however, was writing after the collapse of Napoleon whom he abhorred. Napoleon, in his view, by welding abstractions into the instruments of tyranny, had attempted to cast the nation in his own image. When, on 12 December 1804, Napoleon had himself crowned by Pope Pius VII he formally assumed the role that the Holy Roman emperor had once held. As Consul for Life of the republic, he took the crown from the pope and placed it on his head himself. This famous gesture was more than simple hubris. It embodied the claim that as the supreme representative of the people he was the only person who could effect the transition from republic to empire. Like Charlemagne, whose crown he now wore and who had called himself the

Father of the Europeans, Napoleon's first ambition was to unify a Europe which he saw as one people broken down 'by revolutions and politics'. His idea, he wrote from his final exile on St Helena, had been 'to bring everywhere unity of laws, of principles, of opinions, sentiments, views and interests. Then perhaps it would have been possible to dream for the great European family, the application of the American Congress or of the Amphictyons of Greece.'

The Greek Amphictyonic Council, which had previously inspired both James Madison's image of the future United States in the 1770s and Immanuel Kant's vision of a global cosmopolitan order in the 1790s, had been a loose federation of city-states dedicated to the protection of the temple of Demeter at Anthela near Thermopylae. It did not correspond very closely to the image that many had of the Napoleonic empire, in particular those who were drawn unwillingly and by force into its orbit. But there was a logic in Napoleon's objectives which ran back to the universalistic aspirations expressed in the Declaration of the Rights of Man of 1789. This had set out 'the fundamental principles which must provide the ground for all government' and had gone on to declare that 'the French people [were] the first of all peoples and a model for every nation', or as Napoleon himself later put it rather more bluntly, '*Ce qui est bon pour les français est bon pour tout le monde*' (What is good for the French is good for everybody).

For Napoleon a unified Europe with France at its head was to be only the first step. In his own personal mythology Napoleon was not only the heir to Charlemagne but had also taken up the diadem of Alexander and with it had assumed the historic task of uniting East and West. The first and, as it transpired, the last people to be caught up in this piece of historical mythologizing were the Egyptians. When Napoleon arrived in Egypt in 1798 – significantly on board a ship called *L'Orient* – he came, he claimed, as Alexander had come to the peoples of Bactria, not as a conqueror but as a liberator. More immediately he also hoped that by occupying Egypt he would damage British trade in the eastern Mediterranean and threaten British India. Despite these obvious military objectives, the invasion was certainly unusual. No one else had ever gone on campaign with an entire scientific academy, the Institut d'Égypte. Part conquest, part exploration, the purpose of the Egyptian expedition was to restore a state of true civility to the 'Orient'.

In the words of the massive *Description de l'Égypte* which appeared in twenty-three volumes between 1809 and 1828, and each page of which measured one metre square, Egypt which had 'transmitted its knowledge to so many nations' was now under its Mamlûk and Ottoman rulers 'plunged into barbarism'. From this unhappy condition Napoleon, the 'Mohammed of the West', as Victor Hugo later called him, had come to release it and while he was there to 'make the lives of the inhabitants more pleasant and to procure for them all the advantages of a perfect civilization'.[4] This civilization was to be predominantly French. Yet it was also to be a civilization which would preserve, as had Alexander's, what the French looked upon as the true spirit of the Orient, in this case the wisdom of the Pharaohs in happy alliance with the pieties of Islam. In Napoleon's view it was the French, despite being Christians, and not the Mamlûks who, by restoring to the Egyptians their cultural inheritance, were 'the true Muslims'. In order to get this point across, every-thing the Armée d'Égypte did was explained and justified in precise Qur'anic Arabic, and when the Mohammed of the West departed, he gave strict instructions to his deputy, Jean-Baptise Kléber, to administer Cairo in co-operation with the members of the Institut d'Égypte and local religious leaders.

The occupation did not, however, last long. In June 1801, after a series of battles with local rulers, the Ottomans and the British, the French were finally driven out by a combined British and Ottoman assault. By 1814 Napoleon himself was in exile on the island of Elba, defeated by the combined forces of Russia, Austria, Prussia and Britain and the disillusionment of his own exhausted peoples. His return the following year was spectacular but brief and doomed. On 18 June 1815 at the Battle of Waterloo the new Alexander and with him the vision of a world united beneath the principles of the French revolution suffered its final defeat.[5] Napoleon's had been the most ambitious attempt to create an empire in order to transform a nation, and the final effort prior to Hitler's Third Reich to establish an empire on European soil. Like the Third Reich, the Napoleonic empire did not last for long but at its height in 1812 it contained forty-four million subjects, about 40 per cent of the entire European population. It was also (unlike the Third Reich) to have a lasting influence on the future of the peoples of Europe. The British may have put an end to Napoleon but his vision of a united Europe would resurface in other less bellicose forms, and the European Union today possesses much in common with the declared objectives and political aspirations if not the cultural coerciveness of the Napoleonic dream.

France, however, was by no means the only European nation to employ the idea of empire to unite what was in reality a divided and potentially unstable people. Napoleon's arch-enemy Britain, monarchical and perfidious, employed very similar strategies. The viceregal pageantry with which Governor-General Lord Cornwallis celebrated his victory over Tipu Sultan of Mysore in 1792 combined images of Roman triumphalism with the transfigured image of 'imperial benevolence'. It was meant to enhance his own personal standing and to assure the peoples of India of the good intentions of the British. But it was also intended to enforce the concept of loyalty to the king in the face of the threat of working-class radicalism. Victoria's coronation as Empress of India in 1876 was the most fully-elaborated attempt the modern world has witnessed to recreate the ancient Roman *imperium*. Yet this, too, was meant for home consumption, a largely successful bid by the prime minister Benjamin Disraeli to enhance the faltering status of the monarchy. All such assertions of the power of the nation helped to press home both the legitimacy of its rulers and the strength of its identity. Even as late as 1902 the British coronation ceremony could be praised – in a sentence which ran together Burke's vision of an empire of liberty with nineteenth-century convictions of the racial superiority of the Anglo-Saxons – as the expression of the 'recognition, by a free democracy, of a hereditary crown as a symbol of the worldwide domination of their race'. In this way empire, as the historian Eric Hobsbawm has observed, 'made good ideological cement'.[6] The very existence of colonies could be a source of patriotic pride. 'The people who colonize the most,' wrote the French economist Paul Leroy-Beaulieu in 1874, 'is the first among all peoples.' 'C is for colonies' declared the *ABC for Baby Patriots* published in 1899, in a more belligerent mood:

Rightly we boast,
That of all the great nations
Great Britain has the most.

In order to give the baby patriot a better understanding of what these colonies were and what their submissive inhabitants looked like, during the nineteenth century displays of 'natives' became a regular attraction in the imperial capitals of Europe. The Great Exhibition of 1851 brought to London peoples from every corner of the empire and exhibited them alongside the flora and fauna of their native habitat, so that Eskimos were placed alongside polar bears, and Africans with chimpanzees. As late as 1924–5, the Wembley Exhibition (also in London) included samples of what were tastefully described as 'peoples in residence'. These included Yoruba, Hausa and Fante Mende from West Africa, some Indians, and even 175 Chinese from Hong Kong. Most of them were set up in reconstructions of indigenous housing and could be seen working away at their local crafts and manufactures, the valuable commodities which would eventually flow home in one form or another to the metropolis.

Nor, of course, was the British empire the only one to relish such indirect glimpses of the exotic fringes of its domains. Eighteen 'colonial pavilions' complemented the newly-constructed Eiffel Tower in 1889, and the Paris exhibition of 1900 contained 'colonial villages' in which colourful native peoples could be seen from behind high wire fences going about their daily lives and staring back at those who had come to stare at them. The 1904 St Louis World Fair in Missouri became famous not only as the place where the ice-cream cone was first invented, but for the Philippine Exposition which contained a number of Filipino Villages exhibiting the various peoples of the archipelago, the 'savages' and 'Non Christian tribes', the Negritos and Igorots (whose nudity outraged the puritan sensibilities of the visitors – and attracted them in their thousands), as well as a large contingent of American-trained and dressed Filipino soldiers, there to demonstrate the possibilities for 'evolution' of even the most backward peoples under US colonial patronage.[7]

All of these exhibitions served a double role. They were part of the development of the new social sciences which, since the closing years of the eighteenth century, had begun to exercise a powerful influence not only on the imagination of the élites of Europe but also gradually on the ways in which empire was both conceived and administered. Just as Aotourou and Omai had been brought back as living evidence of the habits and customs of early humankind, so too were their descendants – only now they came in far larger numbers. They were also proof of the benefits which the European policies of 'civilizing' could have. The concept of 'civilizing', and 'civilization' had in one guise or another been an objective of all Europe's imperial ventures since Rome, and it relied upon widely-accepted notions of a universal human nature and law of human evolution. All peoples, it was believed, move from a condition of savagery through one of 'barbarism' until they finally reach the present civilized condition of the European. Along the way their means of production changes from hunting to pastoralism, agriculture and finally commerce; their forms of government evolve from tribalism, through despotism to monarchy; their beliefs grow from simple superstition to true religion and eventually, of course, into Christianity. In the course of their histories, they also put on clothes, acquire arts and sciences, learn how to write and preserve a record of their past, and finally start to build and live in cities.

The vast differences that separated the various peoples of the world could all be explained by a combination of factors. These included climate, terrain, modes of government, or time spent in migration. A people such as the Chinese might be held back for centuries by an inert and despotic mode of government. The American Indians had only developed the rudiments of a political culture because they had had to travel all the way from Mongolia across the Bering Strait to reach their present home. The 'primitive' condition of the Polynesians could be attributed to their isolation from the rest of humankind. However, because all peoples were basically the same, since the human race was a single species and the descendants of a single pair, all could in time acquire the features of civilization which, because of their good fortune, the Europeans had been the first to achieve. Just as the missionaries had assumed that all rational peoples would be able to understand the gospel once it had been explained to them, so the new apostles of civilization believed that the 'backward races' of the world, as they came to be called, were merely waiting for instruction. The peoples of America, Asia and Africa, enthused the marquis de Condorcet in 1793, 'seem to be waiting only to be civilized and to receive from us the means to be so, and find brothers among the Europeans to become their friends and disciples'.[8]

Condorcet's remarks reflect a revised conception of empire as a form of exchange which would come to dominate imperial ideologies in the nineteenth century. The white man's benefits were more than amply compensated for by what Rudyard

Kipling famously called 'the white man's burden'. They, the 'uncivilized', the 'savage', the 'barbarian' would give the Europeans their labour and their raw materials, their 'surplus' as it comfortably came to be called; the Europeans in compensation would bring them enlightenment, technology, Christianity, even cleanliness. In one of the more curious advertisements for the joint virtues of empire and industry, the soap manufacturers Pears issued in 1887 a poster entitled 'The Formula of British Conquest'. It depicted a collection of semi-naked Sudanese, staring in wonder – one is even on his knees in an attitude of prayer – at a rock on which are written the words PEARS' SOAP IS THE BEST. Cleanliness is not only next to godliness. It is one of the defining marks of civilization. And the Europeans could be relied upon to provide it.

The notion that the European imperialists were the agents of progress, preparing those whom Kipling described as the 'new-caught sullen peoples, half devil and half child'[9] to assume one day their allotted place as masters of their own destiny, persisted until the twentieth century. It had been around in one form or another since antiquity. Aristotle had held similar views about the development of peoples and so, too, had Cicero. In its modern form however it was an Enlightenment notion which had been developed by essentially well-meaning cosmopolitans in the salons of Paris, London, Edinburgh and Berlin. It rested upon the overwhelming conviction that all human identity is shaped wholly and solely by the worlds which people inhabit. Even those early and sometimes radical distinctions which Christians had made between believers and non-believers never supposed a division within humankind itself. 'When we pray,' said the thirteenth-century mystic Ramon Llull, 'let us remember the pagans who are of our same blood.' 'Civilization', like Christianity, was a world open to all who chose to enter it.

In the early nineteenth century, however, a darker and more lasting way of understanding difference began to make an appearance: racism. Racism worked with a quite different set of assumptions from the historical evolutionism of the Enlightenment. It assumed that the human family was not one but many. It assumed that those different families were marked out by their appearance, their abilities and, in some quasi-religious sense, by the purposes for which they had been created. And it supposed that those differences, since they were as we would say today 'genetically determined', could not be altered substantially by education, persuasion or example. Some kind of racialism, and certainly implicit forms of racial discrimination, have been a feature of all human societies. But modern racism was different in being based on the new scientific cultures which grew up in Europe at the end of the eighteenth century and which were confident that ultimately everything about the human condition could be explained in terms of biology or physiology. It has always had many faces, and it has always included many and often contradictory theories. All, however, insist that distinctions between peoples are to be found not in culture but in nature, that some races have been granted superior qualities to others, and that racial features can only change by means of biological contact with other races.

In 1841 Jules Joseph Virey, a distinguished and much-respected physician, delivered a lecture to the Académie de médecine in Paris on the biological causes of civilization. Humanity was, he argued, divided into two groups: the 'whites', a term which included all Caucasians; and the 'blacks', who were the Africans, Americans and Asians. The 'whites', he told his audience, 'have attained a more or less perfect stage of civilization', while the 'blacks' struggle for survival in a 'constantly imperfect civilization'. Struggle as they might, the 'blacks' would always remain half-savage, imperfectly civilized. Their destiny was inscribed in the colour of their skin. The reason for this, Virey believed, was that the process of civilization in humankind is akin to that of domestication in animals. Domestic animals, such as cows, and civilized humans have white (or whitish) flesh; untamed animals, such as deer, and uncivilized humans have dark flesh. You only have to compare veal with venison. (Virey passed over in silence the fact that, as sixteenth-century anatomists had discovered, the flesh of all humans is the same colour. Only the skin differs.)

Having thus appropriated humans to the categories to be found in the animal world, Virey was able to draw the obvious conclusion that just as the wild animal was the natural prey of man so the 'black' human was the natural prey of the 'white'. Human beings might not kill and eat other human beings – which would nonetheless seem to be the logical conclusion to draw from his analogy – but it was natural for white humans to enslave black humans. Slavery might seem cruel and abhorrent but such were the ways of nature. 'Is it any more unjust,' he asked 'for the lion to devour the gazelle?' Racism such as Virey's – and it was fairly typical of the cruder range of arguments used both in Britain and in France particularly after the invasion of Algeria in 1830 – made of the Europeans a distinct and special category, especially gifted and ultimately destined to reduce all the other races to some kind of servitude. No one could now say, as a sixteenth-century Spanish Jesuit had once done, that an 'Ethiopian' brought up in Europe would be in all respects save for the colour of his skin a European.[10] Colour of skin and all that was believed to lie underneath it became the whole person.

On Virey's reckoning whites were superior because they were white. But their superiority also had a history. In the 1780s the orientalist Sir William Jones had developed the idea that certain linguistic affinities between Sanskrit and most of what are now called the Indo-European languages implied that all the peoples who spoke those languages must have had a common ancestry. These peoples, the European *Ur-Volk*, he called Aryans. Jones, who was an employee of the East India Company and ranked the sages of ancient India, Valmiki, Vyasa and Kalidasa, as equal to Plato and Pindar, believed that he had established an association between two great but otherwise distinct cultures. The link he had created between ancient Greece and ancient India was linguistic and not racial, but the implications of his belief that a common language supposed a common identity were taken up by later scholars. In particular, the German philologist Max Müller who became Professor of Sanskrit at Oxford in the 1860s and 1870s, developed Jones' ideas into a theory which provided the Aryans with a common racial heritage, a complex migratory history, and an ancestral home in southern Russia. From there they had supposedly spread out and colonized a vast area of land reaching all the way from northern India to western Europe, carrying with them that distinctive way of life, urban and law-governed, which by the late eighteenth century had come to be called 'civilized'. Müller's account became so widely accepted that by the time the

English jurist and Law Member of the Viceroy of India's Council, Henry Maine, came to write his immensely influential *Ancient Law* in 1861 he could declare categorically that civilization was 'nothing more than the name for the old order of the Aryan world'.[11]

At first, racism was limited to broad general distinctions between Europeans, Jews and Arabs, Africans, Chinese, and American Indians, peoples who were obviously distinct in appearance and habitat. Soon, however, as with the older languages of culture and 'national character', it came to be applied to different peoples within Europe itself. The self-styled Count Arthur de Gobineau, often referred to as the father of racist ideology, in *On the Inequality of the Human Races* (1853–5) tried to demonstrate that the Germans and the French aristocracy (whom he assumed to be pure 'Gothic' and thus of Germanic stock) had retained the original virtue of the Aryan peoples. All the rest, mongrelized and bastardized by centuries of interbreeding, had long since abandoned the civilized ways of their remote ancestors.[12]

Gobineau's work was based on a nostalgia for pre-revolutionary France and it had few followers except among backward-looking monarchists and some Germans (a Gobineau Society was founded in Germany in 1894). But by the middle of the nineteenth century a somewhat less extreme and rather less pessimistic racial curtain had been lowered across Europe which followed, roughly, the line of the confessional divide that emerged after the Reformation. In the north were what the liberal philosopher John Stuart Mill, who was also an employee of the East India Company, called the 'self-helping and struggling Anglo-Saxons', in the south the languid, potentially passive and generally despotic Latins – a group which, despite Mill's admiration for the great French philosopher and statesman Alexis de Tocqueville, also included the French.[13] The liberal parliamentarian Sir Charles Dilke in an account of his travels through the British empire, or what he called Greater Britain, remarked that although the Anglo-Saxon peoples were not the same everywhere – climate, environment and upbringing could still take their toll – 'essentially the race continues to be ours'. The future of the world, he claimed, belongs 'to the Anglo-Saxon, to the Russian and the Chinese races' – although the last, he observed, tended to fall under the 'influence of India and the Crown Colonies of Great Britain'. All the others would go to the wall or, like the Maoris, Australian Aborigines, 'Hottentots' and American Indians – those 'dying nations' singled out for extinction by Lord Salisbury in 1898 – vanish altogether.

Ultimately, however, all racial arguments ran into considerable difficulties. If the 'Aryans' were the originators of the peoples of India, Russia and Europe, this made the Indians and the British descendants of a common ancestor. The Indian, as one Indian civil servant observed, 'is like the Englishman, of an Ancient Aryan stock, a fellow subject of the Queen, and an industrious and law abiding citizen', which was why in the 1890s Lord Curzon's government had warned that Indians should on no account be placed in the same category as black Africans for the latter stood 'far below them' in what Curzon called 'the grades of humanity'. What, then, could possibly justify the British occupation of India or what the British saw as their self-evident superiority over its inhabitants? The only possible answer seemed to lie in what enlightened eighteenth-century theorists such as Diderot had eagerly endorsed and nineteenth-century ones most feared: miscegenation.

At some early stage in their history, it was claimed, the Aryan invaders of India had mingled with inferior aboriginal races who were grouped under the headings Dravidian (in southern India) and Turanian, a loose term embracing most non-Indo-European and non-Semitic language groups. Thereafter, racial inter-breeding had weakened the Aryan strain until by the time the British arrived the amount of true Aryan blood that remained in some places was 'infinitesimally small'.[14] The view that interbreeding always resulted in the weakening of the sup-posedly stronger and superior stock was widely held and applied to Africa and America as well as to Asia. But no one could really explain why it did not work the other way round. Why had the Aryans not elevated the Dravidians and Turanians? After all horse-breeding, which provided the model for much racial the-orizing, assumed the predominance of strength rather than weakness. If that were the case with horses, then why not with humans? Racists could never really find answers to such questions. Like the previous cycle of 'barbarism' and 'civ-ilization', racism tended to assume that the hold of the superior peoples over the rest of the world was at best a tenuous one. There was a persistent dread among European colonists that, as Herder had foretold, it would be only a matter of time before the European civilizers and colonizers would themselves become 'natives' – either that or they would perish altogether.

Despite obvious problems of coherence, a belief in a common racial ancestry played a crucial role in the attempt of the British to rule India. Working on the assumption of a common Aryan heritage, they ransacked Sanskrit texts and questioned local religious leaders in an effort to discover a 'purer' form of Hinduism which would be closer to its unsullied Aryan sources and therefore more in keeping, or so they hoped, with their own notions of 'morality'. British India could then be governed in accordance with Hindu laws, or at least with those laws that could be made commensurable with English common law. 'I write and feel,' declared Lord Bentinck, governor-general of India between 1828 and 1835, 'as a legislator for the Hindus and as I believe many enlightened Hindus must feel.'

Bentinck's self-image as the restorer of the ancient Aryan law found its most dramatic expression in the struggle to outlaw sati (suttee), the custom whereby a widow would throw herself, or be pushed by relatives, onto the funeral pyre of her husband so as to perish with him. Sati challenged the concern of the British with 'improving' the Indians at the same time as it pandered to sexual fantasies and nightmares about the exotic Orient. For a society still addicted to public executions and in the process of becoming deeply perplexed about its own sexuality, sati combined sexual prurience with violence in a way that ensured it a great deal of public attention in Britain. Bentinck succeeded in outlawing the practice in 1829 not only on the grounds that it was inherently barbarous and a violation of 'natural justice' but because he had discovered that it was a later corruption of the original Sanskrit law. Its abolition was therefore 'a restorative act' which returned to the Indians their true culture.[15] When a statue of Bentinck by Richard Westmacott was erected in 1835 it showed him gazing into a morally improved future and standing on a drum around which, cast in bronze bas-relief, was a scene of impending sati. A young, remarkably European-looking woman with naked breasts, her sari slipping tantalizingly from her hips, her wailing children torn from her, is being dragged backwards onto the pyre by swarthy, turbaned male relatives. It is a typical piece of Victorian neoclassical eroticism, its images blending the ever-present threat of the (male) 'barbarian' with the feminized 'other' which haunted the overexcited minds of the guardians of the British Raj. Like the climate which rotted leather and turned fine cloth into fungus, and the all-too-potent Indian diseases, Indian sexuality – the writhing dancers of Lucknow, the many-armed goddess Kali – threatened to rot the stout British male from within; his body, in the steaming imagination of Lord Kitchener, commander-in-chief of the British army in India, risked being eaten away by 'slow cankerous and stinking ulcerations'.

The belief in a common ancestry for both Indians and Europeans also implied that beneath the trappings of later non-Aryan elements it might be possible to find in India customs, habits, even institutions that had all but vanished in Europe itself. One of these, which was largely the creation of Henry Maine, was the so-called 'village republic'. Maine persuaded himself that in the traditional, self-sufficient and to some degree self-governing Indian village he had discovered a living instance of what both the ancient Greek *polis* and the German or Scandinavian *mark* had once been. If he was right, then the village republic was an example of the kind of community from which the prevailing social order of the democratic nations of modern Europe had developed. As such, of course, it had to be protected and to some degree preserved.

In the long term, such images of continuity between the European past and the Indian present, and a wish to represent themselves as the more liberal heirs of the Mughal empire, meant that the British in India never attempted to effect very much long-term change in society. Not only did the village republics remain (as they remain to this day) largely unaltered, so too did the various local autocracies to which they belonged. For one of the things Maine seems to have overlooked was that whereas the *polis* and the *mark* had no ultimate overlords, the Indian villages did have. The Indian princely estates were untouched by the Raj and the princes themselves became, in effect, satraps of the British government in Westminster. As Jawaharlal Nehru remarked, it was ironic at least that the British, committed to the progressive amelioration of the Indian peoples into responsible democratic subjects of the crown, should have left so much intact of the backward, static monarchy they had overthrown.

In Africa also, where no notions of a common cultural heritage could apply, the British did their best to avoid much direct intervention in the prevailing social order. They ruled as far as possible through, rather than over, the colonized peoples. It was cheaper, likely to be less troublesome, and fitted well with British notions of empire as a species of paternal custodianship. From this there evolved the doctrine of 'indirect rule'. Here too, the imperial administration was aided by a complex intellectual and scientific (or pseudo-scientific) machine. Just as racialist notions about Aryanism and the studies of Indian culture by Jones and other orientalists had guided the British administration in India, so in Africa the imperial government at the beginning of the twentieth century was influenced by the new science of social anthropology.

As preliterate, preindustrial peoples, the African societies had to be spoken for, and the people who spoke for them were the anthropologists. Something which might be called anthropology had been around since at least the middle of the eighteenth century. But the modern, empirical social science based on extensive first-hand knowledge of the peoples being studied is a creation of the first decades of the twentieth century, and it was in part at least a creature of empire. The most successful and by far the most influential of the anthropologists in Britain (French anthropology was less involved in imperial affairs) were those who belonged to what has come to be called the 'functionalist' school, whose intellectual progenitor was the Polish émigré Bronislaw Malinowski. Malinowski believed that African societies were too fragile and fragmented to accept rapid or dramatic change – something which, in those areas where such changes were attempted, proved to be all too true. The role of the anthropologist was to instruct government in how to make the best of these delicate social worlds and to coax them into the European-dominated future without destroying them in the process. This, Malinowski believed, could only be achieved through understanding how they operated and by working as far as possible through native rulers. The hands-off administration of Africa which came to be called indirect rule was the creation of F. D. Lugard, governor and governor-general of Nigeria between 1912 and 1919, and was the product of long experience rather than anthropological reflection. But it was, Malinowski triumphantly declared, 'a complete surrender to the functional point of view'.

Indirect rule applied, however, only in north and central Africa where the economies were based largely on cash crops and where the climate made settlement unattractive. In southern Africa by contrast, in South Africa itself, Southern Rhodesia (Zimbabwe) and Kenya, the existence of rich arable lands and the discovery of diamonds and precious metals attracted not government agents but private land-speculators and freebooters like Cecil Rhodes. Here, for a while, they enjoyed a freedom of manoeuvre which they could never have had in Asia. When the men of Rhodes' Pioneer Column set out from the Cape Colony in 1890 to occupy what was to become Southern Rhodesia they behaved, leaving aside obvious differences in technology, much as Cortés and Pizarro had done over 300 years before. They seized African land and cattle as and when they chose or required, brutally suppressing all opposition they met first from the Ndebele in 1893–4 and then from the Ndebele and Shona in 1896–7. In southern Africa the lesson of America, even of India, had finally been forgotten. The language of the 'empire of liberty' had been silenced along with any notion of respect for the fragility of the 'primitive'. The conquistador was back. But now he was armed with a Gatling gun.

By the mid-1870s what has come to be called the 'scramble for Africa' among the major, as well as a number of minor, European powers had begun. By 1895 the French had an empire in West Africa three times the size of the British, although Britain managed to secure the major resources in terms of both trade and population. The Germans occupied large areas of East and South-West Africa. King Leopold of Belgium owned, as a private individual since the Belgian parliament wanted nothing to do with it, a region of nearly a million square miles in the Congo Basin which in 1908 became the Belgian Congo. The Italians had established a protectorate over the Indian Ocean coastlands of Somalia; the Portuguese in Angola had transformed what had begun as a costal trading station into a full-scale colony; and the Spanish still clung to Morocco and the island of Fernando Po. By the outbreak of war in 1914 the entire continent – with the exception of a few isolated enclaves, the Republic of Liberia and the Empire of Ethiopia – was under the direct or indirect control of one or another European power.

The French, Dutch, Germans, Spanish, Belgians, Portuguese, Italians, and even briefly the Danes, all had at one time or another a stake in the African continent. But none of them except the Dutch had any significant imperial interests elsewhere in the world. By the second half of the nineteenth century, Britain was alone in having an empire that reached across the world and not only embraced a myriad different peoples and cultures but, while clinging to the ideals of representative government and liberty, included almost every possible kind of social and political community. It was a curious, hybrid beast. 'I know of no example of it either in ancient or modern history,' wrote Disraeli in 1878. 'No Caesar or Charlemagne ever presided over a dominion so peculiar.' It was multiracial and multireligious, diverse in manners and customs, united only in what he called the recognition of 'the commanding spirit of these islands'.[16]

Some kind of answer to Disraeli's puzzlement was provided in a book published in 1883 by the historian John Robert Seeley, called *The Expansion of England*, which rapidly became a bestseller. Seeley argued that the British empire had evolved as a new form of federalism. He did not invoke either Cicero or Cartwright, but his conception of what he now called 'imperialism' was markedly similar to theirs. The empire, as he understood it, was a world federation. His models were the United States which had expanded across a continent in the years after independence and created new, semi-autonomous states without changing either its political system or the allegiance of those states to the federal government, and to a lesser degree the federated states of the massive Russian empire. 'Federalism' for Seeley was yet another expression of what he saw as the genius of the 'Anglo-Saxon' peoples and, more widely, of Europeans in general. In his perhaps prophetic view, federations were destined sooner rather than later to replace what he called the 'country-states' which then dominated the Western world. 'Russia and the United States,' he wrote, 'will surpass in power the states now called great as much as the great country-states of the sixteenth century surpassed Florence.'[17] As Seeley saw it, Britain could either attempt to retain her status as a still-great 'country-state' and eventually, like Spain and Portugal, pass into national insignificance, or else transform herself and her empire from a metropolis surrounded by a number of divergent and distinct colonies into a federal superpower.[18] To do that, of course, she would have to grant a far greater measure of independence to those colonies than they currently enjoyed and that, Seeley recognized, as Adam Smith had done over a century earlier, no imperial power was ever likely to do. In many respects Seeley's vision of Britain's options has turned out to be remarkably precise. Except, of course, that as the 'country-state' now slowly loses its enduring pre-eminence, the form of federation that has arisen to replace it is not British but European.

Whatever its ultimate future, the British empire in the early twentieth century remained committed to the view that the justification for its survival was its mission to 'civilize' the 'barbarian' and in so doing to bring the peoples of the world together into a single worldwide community. Implicit in all this was the notion that one day, in however distant a future, the colonized peoples of the world would indeed become 'civilized'. When that happened, they would logically have to be given back control of their own lives. Lord Macaulay in his speech on the renewal in 1833 of the East India Company's charter had declared that 'by good government we may educate our subjects into a capacity for better government; that having become instructed in European knowledge they may, in some future age, demand European institutions'. He did not know when it would come but he declared that when it did 'it will be the proudest day in English history'.[19]

11 *Ending*

The rapid exploration of the Pacific and the settlement by the British in Australia and New Zealand had by the end of the eighteenth century extended the cordon of European influence and maritime power around the entire globe. The Europeans were now well on their way to establishing the hegemony which would survive until the middle of the twentieth century. Their only remaining competitors were China and the Ottoman empire. Although visibly failing even by the end of the eighteenth century, they were still powerful enough to command respect as independent powers well into the nineteenth. The Ottoman sultanate resisted European incursions by playing off one power against another in what came to be called the 'Great Game', and staggered on until the end of the nineteenth century. By 1900, however, little remained of the ancient sultanate and in 1908 it was seized by a group of liberal reformers known collectively as the Young Turks who attempted to transform it into a modern secular republic.[1]

China, although it was regarded as a valued and powerful trading partner, was already beginning to look vulnerable to rapacious English eyes when Lord George Macartney made his famous visit on behalf of the East India Company and George III in 1793. Macartney is best remembered today for his celebrated refusal to perform the traditional kowtow before the emperor.[2]

His defiance was not merely a question of personal honour. Ambassadors can be relied upon to set personal dignity aside when called upon to do so, and Macartney was a good ambassador. His refusal to grovel before the Son of Heaven was rather a measure of his conviction that what he looked upon as a suspicious, introverted civilization could not long resist the raw power of free trade – nor ultimately, although this still lay some distance in the future, the power of western technology. The Middle Kingdom was clearly a society which had grown ancient and moribund. It now stood, said Herder, 'as an old ruin on the verge of the World'.[3] One push and over it would go. And, of course, the innovative, unceremonial, individualistic Europeans were there to do the pushing.

Within a few years the Europeans, the British and French in particular, were making increasingly intemperate demands that the Chinese open their doors to 'foreign devils', demands which culminated in the so-called Opium Wars of 1839–42. Britain extended its base at Hong Kong and virtually detached Tibet which it considered to be properly a part of British India (thus creating a dispute over the status and sovereignty of the mountain kingdom which still rages today). In 1859 the British also established the Imperial Maritime Customs, a vast bureaucracy nominally under the control of the emperor but acting largely in British commercial interests. Germany set up bases in the north of the country while the French, who had already occupied Indonesia, extended their influence over the south.

In 1900, Britain, France, Russia, Italy, Germany, the USA and Japan (which had already seized Korea and Taiwan) joined forces to put down the so-called Boxer Rebellion and loot Beijing. In 1911, as a direct consequence of these incursions, the Chinese empire, which had survived since the days of Genghis Khan, collapsed before an internal rebellion which delivered it into the hands of a number of regional commanders known in the West as warlords under whose control it remained until the communist takeover in 1949. For both the West and the newly communist East, imperial China no longer represented (as it had done to so many in the eighteenth century when all things Chinese were in vogue) an example of enviable political stability as the only empire in the history of the world to have endured for centuries. It became instead an example of 'Oriental despotism', of all that was most damaging to the human spirit in the power of tradition, hierarchy, and veneration of the past.

The final demise of the mighty Chinese empire left the world in the hands of the major European powers, Russia and the United States. In the year 1800 they occupied or controlled some 35 per cent of the surface of the planet, by 1878 67 per cent, and by 1914 over 84 per cent.[4] Before long, however, as with all previous imperial orders, this virtual hegemony began to falter. By 1945, after two world wars, fought largely between Western powers for Western ends – 'Europe's two great civil wars', the Spanish statesman Salvador de Madariaga once called them – it was obviously nearing its end. The new European empires of the twentieth century, the would-be empires of Hitler and Mussolini, rose and fell in the space of a very few years. The empire which was the USSR, an extension to the west of the older empire of the tsars, fell with the ideology which had sustained it although it survives, fitful and divided, to the east. The European overseas empires all disappeared between 1947 and the late 1960s. Britain still has fourteen colonies, although they are now officially described as 'dependent territories' – and, more contentiously, continues to rule over the province of Northern Ireland. The Commonwealth lives on as a tattered coda to Burke's 'empire of liberty'. France has overseas provinces in the Pacific and the Indian Ocean. Spain still clings to Ceuta and Melilla on the North African coast. But these are mostly just fading memories.

The fall of the modern European empires was as rapid as their rise had been. And in most places the reasons for their downfall were similar. Ultimately, all had maintained their rule through acquiescence rather than by force or the threat of force. True, there had been some nasty episodes. But brutal and unwarranted as might have been, say, the suppression of the so-called Indian Mutiny of 1857, it failed in the long run to alter substantially the balance of power between the British and their Indian subjects. What had applied to the Roman empire also applied to the British, French, German and, ultimately, even the Russian empires: subject peoples were only willing to remain in subjection so long as at least a significant number of them could see some benefit in doing so. Furthermore, unlike any of the previous empires, those which had grown up after the beginning of the nineteenth century had rarely, except in southern Africa, exported many of their own peoples or created substantial creole élites capable of resisting native insurgency when it finally came.

Resistance to any kind of rule requires organization and courage. In the case of resistance to colonial rule, it also requires some vision of a better future in a postcolonial world. It requires an ideology capable of mobilizing those who might otherwise accept the status quo as inevitable. Ironically, this was provided by the same refashioning of society that had been the driving force behind most modern imperialism, namely nationalism. Of all Lord Macaulay's 'European institutions' the only one that most colonial peoples in the twentieth century have consistently demanded is the independent nation-state.

The imperial powers had provided indigenous élites with as much education as they saw fit in order to run the lower reaches of their empires for them. In so doing they had also armed them with modernizing ideals and Western notions of national self-determination. From Ireland to Java, the nation seemed to offer what has been called by the political scientist Benedict Anderson an 'imagined community' – a community which, although it has none of the properties that older face-to-face societies like the village or parish once offered, nevertheless holds out the prospect of belonging to a larger and potentially more powerful grouping.[5]

In most cases, if not all, such communities did not already exist. They had to be created. To achieve this it was widely believed that the territories they occupied had to correspond to the language and ethnic group of the majority of their inhabitants. In extreme cases those who spoke some other language or belonged to another ethnic group would have to be either deported or, if they would not or could not go, annihilated. Ethnic cleansing is by no means an invention of the post-Soviet world. Above all, of course, the nation had to be self-governing. The claim that national self-determination could only be achieved with full state independence – a belief to which Basque and Corsican extremists still cling – had emerged in the 1870s as an ideal during the struggle for national recognition within Europe itself as various nationalities, Italians, Germans, Irish and Polish, sought independence from the Austro-Hungarian, British and Russian empires. It was only a matter of time before the same ideals and expectations took root in Europe's overseas dependencies.

And when they did the consequences were devastating. Within a very brief space of time, from the end of the First World War until the mid-1960s, the nationalisms of the formerly dependent peoples had swept the once-massive imperial edifices away. In some places, the imperialists recognized that their time was up and got out while they could with some dignity and not too much expense. The British scuttled away from most of their possessions in Africa and the Caribbean, leaving behind them unstable island economies which have only been saved, if saved they have been, by the arrival of American tourism. Portuguese Goa was finally occupied by Indian troops in 1961. Hong Kong, the last British colony of any size, was handed back to China in 1997, with a ceremony like something out of Gilbert and Sullivan to mark the final going-down of the British sun. In contrast, Macao, the last Portuguese factory in Asia, went two years later almost without anyone noticing. In others places – the Belgian Congo, Algeria, Cyprus, Rhodesia (seized by its white settler population in 1965), Angola, Mozambique – the departure was brutal and protracted. Colonial wars, wars of independence, wars by peoples to regain their status as peoples, were a constant feature of the first sixty or seventy years of the twentieth century and the hostilities they have created are likely to survive well into the first half of the twenty-first.

The processes of decolonization have left in their wake not only bitter memories and undying enmities. They have also created what sometimes appear to be insuperable dilemmas for the world's new nations. For not only is the nation a relatively new and entirely European conception, it is also the case that few of the former imperial districts from which most post-colonial nations have been constructed had any existence prior to the arrival of the Europeans. This was also true in the ancient world. Spain, Britain and Gaul were all in various ways creations of Rome. So, too, was Italy itself. Spanish vice-regal divisions lie behind the modern frontiers of the republics of Spanish America. The modern states of Eastern and Central Europe took shape under the aegis of the Holy Roman empire, and their present distribution of peoples is in large part the creation of the Austro-Hungarian empire, the empire of the Tsars, or the Soviet Union.

Nowhere is this effect as marked, and nowhere have its consequences been as far-reaching, as in the European empires in Asia and Africa. Here imperial foundations brought together peoples who shared very little with one another. Sometimes this was done simply by drawing boundary lines around the territories of a number of different and even hostile groups, sometimes through either forced or voluntary migration. This is most tragically obvious in Africa. Africa, as its postcolonial history has demonstrated all too brutally, is a land violated not just by the activities of European freebooters but by a false conception of ethnicity. Unlike India or much of Asia, or even ancient Mexico and Peru, sub-Saharan Africa before the arrival of the Europeans had very few very large-scale societies. One of the tragic consequences of indirect rule (for which the anthropologists cannot be held responsible) was the assumption that Africans were divided into what, in honour of some supposed affinity with early European societies, were called tribes. Most of these were either too large or too small to capture the complex ethnic divisions of most parts of the continent. The Bangala of Zaire, the Baluyia and Kikuyu of Kenya, the Bagisu of Uganda, and the Yoruba and Ibo of Nigeria were all colonial inventions. The Ibo were a New World fiction created by lumping together into a single ethnic and hence tribal group all slaves speaking any one of the (numerous) Ibo dialects. Such categorizations made the district officer's task easier. But as the division between the administrative areas of British, French, Belgian and German Africa hardened, they in their turn became the boundary lines of the new post-independence African states. The long-term consequences of this process proved to be disastrous. Ethnic divisions and conflict which could never have existed before the coming of the Europeans rapidly became, and have remained, the dominant feature of the continent.

Nearly all the modern postcolonial states have been in this way the creations of former imperial administrations. Today schoolchildren from Bulawayo still gather at the tomb of Cecil Rhodes in the Matopos Hills in south-eastern Zimbabwe just as they did when their country was Rhodesia. They do so not because their teachers and parents have any fond memories of British rule but because without Rhodes there would have been no modern nation for them to inherit.[6] Attempts to associate modern Zimbabwe in anything but name with the Munhumatapa empire which flourished in the high veldt in the sixteenth century remain unpersuasive as a national foundation. Although the historical connection is an obvious source of pride, as are the great ruins of Zimbabwe itself, modern Zimbabwe is the nation that Rhodes created and President Mugabe has inherited.

Inevitably, colonial peoples have also discovered that anti-colonialism and collective identity are not the same thing. It was much easier for Tamils, Brahmins, Bengalis, Sikhs, Malays, Nilotes or Ashantis to recognize that they were not Englishmen than it was for them to imagine themselves to be Singhalese, Indians, Pakistanis, Malayasians, Sudanese or Ghanaians.[7] In the early nineteenth century the 'liberator' of Peru, San Martín, in an effort to create a modern Peruvian nation which would incorporate both the white creole population and the former subjects of the Inca empire, issued an edict 'baptizing' all Quechua-speaking Indians as Peruvians. At one time or another all nationalists have had recourse to similarly desperate measures. And every nationalist has had good cause to echo the remark supposedly made by Ferdinando Martino, Italian minister of public instruction, in 1896, 'We have made Italy, now we must make the Italians.'[8]

Making Italians, or Indians or Cypriots or Malaysians, has often proved to be an impossible task. Once the imperial regime has been shaken off, once the new nation has been called into existence, complete with a collective identity marked by flags, national anthem, currency and postage, once a political élite has emerged or has been hastily assembled, once the imperialists and the settlers who still have somewhere to go have gone 'home' – then the old divisions which the empire had stifled and new ones which it had inevitably and sometimes intentionally created have further split the 'new' nations into ever smaller national and ethnic groupings. India, Pakistan, Nigeria, Cyprus, Indonesia, Malaysia have all since the end of British rule divided and subdivided. The same has been true of Vietnam, much of Central Africa after the expulsion of the French, and parts of

West Africa following the departure of the Portuguese. New nations can be brought into being with the flourish of a pen. New peoples take far longer to gestate.

Nor are former colonies the only states to experience this process. In Europe itself, processes that began on the edges of the empire at the end of the eighteenth century have in the twenty-first crept back to transform the metropolis itself, just as in their different ways Montesquieu and Tocqueville warned that they would. Spain, which the ministers of Philip III and IV in the seventeenth century, the enlightened monarch Charles III in the eighteenth, the liberals in the nineteenth and then, with savage ferocity, General Franco in the twentieth, all tried to fuse together out of Catalans, Basques, Castilians, Adalusians, Galicians, has now all but fallen apart. It is ruled over by a monarch who holds power in the name of the nation but, as he himself has said, that nation has in a little over twenty years become the first federal state of the new federal Europe. Even the United Kingdom, which although only united since the beginning of the eighteenth century seemed nevertheless to have been stable for far longer than any other European nation, is inexorably dissolving back into its component parts. 'Internal decolonization' it has been called, and there is no knowing where it will stop, no knowing what in the future might be the ideal unit that we choose to call a 'people'.

Creoles, indigenes and local separatists are not the only groups to make demands on the steadily dissolving body of empire. In a world in which the West no longer clings quite so self-confidently to its belief in the superiority of its way of life, in which attitudes towards the developing world in general have become far more ambiguous, the remaining aboriginal peoples of the world, in the Americas, Australia and New Zealand, have begun to insist on some measure of recognition. Creole states, from Argentina (which until thirty years ago denied the existence of any significant preconquest groups) to Canada, have modified their constitutions and re-examined original treaties of settlement.

Perhaps the most celebrated attempt by an indigenous group to reclaim its territory and its right to historical recognition is what has come to be called the 'Mabo Case'. In 1982, three representatives of the Meriam peoples living in the Murray Islands in the Torres Straits, Eddie Mabo, David Passi and James Rice, brought an action in the Australian High Court against the State of Queensland, claiming that 'the Meriam people were entitled to the Islands as owners, possessors, occupiers and as persons entitled to enjoy the Islands', and that 'the Islands were not and never had been "Crown Land"'. In order to make their case, they went on to argue that the claim made in 1788, whereby Australia had been declared to be *terra nullius* – 'unoccupied land' – and could thus be seized by anyone who chose to, had been invalid. In 1992, the Australian High Court ruled in their favour, thus depriving the Commonwealth of Australia of its sovereignty not merely over the Murray Islands but, by implication, over the entire continent. This was followed in December 1993 by the Native Title Act which, although it stopped short of handing back Australia to its aboriginal inhabitants, did set up measures to redress what the judges of the High Court called 'the national legacy of unutterable shame' which was, in their view, the history of the dealing of European settlers with the Aboriginals.

For many it has been a cathartic experience, a forced recognition that the creole nations that have evolved out of the
disappearance of the old European empires have never been one
and united. So far, few indigenous peoples have attempted full
autonomy from the nations by which they are encompassed.
(The Inuit nation created in northern Canada in 1999 is, despite
the ceremony with which it was inaugurated and the claims it
has made for itself, little more than a self-administered
province.) All aboriginal peoples are inescapably peoples of two
worlds. They are Mi'Kmaq and Canadian, Maori and New Zea-
lander. They share two cultures and may, as has happened on a
number of occasions, claim protection from one culture under
the laws of the other. No one resists the idea that cultures are
porous and subject to periodic reinvention so fiercely as the
spokespersons of aboriginal peoples. This is hardly surprising
since so much of their claim depends upon an appeal to continuing cultural difference. Yet few cultures are as poly-
morphous as they are. Everywhere in the world they nestle
within other cultures, predominantly of European origin, where
they constitute the minority. You cannot shed hundreds of
years of frequently oppressive and subservient coexistence by
nostalgia alone.

The difficulties faced by aboriginal peoples are, paradoxically,
not unlike those shared by other groups which, rather than
attempting to survive in their former homelands, have fled to
the metropolises of the empires by which they had once been
occupied. Whereas European settlers once flowed out to
America, Africa and Asia, Asians, Africans and the peoples of
the Caribbean are in increasing numbers flowing back to Europe.
These are not, as they are so often represented, isolated immi-

grant groups. They are full-scale migrations, peoples on the move, of a kind that Europe has not experienced since the final days of the Roman empire. Large communities have grown up which are in some cases very nearly autonomous – Bradford, in England, the Barbès district of Paris, and Chinatowns just about anywhere – and cling fiercely to the lifeways, cultural habits, beliefs, not to mention dress, languages and food of their original homelands. Yet even within these enclaves cultures cannot remain self-contained for long. The first generation may attempt as far as it is able to insulate itself from the surrounding, alien world. But the next generally want something more. While still recognizing themselves to be Pakistani or Algerian or Moroccan, they also and perhaps most clearly see themselves as British or French or Spanish. In most of the former European imperial capitals from London to Lisbon intermingling and intermarriage have gone a long way towards creating truly multiethnic communities. The frontier and the metropolis are no longer as distinct as they once were, and in the future the differences are likely to diminish even further.

While the memories of empire fade or are transformed at least within Europe itself, the idea of the nation, which had done so much, if only as an aspiration, to bring about their demise, is itself under threat. In recent years there has been much talk of globalization and the end of the nation-state. To most observers, however, it must seem that the nation-state still has a lot of life left in it. Peoples think of themselves overwhelmingly in nationalist terms. Those who do not are generally, as they have always been, the wealthy, the privileged, the intellectual. Diderot could afford to tell David Hume in 1768, 'You belong to all the nations of the earth and you never ask a man for his place of birth. I flatter myself that I am like you, a citizen of the great city of the world,' because while Diderot knew that he was also French and Hume knew himself to be what he called a 'North Briton' both of them also belonged to a cosy, self-sustaining universe which in their day was called 'the republic of letters' – a fictional, transcendental nation of the mind.[9] Today, the equivalent sentiments are more likely to be expressed by those who sit at the front in aeroplanes, international bankers and their friends, than among the intelligentsia. Cosmo-politanism has generally been a luxury that only aristocracies of one kind or another can really afford.

Yet for all the persistence of national sentiments there are signs that, as peoples once formed themselves into empires and thence into nations, they are in some parts of the world becoming peoples again. The European Union, which to so many of its enemies looks like an empire, is one arena in which the nation-state is being slowly and sometimes painfully trans-formed into a confederation. For all the problems it has encoun-tered, it has demonstrated that sovereignty and cultural identity do not need to be inseparable and that it is possible to live by laws drafted by a multinational executive while remaining culturally tied just as firmly as before to local and national allegiances. More significantly perhaps, Europe is rapidly becoming an arena where being French, for instance, is no longer such a mystery to those who are British, or vice versa – where different cultural lives complement one another whereas before they were only a source of conflict. The outbursts of bloody chauvinism unleashed upon Eastern Europe after the collapse of the Soviet Union, and the European Union's apparent powerlessness in the face of them, might be taken as a depressing indication that what Sigmund Freud so tellingly called 'the narcissism of small differences' is still an enduring human passion. But for all that, as new generations of peoples grow up who are willing to think of themselves as Europeans, as well as German or Dutch or Portuguese, it is still possible to hope that nationalism as the expression of solidarity formed through the hatred of difference is steadily if slowly in retreat.

These changes, and it is impossible to say how far and how fast they will reach, have all occurred in a rapidly changing world, a world that has become 'global'. On closer examination, if we ignore the omnipresent fast-food chains and video games which are to be found across the planet from Belfast to Beijing, globalization turns out to be relatively restricted. It is a term applied more to economies than to culture or politics and, as the World Bank recently pointed out, the world economy is less unified today than it was a hundred years ago. Globalization has, however, become a scare-word which for many describes a vaster and infinitely more menacing universal empire than any of those that have preceded it.[10] Empires are no more, the argument goes, but the habits and customs which sustained those of Europe for so long are now being smuggled back in with markets, international funding agencies and well-meaning but generally misguided non-governmental organizations taking the place of armies, administrators and priests.

In one sense, this is historically misleading. Volkswagen, the World Bank, the IMF or the World Wide Fund for Nature are not easily identifiable as 'imperialist' even if the language they use and the behaviour of their employees frequently are. They do not serve a central state and their long-term objectives are only incidentally political. Yet it is clearly true, as the peoples of the developing world have protested so often and so bitterly, that the legacies of the older empires have not entirely gone away. The surrender of colonies, the undoing of institutions, even the abandonment of an enduring ideology do not always lead to the renunciation of a creed, a conviction, a way of life.

There remains an assumption that has been with us since the days of Alexander the Great that certain values, the values 'we' treasure, are not merely the expression of our desires and preferences but are in some larger sense the obvious and necessary values of humankind. Above all, the modern heirs of Alexander tend to assume that a rule of law which respects individual rights and liberal democratic government (as practised in the United States) is a universal and not, as it most surely is, the creation of Graeco-Roman christendom. In 1995 the United Nations published a document called *Our Global Neighbourhood*. Its authors set out to explain that although international law – the 'law of nations' – was historically 'made in Europe by European jurists to serve European ends' and was 'based on Christian values and designed to advance Western expansion', it nevertheless came up with the right answers because despite its origins it was responsible for the creation of a universal conception of the person. Therefore, they insist, 'no longer is it credible for a state to turn its back on international law, alleging a bias towards European values and influence'. All that humankind now requires, they conclude, in order to bring about that elusive but eternal dream of 'perpetual peace' is a 'global citizenship' based on 'a strong commitment to principles of equity and democracy grounded in civil society'.[11]

It is not hard to see beneath this, well-intentioned though it evidently is, something very similar to the Roman notion of the *civitas*. The law of nations – or, as one American political philosopher, John Rawls, has tried to redefine it, the 'law of peoples' – remains, just as it was for the Roman emperor Caracalla, a universal creed.[12] It may well be that as we move forward into the new millennium and better and faster systems of communication shrink our world we do require some common code that will be able to unite us all, if only at times of crisis. At present there seems to be none on offer other than the law of nations. We would do well, however, to remember in our multicultural enthusiasm that this, like all forms of universalism, was once created in order to make a group of peoples into an empire.

Droctulft's journey with which this book began – and the journeys of all the world's Droctulfts – is nearing its end. Byzantium is no more and Ravenna has become an industrial nightmare linked to a seedy seaside resort. Although he could hardly have guessed that it would turn out this way, the 'civilization' for which Droctulft abandoned one life and sacrificed another has now reached, almost, into the furthermost recesses of the world. The Englishwoman, the 'captive' to whom Borges' grandmother had spoken that evening on the Pampas a little over a century ago, has become, along with the peoples who seized her as an infant, a relic, a figure from an infinitely remote past. 'Barbarism' exists as truly as it ever did but it no longer has a home. Now we do not struggle, as Droctulft did, with invaders. We struggle only with ourselves.

Notes

INTRODUCTION

1 *De Consulatu Stilichonis*, III, 135–70.
2 Review of Herder's *'Ideas on the Philosophy of the History of Mankind'*, in *Kant: Political Writings*, ed. Hans Reiss (Cambridge, 1991), p. 220.
3 *Corpus Hermeticum*, ed. A. J. Festugière and Arthur Darby Knock (Paris, 1954), IV Fr. 23, pp. 14–16.
4 See the essays in Maurice Duverger (ed.), *Le concept d'empire* (Paris, 1980).
5 J. S. Richardson, *'Imperium Romanum*: Empire and the Language of Power', *Journal of Roman Studies*, LXXXI (1991), 1–9.
6 See Hugh Tinker, *A New System of Slavery: The Export of Indian Labour Overseas 1830–1920* (London, 1974).
7 Sunil Khilnani, *The Idea of India* (New York, 1997), p. 118.
8 *Novum Organum*, in *The Works of Francis Bacon*, ed. James Spedding, R. L. Ellis and D. D. Heath (London, 1857–74), IV, p. 92.

1. THE FIRST WORLD CONQUEROR

1 François Hartogh, *Mémoires d'Ulysse: Récits sur la frontière en Grèce ancienne* (Paris, 1996), pp. 12–13.
2 John Boardman, *The Greeks Overseas: Their Early Colonies and Trade* (New York and London, 1980).
3 Bartolomé de Las Casas, *A Short Account of the Destruction of the Indies*, trans. Nigel Griffin (London and New York, 1992), p. 15.
4 *The Fortunes of Alexander*, 327 ff.
5 Inga Clendinnen, ' "Fierce and Unnatural Cruelty": Cortés and the Conquest of Mexico', in *New World Encounters*, ed. Stephen Green-

blatt (Berkeley, Los Angeles and London, 1993), pp. 12–47.

6 Jared Diamond, *Guns, Germs, and Steel: The Fate of Human Societies* (New York and London, 1999), pp. 67–81.

7 The best modern account of Alexander's life and campaigns is A. B. Bosworth, *Conquest and Empire: The Reign of Alexander the Great* (Cambridge, 1988).

8 *Florida*, VII.

9 Ibid.

10 Plutarch, *Parallel Lives*, 'Pompey', 2.2; and Sallust, *Historiae*, 3.88 M.

11 Quoted by Robin Lane Fox, *The Search for Alexander* (Boston, 1980), p. 23.

12 *The Fortunes of Alexander*, 328b.

13 *Politics*, 1252 b 4.

14 *The Fortunes of Alexander*, 328b.

15 *Quaestiones naturales* VI, 23, and *Epistolae* 91.17.

16 The standard work is George Cary, *The Medieval Alexander* (Cambridge, 1956).

17 *The 'Alexandreis' of Walter of Châtillon: A Twelfth-Century Epic*, trans. David Townsend (Philadelphia, 1996), Book X.

2. THE EMPIRE OF THE ROMAN PEOPLE

1 The story is told by Aulus Gellius, *Noctes Atticae*, iv, 8.

2 D. O. Thomas (ed.), *Richard Price: Political Writings* (Cambridge, 1991), p. 38.

3 See Andrew Lintott, *Imperium Romanum: Politics and Administration* (London and New York, 1993).

4 *De Officiis*, 1.38.

5 *The Reason of State* [*Della ragion di stato*], trans. P. J. and D. P. Waley (London, 1956), pp. 6–7.

6 Quoted in P. A. Garney, 'Laus Imperii', in *Imperialism in the Ancient World*, ed. P. A. Garney and C. R. Whittaker (Cambridge, 1978), p. 168.

7 *De Legibus*, I, x, 29; xii, 33.

8 *Institutes*, Proemium.

9 S. Albert, *Bellum Iustum*, Frankfurter Althistorische Studien, 10 (Kallmunz, 1980).

10 *De Officiis*, 1.34–5: 'There are two types of conflict: the one proceeds by debate, the other by force. Since the former is the proper concern of man, but the latter of beasts, one should only resort to the latter if one may not employ the former.'

11 *De Republica*, 3.34.

12 *De Legibus*, 1. xxii. 4.

13 'Lectures on Law: Citizens and Aliens', in *The Works of James Wilson*, ed. Robert Green McCloskey (Cambridge, Mass., 1967) II, p. 581.

14 *Discorsi*, II, 2.

15 *De Officiis*, 2.27.

16 *De Otio*, 4.1.

17 Burton Stein, 'Vijayanagara', in *The New Cambridge History of India* (Cambridge, 1989), I, 2.

18 *De Consulatu Stilichonis*, III, 135–70. St Augustine's comment on Honorius is quoted by Peter Brown, *Augustine of Hippo: A Biography* (London, 1976), p. 291. See Richard Koebner, *Empire* (Cambridge, 1961), pp. 14–19.

19 Ernest Barker, 'The Conception of Empire', in *The Legacy of Rome*, ed. Cyril Bailey (Oxford, 1923), p. 53.

20 *De Republica*, VI, 19–20.

21 *Ab urbe condita libri*, XXXVIII, 60.5.

22 Claude Nicolet, *L'Inventaire du monde: géographie et politique aux origines de l'empire romain* (Paris, 1988).

23 This point is made by Mark Elvin, *The Pattern of the Chinese Past: A Social and Economic Interpretation* (Stanford, Ca., 1973), pp. 18–22.

24 *Ab urbe condita libri*, XXXVII, 35.

25 Henry Chadwick, 'Envoi: On Taking Leave of Antiquity', in *The Oxford History of the Classical World*, ed. John Boardman, Jasper Griffin and Oswyn Murray (Oxford and New York, 1986), p. 808.

26 Ramsay MacMullen, *Christianizing the Roman Empire A.D. 100–400* (New Haven and London, 1984).

27 For a general history of the empire see Michael Grant, *Historical Rome* (Englewood Cliffs, N.J., 1978).

3. UNIVERSAL EMPIRE

1 Marie Tanner, *The Last Descendant of Aeneas: The Habsburgs and the Mythic Image of the Emperor* (New Haven and London, 1993).

2 *Historia imperial y caesarea, en la qual en summa se contiene las vidas y hechos de todos los caesares imperadores de Roma desde Julio Caesar hasta el Emperador Carlos Quinto* (Antwerp, 1561), sig. 1ᵛ.

3 C. A. Bayly, *Imperial Meridian: The British Empire and the World 1780–1830* (Harlow, 1989), pp. 19–34.

4. CONQUERING THE OCEAN

1 For an authoritative account of Henry's life see Peter Russell, *Prince Henry 'The Navigator': A Life* (New Haven and London, 2000).

2 See Sanjay Subrahmanyam, *The Career and Legend of Vasco da Gama* (Cambridge, 1997).

3 On Columbus' life see Felipe Fernández Armesto, *Columbus* (New York and London, 1991).

4 *An Inquiry into the Nature and Causes of the Wealth of Nations*, ed. R. H. Campbell and A. S. Skinner (Oxford, 1976), p. 560.

5. SPREADING THE WORD

1 *De Civitate Dei*, V, 15.

2 Colossians, 11.

3 *Histoire d'un voyage faict en la terre du Bresil autrement dite Amerique* (Geneva, 1578).

4 The story is told, at length, by Bartolomé de Las Casas, *Historia de las Indias*, ed. Augustín Millares Carlo (Mexico and Buenos Aires, 1951), II, pp. 441–4.

5 *A Short Account of the Destruction of the Indies*, trans. Nigel Griffin (London and New York, 1992).

6 See Anthony Pagden, *The Fall of Natural Man: The American Indian and the Origins of Comparative Ethnology* (Cambridge, 1982), pp. 109–45.

7 *Boswell's Life of Johnson*, ed. G. B. Hill (Oxford, 1934), I, 45.

8 Quoted in *A Short Account of the Destruction of the Indies*, p. xiv.

6. THE DECLINE OF THE IBERIAN WORLD

1 Geoffrey Parker, 'David or Goliath? Philip II and His World in the 1580s', in *Spain, Europe and the Atlantic World: Essays in Honour of John H. Elliott*, ed. Richard Kagan and Geoffrey Parker (Cambridge, 1995), pp. 254–5.

2 See J. H. Elliott, *Spain and its World 1500–1700* (New Haven and London, 1989), pp. 241–62.

3 *An Inquiry into the Nature and Causes of the Wealth of Nations*, ed. R. H. Campbell and A. S. Skinner (Oxford, 1976), p. 563.

4 The best account of the Portuguese empire is A. J. R. Russell-Wood, *The Portuguese Empire, 1415–1808: A World on the Move* (Baltimore and London, 1992).

7. EMPIRES OF LIBERTY, EMPIRES OF TRADE

1 H. P. Biggar, *A Collection of Documents Relating to Jacques Cartier and the Sieur de Roberval*, Publications of the Public Archives of Canada, No. 14 (Ottawa, 1930), p. 128.

2 Stephen Greenblatt, *Marvellous Possessions: The Wonder of the New World* (Oxford, 1991), pp. 109–18.

3 *Judicious and Select Essays and Observations* (London, 1667), p. 20.

4 Anthony Pagden, *Lords of All the World: Ideologies of Empire in Spain, Britain and France, c. 1500–c. 1800* (New Haven and London, 1995), pp. 178–200.

5 Quoted in Steven Pincus, 'The English Debate over Universal Monarchy', in *A Union for Empire: Political Thought and the British Union of 1707*, ed. John Robertson (Cambridge, 1995), p. 42.

6 'A Discourse on Government with Relation to Militias', in *The Political Works of Andrew Fletcher* (London, 1737), p. 66.

7 James Axtell, *The Invasion Within: The Contest of Cultures in Colonial North America* (New York and Oxford, 1985), p. 133.

8 'Philo-Caledon', *A Defence of the Scots Settlement in Darien with an Answer to the Spanish Memorial against it* (Edinburgh, 1699), p. 24.

9 See Richard White, *The Middle Ground: Indians, Empires and Republics in the Great Lakes Region 1650–1815* (Cambridge, 1991).

10 *Speech of Edmund Burke Esq. on Moving his Resolution for Conciliation with the Colonies* (London, 1775), p. 48.

11 *An Inquiry into the Nature and Causes of the Wealth of Nations*, ed. R. H. Campbell and A. S. Skinner (Oxford, 1976), p. 61.

12 *The Writings and Speeches of Edmund Burke*, ed. Paul Langford (Oxford, 1981), II, p. 194.

13 David Armitage, 'The British Conception of Empire in the Eighteenth Century', in *Imperium/Empire/Reich: Ein Konzept politischer Herrschaft im deutsch-britischen Vergleich*, ed. Franz Bosbach and Hermann Hiery (Munich, 1999), pp. 91–107.

14 See in particular, P. J. Marshall, 'The British in Asia: Trade to Dominion, 1700–1765', in *The Oxford History of the British Empire*, Vol. II, *The Eighteenth Century*, ed. P. J. Marshall (Oxford, 1998), pp. 487–507.

15 Quoted in Rajat Kanta Ray, 'Indian Society and the Establishment of British Supremacy, 1765–1818', in ibid., p. 514.

16 *Political Writings*, ed. D. O. Thomas (Cambridge, 1991), p. 71.

17 *The Speeches of the Right Hon. Edmund Burke*, Vol. V, 'India, Madras and Bengal, 1774–1785', ed. P. J. Marshall (Oxford, 1981), p. 385.

18 See P. J. Marshall, *The Impeachment of Warren Hastings* (Oxford, 1965).

19 David Bromwich (ed.), *On Empire, Liberty and Reform: Speeches and Letters of Edmund Burke* (New Haven and London, 2000), pp. 15–16.

8. SLAVERY

1 See M. I. Finley ed. *Classical Slavery* (London and Totowa, N.J., 1987) and *Ancient Slavery and Modern Ideology* (New York, 1980).

2 Gomes Eanes de Zurara, *Crónica dos feitos na conquista de Guiné*, ed. Torquato de Sousa Soares (Lisbon, 1961), I, pp. 145–8.

3 See Robin Blackburn, *The Making of New World Slavery: From the Baroque to the Modern 1492–1800* (London, 1997).

4 Quoted in Anthony Pagden, *Lords of All the World: Ideologies of Empire in Spain, Britain and France, c. 1500–c. 1800* (New Haven and London, 1995), p. 171.

5 See Philip Curtin, *The African Slave Trade: A Census* (Madison, 1969).

6 *Politics*, 1254 b 27ff.

7 See Anthony Pagden, *The Fall of Natural Man: The American Indian and the Origins of Comparative Ethnology* (Cambridge, 1982), pp. 27–56.

8 Letter to Fray Bernardo de Vique O.P., in *Political Writings*, ed. Anthony Pagden and Jeremy Lawrance (Cambridge, 1991), pp. 334–5.

9 See David Eltis, *Economic Growth and the Ending of the Atlantic Slave Trade* (New York and London, 1987).

10 J. D. Farge, *A History of Africa* (London, Melbourne, Auckland and Johannesburg, 1978), pp. 339–40.

11 See Robin Blackburn, *The Overthrow of Colonial Slavery 1776–1848* (London and New York, 1998).

12 Quoted in Hugh Thomas, *The Slave Trade: The Story of the Atlantic Slave Trade: 1440–1870* (New York, 1997), pp. 789.

9. THE FINAL FRONTIER

1 Louis-Antoine de Bougainville, *Voyage autour du monde par la frégate la Boudeuse et la flûte l'Etoile; en 1766, 1767, 1768 and 1769* (Paris, 1980), pp. 133–70.

2 Bernard Smith, *European Vision and the South Pacific* (New Haven and London, 1985), p. 130.

3 *Histoire des navigations aux terres australes* (Paris, 1756), I, pp. 17–19.

4 *The Journals of Captain James Cook on his Voyages of Discovery*, ed. J. C. Beaglehole (Cambridge, 1955–67), Vol. I, 'The Voyage of the Endeavour, 1768–1771', p. 514.

5 Ibid., pp. cclxxx–cclxxxiii.

6 *European Vision and the South Pacific*, pp. 114–15.

7 *The Journals of Captain James Cook on his Voyages of Discovery*, Vol. III, 'The Voyage of the Resolution and Discovery, 1776–1779', pp. 239–59.

8 Bernard Smith, *Imagining the Pacific: In the Wake of the Cook Voyages* (New Haven and London, 1992), pp. 225–40.

10. EMPIRE, RACE AND NATION

1 *Outlines of a Philosophy of the History of Man* [*Ideen zur Philosophie der Geschichte der Menschheit*], trans. T. Churchill (London, 1800), p. 224.

2 See Anthony Pagden, *European Encounters with the New World: From Renaissance to Romanticism* (New Haven and London, 1993), pp. 172–9.

3 Richard Koebner, *Empire* (Cambridge, 1961), p. 277.

4 Edward Said, *Orientalism* (New York and London, 1979), pp. 81–5.

5 Henry Laurens, Charles C. Gillispie, Jean-Claude Golvin and Claude Traunecker, *L'Expédition d'Egypte: 1798–1801* (Paris, 1989).

6 *The Age of Empire, 1875–1914* (London, 1987), p. 70.

7 Paul Kramer, 'Making Concessions: Race and Empire Revisited at the Philippine Exposition, St Louis, 1901–1905', *Radical History Review*, 73 (1999), pp. 75–114.

8 *Esquisse d'un tableau historique des progress de l'esprit humain* (Paris, 1793), pp. 335–7.

9 *A Choice of Kipling's Verse, Selected with an Essay on Rudyard Kipling by T. S. Eliot* (London, 1963), p. 136.

10 On Virey see Anthony Pagden, 'The "Defence of Civilization" in Eighteenth-Century Social Theory', *History of the Human Sciences*, 1 (1988), pp. 33–45.

11 See, in general, Leon Poliakov, *The Aryan Myth: A History of Racist and Nationalist Ideas in Europe*, trans. E. Howard (London, 1974).

12 John Burrow, *The Crisis of Reason: European Thought, 1848–1914* (New Haven and London, 2000), pp. 106–7.

13 *Utilitarianism, Liberty, Representative Government*, ed. Geraint Williams (London, 1993), pp. 197–227.

14 George Campbell, *Memories of My Indian Career* (London, 1893), I, p. 59.

15 Lata Man, 'Contentious Traditions: The Debate on Sati in Colonial India,' in *Recasting Women: Essays on Indian Colonial History*, ed. Kumkum Sangari and Sudesh Vaid (New Brunswick, 1990), pp. 88–126.

16 Quoted in Richard Koebner and Helmut Dan Schmidt, *Imperialism: The Story and Significance of a Political Word, 1840–1960* (Cambridge, 1964), pp. 136–7.

17 J. R. Seeley, *The Expansion of England* (London, 1925), p. 350.

18 See Koebner and Schmidt, *Imperialism*, pp. 173–5.

19 Quoted by Thomas R. Metcalf, *Ideologies of the Raj*, Vol. II. 4 of *The New Cambridge History of India* (Cambridge, 1994), p. 34.

11. ENDING

1 See Efraim Karsh and Inari Karsh, *Empires of the Sand: The Struggle for Mastery in the Middle East 1789–1923* (Cambridge, Mass., and London, 1999).

2 Jonathan D. Spence, *The Chan's Great Continent: China in Western Eyes* (New York and London, 1998), p. 101.

3 Quoted ibid., pp. 99–100.

4 Paul Kennedy, *The Rise and Fall of the Great Powers* (New York, 1987), pp. 148–9.

5 *Imagined Communities: Reflections on the Origins and Spread of Nationalism*, rev. edn (London, 1991).

6 Recorded by Peter Fry in 'Spirits of the Hills', *Times Literary Supplement*, 7 April 2000, p. 22.

7 Anthony D. Smith, *National Identity* (London and New York, 1991).

8 Cf. J. C. Lescure, 'Faire les Italiens', in *L'Europe des nationalismes aux nations* (Paris, 1996), II, p. 9. The remark has also been attributed to Carlo Cattaneo and Massimo d'Azeglio.

9 *Correspondence*, ed. G. Roth (Paris, 1955), VIII, p. 16.

10 For the most recent, overstated and hysterical expression of this fear, see Michael Hardt and Antonio Negri, *Empire* (Cambridge, Mass., and London, 2000).

11 *Our Global Neighbourhood: The Report of the Commission on Global Governance*, with an introduction by Nelson Mandela (Oxford, 1995).

12 John Rawls, *The Law of Peoples* (Cambridge, Mass., and London, 1991).

Bibliography

Albert, S., *Bellum Iustum*, Frankfurter Althistorische Studien, 10 (Kallmunz, 1980).

Anderson, Benedict, *Imagined Communities: Reflections on the Origins and Spread of Nationalism*, rev. edn (London, 1991).

Armitage, David, 'The British Conception of Empire in the Eighteenth Century', in *Imperium/Empire/Reich: Ein Konzept politischer Herrschaft im deutsch-britischen Vergleich*, ed. Franz Bosbach and Hermann Hiery (Munich, 1999).

Axtell, James, *The Invasion Within: The Contest of Cultures in Colonial North America* (New York and Oxford, 1985).

Bacon, Francis, *The Works of Francis Bacon*, eds. James Spedding, R. L. Ellis and D. D. Heath, 14 vols (London, 1857–74).

Bailey, Cyril (ed.), *The Legacy of Rome* (Oxford, 1923).

Barker, Ernest, 'The Conception of Empire', in *The Legacy of Rome*, ed. Cyril Bailey (Oxford, 1923).

Bayly, C. A., *Imperial Meridian: The British Empire and the World 1780–1830* (Harlow, 1989).

Blackburn, Robin, *The Making of New World Slavery: From the Baroque to the Modern 1492–1800* (London, 1997).

——, *The Overthrow of Colonial Slavery 1776–1848* (London, 1988).

Boardman, John, *The Greeks Overseas: Their Early Colonies and Trade* (New York and London, 1980).

Boardman, John, Jasper Griffin and Oswyn Murray (eds.), *The Oxford History of the Classical World* (Oxford and New York, 1986).

Bosworth, A. B., *Conquest and Empire: The Reign of Alexander the Great* (Cambridge, 1988).

Botero, Giovanni, *The Reason of State* [*Della ragion di stato*], trans. P. J. and D. P. Waley (London, 1956).

Bougainville, Louis-Antoine de, *Voyage autour du monde par la frégate la Boudeuse et la flûte l'Étoile; en 1766, 1767, 1768 and 1769* (Paris, 1980).

Boxer, Charles, *The Dutch Seaborne Empire, 1600–1800* (New York and London, 1970).

Bromwich, David (ed.), *On Empire, Liberty and Reform: Speeches and Letters of Edmund Burke* (New Haven and London, 2000).

Brown, Peter, *Augustine of Hippo: A Biography* (London, 1976).

Burke, Edmund, *Speech of Edmund Burke Esq. on Moving His Resolution for Conciliation with the Colonies* (London, 1775).

——, *The Speeches of the Right Hon. Edmund Burke*, Vol. V 'India, Madras and Bengal, 1774–1785', ed. P. J. Marshall (Oxford, 1981).

——, *The Writings and Speeches of Edmund Burke*, ed. Paul Langford (Oxford, 1981).

Burrow, John, *The Crisis of Reason: European Thought, 1848–1914* (New Haven and London, 2000).

Cambridge History of Africa, general eds. J. D. Fage and Roland Oliver, 8 vols (Cambridge and New York, 1975–86).

Campbell, George, *Memories of My Indian Career*, 2 vols (London, 1893).

Cary, George, *The Medieval Alexander* (Cambridge, 1956).

Condorcet, Marie-Jean, marquis de, *Esquisse d'un tableau historique des progress de l'esprit humain* (Paris, 1793).

Cook, James, *The Journals of Captain James Cook on his Voyages of Discovery*, ed. J. C. Beaglehole, 3 vols (Cambridge, 1955–67).

Corpus Hermeticum, eds. A. J. Festugière and Arthur Darby Knock (Paris, 1954).

Curtin, Philip, *The Image of Africa: British Ideas and Action, 1780–1850* (Madison, 1964).

——, *The African Slave Trade: A Census* (Madison, 1969).

De Brosses, Charles, *Histoire des navigations aux terres australes*, 2 vols (Paris, 1756).

Diamond, Jared, *Guns, Germs, and Steel: The Fate of Human Societies* (New York and London, 1999).

Duverger, Maurice (ed.), *Le concept d'empire* (Paris, 1980).

Edney, Mathew H., *Mapping an Empire: The Geographical Construction of British India 1765–1843* (Chicago and London, 1997).

Elliott, J. H., *Imperial Spain, 1469–1716* (London, 1963).

——, *Spain and its World 1500–1700* (New Haven and London, 1989).

Eltis, David, *Economic Growth and the Ending of the Atlantic Slave Trade* (New York and London, 1987).

Elvin, Mark, *The Pattern of the Chinese Past: A Social and Economic Interpretation* (Stanford, Ca., 1973).

Farge, J. D., *A History of Africa* (London, Melbourne, Auckland, and Johannesburg, 1978).

Fernández Armesto, Felipe, *Columbus* (New York and London, 1991).

Finley, M. I., *Ancient Slavery and Modern Ideology* (New York, 1980).

—— (ed.), *Classical Slavery* (London and Totowa, N.J., 1987).

Fletcher, Andrew, *The Political Works of Andrew Fletcher* (London, 1737).

Fox, Robin Lane, *The Search for Alexander* (Boston, 1980).

Garney, P. A., and C. R. Whittaker (eds.), *Imperialism in the Ancient World* (Cambridge, 1978).

Grant, Michael, *Historical Rome* (Englewood Cliffs, N.J., 1978).

Greenblatt, Stephen, *Marvellous Possessions: The Wonder of the New World* (Oxford, 1991).

—— (ed.), *New World Encounters* (Berkeley, Los Angeles and London, 1993).

Hardt, Michael, and Antonio Negri, *Empire* (Cambridge, Mass., and London, 2000).

Hartogh, François, *Mémoires d'Ulysse: Récits sur la frontière en Grèce ancienne* (Paris, 1996).

Herder, Johann Gottfried von, *Outlines of a Philosophy of the History of Man* [*Ideen zur Philosophie der Geschichte der Menschheit*], trans. T. Churchill (London, 1800).

Hobsbawm, Eric, *The Age of Empire, 1875–1914* (London, 1987).

Kagan, Richard, and Geoffrey Parker (eds.), *Spain, Europe and the Atlantic World: Essays in Honour of John H. Elliott* (Cambridge, 1995).

Kant, Immanuel, *Political Writings*, ed. Hans Reiss (Cambridge, 1991).

Karsh, Efraim, and Inari Karsh, *Empires of the Sand: The Struggle for Mastery in the Middle East 1789–1923* (Cambridge, Mass., and London, 1999).

Kennedy, Paul, *The Rise and Fall of the Great Powers* (New York, 1987).

Khilnani, Sunil, *The Idea of India* (New York, 1997).

Kipling, Rudyard, *A Choice of Kipling's Verse, Selected with an Essay on Rudyard Kipling by T. S. Eliot* (London, 1963).

Koebner, Richard, *Empire* (Cambridge, 1961).

——, and Helmut Dan Schmidt, *Imperialism: The Story and Significance of a Political Word, 1840–1960* (Cambridge, 1964).

Kramer, Paul, 'Making Concessions: Race and Empire Revisited at the Philippine Exposition, St Louis, 1901–1905', *Radical History Review*, 73 (1999).

Las Casas, Bartolomé de, *Historia de las Indias*, ed. Augustín Millares Carlo, 3 vols (Mexico and Buenos Aires, 1951).

——, *A Short Account of the Destruction of the Indies*, trans. Nigel Griffin (London and New York, 1992).

Laurens, Henry, Charles C. Gillispie, Jean-Claude Golvin and Claude Traunecker, *L'Expédition d'Egypte: 1798–1801* (Paris, 1989).

Léry, Jean de, *Histoire d'un voyage faict en la terre du Bresil autrement dite Amerique* (Geneva, 1578).

Lintott, Andrew, *Imperium Romanum: Politics and Administration* (London and New York, 1993).

MacMullen, Ramsay, *Christianizing the Roman Empire A.D. 100–400* (New Haven and London, 1984).

Marshall, P. J., *The Impeachment of Warren Hastings* (Oxford, 1965).

Metcalf, Thomas R., *Ideologies of the Raj*, Vol. II. 4 of *The New Cambridge History of India* (Cambridge, 1994).

Mexia, Pedro de, *Historia imperial y caesarea, en la qual en summa se contiene las vidas y hechos de todos los caesares imperadores de Roma desde Julio Caesar hasta el Emperador Carlos Quinto* (Antwerp, 1561).

Mill, John Stuart, *Utilitarianism, Liberty, Representative Government*, ed. Geraint Williams (London, 1993).

Mommsen, Wolfgang, *Theories of Imperialism*, trans. P. S. Falla (Chicago, 1980).

Nicolet, Claude, *L'inventaire du monde: géographie et politique aux origines de l'empire romain* (Paris, 1988).

Our Global Neighbourhood: The Report of the Commission on Global Governance, with an introduction by Nelson Mandela (Oxford, 1995).

Oxford History of the British Empire, general ed. Roger Louis, 5 vols (Oxford and New York, 1998–9).

Pagden, Anthony, *The Fall of Natural Man: The American Indian and the Origins of Comparative Ethnology* (Cambridge, 1982).

——, 'The "Defence of Civilization" in Eighteenth-Century Social Theory', *History of the Human Sciences*, 1 (1988).

——, *European Encounters with the New World: From Renaissance to Romanticism* (New Haven and London, 1993).

——, *Lords of All the World: Ideologies of Empire in Spain, Britain and France, c. 1500–c. 1800* (New Haven and London, 1995).

Parker, Geoffrey, *Spain in the Netherlands, 1559–1659* (London, 1979).

Poliakov, Leon, *The Aryan Myth: A History of Racist and Nationalist Ideas in Europe*, trans. E. Howard (London, 1974).

Price, Richard, *Political Writings*, ed. D. O. Thomas (Cambridge, 1991).

Raleigh, Sir Walter, *Judicious and Select Essays and Observations* (London, 1667).

Rawls, John, *The Law of Peoples* (Cambridge, Mass., and London, 1991).

Richardson, J. S., '*Imperium Romanum*: Empire and the Language of Power', *Journal of Roman Studies*, LXXXI (1991).

Robertson, John (ed.), *A Union for Empire: Political Thought and the British Union of 1707* (Cambridge, 1995).

Russell, Peter, *Prince Henry 'The Navigator': A Life* (New Haven and London, 2000).

Russell-Wood, A. J. R., *The Portuguese Empire, 1415–1808: A World on the Move* (Baltimore and London, 1992).

Said, Edward, *Orientalism* (New York and London, 1979).

——, *Culture and Imperialism* (New York and London, 1993).

Sangari, Kumkum, and Sudesh Vaid (eds.), *Recasting Women: Essays on Indian Colonial History* (New Brunswick, 1990).

Scammell, G. V., *The World Encompassed* (London and New York, 1981).

Schumpeter, Joseph, *Imperialism and Social Classes*, trans. Heinz Norden (Oxford, 1951).

Seeley, J. R., *The Expansion of England* (London, 1925).

Smith, Adam, *An Inquiry into the Nature and Causes of the Wealth of Nations*, ed. R. H. Campbell and A. S. Skinner, 2 vols (Oxford, 1976).

Smith, Anthony D., *National Identity* (London and New York, 1991).

Smith, Bernard, *European Vision and the South Pacific* (New Haven and London, 1985).

——, *Imagining the Pacific: In the Wake of the Cook Voyages* (New Haven and London, 1992).

Spence, Jonathan D., *The Chan's Great Continent: China in Western Eyes* (New York and London, 1998).

Stein, Burton, *Vijayanagara*, Vol. I. 2. of *The New Cambridge History of India* (Cambridge, 1989).

Subrahmanyam, Sanjay, *The Career and Legend of Vasco da Gama* (Cambridge, 1997).

Tanner, Marie, *The Last Descendant of Aeneas: The Habsburgs and the Mythic Image of the Emperor* (New Haven and London, 1993).

Thomas, Hugh, *The Slave Trade: The Story of the Atlantic Slave Trade: 1440–1870* (New York, 1997).

Tinker, Hugh, *A New System of Slavery: The Export of Indian Labour Overseas 1830–1920* (London, 1974).

Trudel, Marcel, *The Beginnings of New France, 1524–1663*, trans. Patricia Claxton (Toronto, 1973).

Vitoria, Francisco de, *Political Writings*, ed. Anthony Pagden and Jeremy Lawrance (Cambridge, 1991).

Walter of Châtillon, *The 'Alexandreis' of Walter of Châtillon: A Twelfth-Century Epic*, trans. David Townsend (Philadelphia, 1996).

White, Richard, *The Middle Ground: Indians, Empires and Republics in the Great Lakes Region 1650–1815* (Cambridge, 1991).

Williams, Robert A., *The American Indian in Western Legal Thought: The Discourses of Conquest* (New York and Oxford, 1990).

Wood, Gordon, *The Creation of the American Republic 1776–1787* (New York and London, 1972).

Zurara, Gomes Eanes de, *Crónica dos feitos na conquista de Guiné*, ed. Torquato de Sousa Soares (Lisbon, 1961).

Key Figures

Alexander III of Macedon (356–323 BC) called 'the Great', Greek monarch, creator of a vast empire which reached from the Adriatic to the Indus, from the Punjab to the Sudan, the subject of a number of mythical tales about his courage and wisdom, and a hero for many later empire-builders, among others Pompey, Trajan and Napoleon.

Apuleius (c. 125–c. 170) writer and orator, best known for the *Golden Ass*, the only surviving complete Latin novel, as well as a miscellany of declamations, narrative descriptions and anecdotes called the *Florida*.

Aristotle (384–322 BC) Greek philosopher, logician, epistemologist, political theorist, aesthetician, biologist, astronomer. Aristotle not only practised these subjects but in a sense he invented most of them. He had been a pupil of Plato and was the tutor to Alexander the Great (*q.v.*).

Augustine of Hippo, Saint (354–430) one of the Fathers of the church who eventually became Bishop of Hippo in North Africa. He was the author of, among many other works, *The City of God*, and exercised a profound influence on the development of Christian theology.

Augustus (63 BC–AD 14) emperor of Rome, the first to assume the title *princeps* (first among men) and virtual creator of the system and ideology, known as the principate, which dominated the empire during the first three centuries of the Christian era.

Bacon, Francis (1561–1626) English philosopher, scientist and statesman, author among a vast body of writings of the highly influential *Great Instauration* and of series of essays in the manner of Michel de Montaigne.

Bentinck, Lord William (1774–1839) governor-general of Bengal (1828–33) and of India (1833–5), a liberal reformer who attempted to govern India according to Hindu laws, opened up judicial post to Indians and abolished sati, the Hindu practice of widow-burning.

Bolívar, Simón (1783–1830) called 'The Liberator', soldier-statesman and liberator of much of South America from the Spanish.

Borges, Jorge Luis (1899–1986) Argentine poet, writer, essayist, librarian.

Bougainville, Count Louis Antoine de (1729–1811) French mathematician and explorer, and the first Frenchman to circumnavigate the globe. Best known for his description of the pleasures to be found on the island of Tahiti and for having brought the first Bougainvillea to Europe, a plant which is named after him.

Burke, Edmund (1729–97) Irish philosopher, pamphleteer, orator and Whig member of parliament. He pleaded the American case during the War of Independence and organized the impeachment trial of Warren Hastings (q.v.). His best-known work, *Reflections on the Revolution in France*, was a fierce and excoriating denunciation of the ideology of the French revolution.

Caesar, Julius (100–44 BC) Roman military leader, conqueror of Gaul and Britain and responsible for the beginning of the end of the Roman republic for which he was assassinated by republican patriots.

Charles I, 'Charlemagne' (742–814) king of the Franks. With the exception of Asturias in Spain, southern Italy and the British Isles, he united almost all the Christian lands in Western Europe. Crowned emperor in 800.

Charles V, Holy Roman Emperor (1500–58) united the kingdoms of Spain, the Netherlands, much of Italy, and all of Central and South America. His was, as the Italian poet Ariosto said of it, an empire 'on which the sun never set'. He abdicated in favour of his son Philip II in 1556.

Cicero, Marcus Tullius (106–43 BC) Roman jurist, orator and philosopher. He wrote treatises on law, politics – the best known being *On*

Duties (*De Officiis*) – and rhetoric, and a large number of speeches which he delivered to the Roman senate. Cicero was a staunch republican and was executed in 43 BC.

Claudian (**Claudius Claudianus**, 370–404) Latin poet and panegyrist.

Columbus, Christopher (**Cristoforo Colombo**, 1451–1506) Genoese navigator who in 1492 became the first historically significant European to set foot in the Americas. Columbus made three subsequent voyages to America, in 1493, 1498 and 1506, and occupied most of Hispaniola (now Haiti and the Dominican Republic). Although by the time of his return from his second voyage, during which he sailed into the Gulf of Paria (Venezuela), it was obvious to almost everyone in Europe that he had come across a 'New World', Columbus insisted until his death that the eastern seaboard of America was in fact the western extremity of Asia.

Constant, Benjamin (1767–1830) Franco-Swiss liberal political theorist and novelist. Passionate in his denunciation of the Napoleonic empire, he became a deputy in the French parliament in 1819 after the fall of Napoleon (*q.v.*), and president of the Council of State in 1830. He is best remembered today for *The Spirit of Conquest and Usurpation and their Relation to European Civilization*, *Principles of Politics Applicable to all Representative Governments*, the *Liberty of the Ancients Compared with that of the Moderns*, and the novel *Adolph*.

Constantine the Great (*c.* 280–337) Roman emperor responsible for the creation of Constantinople (now Istanbul) and for making Christianity the official religion of the empire.

Cook, Captain James (1728–79) English navigator. He made three voyages to the Pacific between 1768 and 1779 during which he circumnavigated Australia and charted much of its coastline. His accounts of his journeys earned him an enormous following in Europe and his death on the beach at Hawaii on his final voyage, at the hands of Hawaiians who may or may not have taken him for their god Lono, has been the subject of a prolonged and heated debate ever since.

Cortés, Hernán (1485–1547) Spanish conquistador who between 1519 and 1521 overran the Aztec empire. He also founded the city of Mexico, created the Spanish settlement of New Spain, and led the first major expedition to Honduras.

Cyrus the Great (r. 559–c. 529 BC) Persian emperor, founder of the Achaemenid empire.

Darius I (550–486 BC) called 'the Great', Persian emperor who extended the empire from the Indus Valley to Macedonia. He began the construction of the great palace at Persepolis and may have been responsible for establishing Zoroastrianism as the official religion.

Diderot, Denis (1713–84) French philosopher, essayist, short-story writer, dramatist and editor, with Jean d'Alembert, of the *Encyclopédie*. He contributed extensively to the Abbé Raynal's (q.v.) massive *Philosophical and Political History of the Two Indies*, one of the most violent condemnations of European colonialism in the eighteenth century, and wrote a fictional supplement to Bougainville's (q.v.) account of his experiences on Tahiti which helped create the myth of the 'noble savage' in the eighteenth century.

Gama, Vasco da (1460–1524) Portuguese navigator who in 1497 was the first European to sail around the Cape of Good Hope and thus establish a sea-route between Europe and India.

Gibbon, Edward (1737–94) one of the greatest of the eighteenth-century historians, best known for *The Decline and Fall of the Roman Empire*, first published in 1776.

Gobineau, Joseph-Arthur, self-styled Comte de (1816–82) French diplomat and social theorist. He wrote a number of stories, histories and literary criticism but is best known for his *Essay on the Inequality of the Human Races* of 1853–5 which is regarded as one of the founding documents of modern racism.

Hakluyt, Richard (1552–1616) English historian and geographer, and propagandist for English maritime expansion, best known as the compiler of the *Principal Naviations, Voyages and Discoveries of the English Nation*.

Hastings, Warren (1732–1818) governor-general of India from 1774–85. On his return to Britain, Hastings was impeached at the instigation of

Edmund Burke (q.v.) for misconduct. His trial dragged on from 1788 until 1795 when he was acquitted.

Henry, Prince, of Portugal (1394–1460) sometimes called 'the Navigator', Portuguese prince who sponsored the earlier European voyages down the coast of West Africa, played a decisive role in European involvement in the African slave trade, and opened the way for all future European overseas expansion.

Herder, Johann Gottfried von (1744–1803) German philosopher, historian, theologian, linguist and poet, former pupil of Kant (q.v.) and often claimed to be the intellectual founder of modern German nationalism. Best known for *Reflections on the Philosoply of the History of Mankind*, and *Yet Another Philosophy of History*.

Herodotus of Halicarnassus (c. 484–420 BC) Greek historian and author of the earliest historical narrative we possess, which is largely concerned with the wars between the Greeks and the Persians.

Hume, David (1711–76) Scottish or 'North Briton' sceptical philosopher, essayist and historian, author of *A Treatise of Human Nature*, *An Enquiry Concerning Human Understanding*, and the multi-volume *History of England*.

Jones, Sir William (1746–94) British orientalist and judge. He was the first man to suggest an association between Greek and Sanskrit, and the existence of an Indo-European family of languages. His *Institutes of Hindu Laws* (1794) greatly influenced British attempts to make the British and Hindu legal systems compatible.

Kant, Immanuel (1632–1704) German philosopher, author of the *Critique of Pure Reason*, the *Critique of Practical Reason* and the *Critique of Judgement* (among many other works) which were responsible for the creation of a system of ethics which still dominates Western liberal ways of thinking.

Las Casas, Bartolomé de (1474?–1566) Spanish Dominican, Bishop of Chiapas in Mexico and 'Apostle to the Indians'. The fiercest and best-known champion of the rights of the American Indians in the sixteenth century, he was a prolific writer and tireless agitator whose efforts had considerable impact on the Spanish administration of the Americas.

Livy (Titus Livius, 59 BC–AD 17) Roman historian, his *Ab urbe condita libri* ('Books from the Foundation of the City') is a celebration of the rise of the empire, in much the same way as is Virgil's (*q.v.*) *Aeneid*.

Locke, John (1632–1704) English philosopher, best known as the author of *An Essay on Human Understanding* and *Two Treatises on Government*. Locke was involved in the settlement of the Carolinas for which he wrote a constitution, and was a shareholder in the Royal Africa Company.

Machiavelli, Niccolò (1469–1527) Florentine political theorist, playwright, diplomat and author, most famously, of *The Prince* and the *Discourses on Livy*.

Magellan, Fernando (Fernão de Magalhães, 1480–1521) Portuguese navigator, left Spain in 1519, discovered the Straits of Magellan and crossed the Pacific. He was killed in the Philippines, but one ship of his fleet returned to Spain in 1522 having completed the circumnavigation of the world.

Maine, Sir Henry (1822–88) English jurist, member of the Law Council of the governor-general of India, responsible for codifying Indian law, first professor of comparative jurisprudence at the University of Oxford, and author of the influential *Ancient Law*.

Malinowski, Bronislaw (1884–1942) Polish anthropologist who spent much of his professional life in London. He was a prolific writer who is generally identified as one of the founders of the 'functionalist' school of British social anthropology.

Mill, John Stuart (1806–73) English utilitarian philosopher, liberal and political economist. Best known for his *Principles of Political Economy* and the essay *On Liberty*.

Montesquieu, Charles-Louis de Secondat, baron de (1689–1755) French jurist and philosopher, the author of *The Sprit of the Laws*, an encyclopaedic study of the social habits and legal systems of the world, which is often considered to be the first work of comparative sociology.

Müller, Max (1823–1900) German orientalist and linguist who spent most of his professional life at Oxford University. His main achievement was the fifty-one volumes of the *Sacred Books of the East* (1879–1904). He also did much to develop the idea of an Aryan race from which the peoples of both India and Europe are descended.

Napoleon Bonaparte (1769–1821) French general, First Consul (1799–1804) and Emperor of the French (1804–14/15). Napoleon attempted to impose the principles of the French revolution upon the whole of Europe. He failed but he helped create the Europe of nations which exists to this day. He also transformed France itself, revised the entire legal system (the Napoleonic Code) and reorganized the system of administration and education.

Ovid (43 BC–AD 17/18) Roman poet, author of the *Metamorphoses*.

Philip II (382–336 BC) king of Macedon and father of Alexander the Great (*q.v.*). He created the formidable Macedonian army with which in August 338 at Chaeronea he won a crushing victory over an alliance of southern Greek cities led by Athens and Thebes. This made Macedon an unchallenged superpower and prepared the way for his son's conquests in Persia.

Philip II (1527–98) king of Spain from 1556 and from 1580 king of Portugal. During his reign the Spanish-Portuguese empire, known collectively as the Catholic Monarchy, achieved its greatest power and extent.

Pizarro, Francisco (c. 1475–1541) Spanish conquistador who between 1530 and 1533 destroyed the empire of the Incas.

Plutarch (c. 46–120) Roman philosopher, essayist and historian, author of an admiring yet perceptive *Life of Alexander*, best known for his exemplary biographical sketches, the *Parallel Lives*, and a series of ethical reflections, the *Moralia*.

Polybius (c. 200–c. 118 BC) Greek historian of Rome's rise to Mediterranean dominion.

Raleigh, Sir Walter (1554?–1618) English seaman, adventurer and writer. In 1585 and 1589 he attempted to found a colony on Roanoke Island, which he named Virginia, and in 1595 led an expedition to Guiana in search of the legendary El Dorado (described in fanciful terms in *The*

Discoverie of Guiana of 1596). He returned again in 1616, promising King James I a new Peru. He failed and in 1618 was executed.

Raynal, Guillaume-Thomas, Abbé (1713–96) French historian, social theorist, journalist and pamphleteer. He is best known as the author of the *Philosophical and Political History of the Two Indies*, first published in 1772, a history and fierce critique of European colonization. A later and much enlarged version published in 1780 contained long passages by Denis Diderot (*q.v.*) and others. It was immensely popular, went through thirty editions between 1772 and 1789 and was translated into every major European language.

Scipio Africanus Major, Publius Cornelius (236–184 BC) noted Roman general who defeated the Carthaginian leader Hannibal at the battle of Zama (probably modern Jama) in 202 and occupied part of North Africa, for which he received the sobriquet 'Africanus'. He also led a Roman army against the Seleucid emperor Antiochus the Great in what is now Syria.

Seneca, Lucius Annaeus (*c.* 4/5 BC–AD 65) tragedian, philosopher and tutor to the emperor Nero. He was one of the most important of the Roman Stoics.

Smith, Adam (*c.* 1723–90) Scottish philosopher and political economist, best known for *The Wealth of Nations*, which still exercises a considerable influence over economic thinking, and *The Theory of Moral Sentiments*.

Soto, Domingo de (1494–1560) Spanish theologian, pupil and successor to Francisco de Vitoria (*q.v.*). His *On Justice and Right* became a standard work in sixteenth- and seventeenth-century European universities. Like Vitoria, he questioned the Spanish crown's claim to be the legitimate ruler of the Americas.

Thucydides (*c.* 460–400 BC), with Herodotus (*q.v.*), the greatest of the Greek historians and author of a history of the Peloponnesian war between Athens and Sparta between 431 and 404 BC.

Tocqueville, Alexis de (1805–59) French liberal political philosopher and statesman, best known as the author of *Democracy in America* and the *Old Regime and the Revolution*.

Trajan (Marcus Ulpius Trajanus, 53–117) Roman emperor during whose rule the empire reached its greatest extent.

Vieira, Antonio (1608–97) Jesuit missionary, orator and diplomat, often thought to be the originator of the Brazilian national mystique of the single nation of mixed bloods, European, African and Amerindian.

Virey, Jules-Joseph noted French physician, author of two works, the *Natural History of the Human Species* (1824) and 'On the Causes of Sociability in Animals and Civilization in Men' (1841), which claimed that there existed marked physiological differences between different races which determined their aptitude for 'civilization'.

Virgil (70–19 BC) Roman poet, best known for his epic on the founding of Rome, the *Aeneid*.

Vitoria, Francisco de (*c.* 1485–1546) Spanish theologian, author of a number of writings questioning the legitimacy of the Spanish conquest of America which had a lasting influence on the subsequent creation of international law.

Xerxes I (Khshaiarsha, *c.* 519–465 BC) son of Darius I (*q.v.*), king of Persia from 486 BC. In 480 he led a massive army into Greece, laid waste to most of Attica and burned the Acropolis in Athens; but his fleet was destroyed at Salamis in September 480 in a battle which decided the future of the Greek world.

Chronology

513 BC	Darius I, Persian emperor, crosses the Bosphorus into Europe
480 BC	Battle of Salamis; Greeks destroy the Persian fleet, thus averting a full-scale invasion
334 BC	Alexander the Great crosses the Dardenelles and begins the destruction of the Persian empire
323 BC	death of Alexander the Great
168 BC	Battle of Pydna; Roman armies put an end to the Macedonian monarchy
44 BC	assassination of Julius Caesar
27 BC	creation of the Roman principate under Octavian
AD 212	the Roman emperor Caracalla extends citizenship to all free inhabitants of the empire
324	Constantine the Great founds a new capital at Byzantium and names it Constantinople
410	Alaric the Goth sacks Rome; Roman rule comes to an end in the West
528	Justinian, emperor in the East, begins the codification of all Roman law
800	Charles I ('Charlemagne'), king of the Franks, crowned by the pope as emperor
1071	Seljuk Turks take Jerusalem
1095–1291	eight major crusades, armed expeditions under the aegis of the papacy, attempt unsuccessfully to recover Jerusalem
1405–33	voyages of the treasure fleet of the admiral Zheng He
1453	Ottoman Turks seize Constantinople, rename it Istanbul and put an end to the Byzantine empire

1492	Christopher Columbus' first transatlantic voyage
1498–9	Vasco da Gama sails to India via the Cape of Good Hope
1519	Charles of Habsburg elected Holy Roman emperor
1519–22	Spanish fleet under Fernão de Magalhães (Magellan) completes first circumnavigation of the globe
1521	Spanish forces under Hernán Cortés overthrow the Aztec empire; Martin Luther appears before the Diet of Worms
1529	Ottoman army of Suleiman the Magnificent lays siege to Vienna
1533	Francisco Pizarro seizes the Inca capital of Cuzco
1534	first voyage of Jacques Cartier to the Gulf of St Lawrence
1580	Philip II of Spain conquers Portugal thus uniting the empires of the two kingdoms
1581	Dutch declare independence from Spain
1583	Sir Walter Raleigh's expedition to Guiana
1600	charter of the East India Company
1607	English settlement at Jamestown
1618	outbreak of the Thirty Years War
1620	voyage of the *Mayflower*
1648	conclusion of the Thirty Years War, Treaty of Westphalia, creation of the system of European states
1668	East India Company takes over Bombay
1690	English settlement at Calcutta
1756	outbreak of Seven Years War
1760	New France surrenders to the British
1763	Peace of Paris brings Seven Years War to an end, leaving Britain in possession of most of North America
1768	Captain Cook's first voyage
1771	publication of Antoine de Bougainville's *Voyage autour du monde*
1772	Cook's second voyage
1776	Declaration of American Independence; publication of Adam Smith's *The Wealth of Nations*, Edward Gibbon's *Decline and Fall of the Roman Empire*; start of Cook's last voyage
1779	death of Cook in Hawaii

1788–95	trial of Warren Hastings, governor of Bengal
1789	beginning of the French revolution
1791	slave revolt in Santo Domingo
1793	Lord Macartney's embassy to China
1803	beginning of the Napoleonic Wars
1806	Holy Roman empire comes to an end
1807	abolition of the slave trade in the British Empire
1810–21	Spanish-American Wars of Independence
1815	Battle of Waterloo, end of Napoleonic Wars, Napoleon exiled to the island of St Helena; Britain takes control of the Cape Colony (South Africa) from the Dutch
1829	sati abolished
1830	French occupy Algeria
1839–42	Opium War between Britain and China
1853	David Livingstone crosses the continent of Africa
1858	abolition of the East India Company
1859	publication of Charles Darwin's *On the Origin of Species*
1869	opening of the Suez Canal
1876	Queen Victoria becomes empress of India
1888	abolition of slavery in Brazil
1890	Cecil Rhodes made prime minister of Cape Colony
1900	Boxer 'rebellion' in China
1908	end of the Ottoman sultanate and creation of the modern Turkish republic
1911	abolition of the Chinese monarchy
1914–18	First World War
1917	creation of the USSR
1939–45	Second World War
1944	Bretton Woods Conference establishes World Bank and International Monetary Fund
1945	establishment of the United Nations
1947	partition and independence of India and Pakistan
1948	independence of Ceylon, renamed Sri Lanka in 1972
1949	establishment of the People's Republic of China
1957–66	independence of the Sudan, the Gold Coast (Ghana), Malaya, Nigeria, Cyprus, Jamaica, Trinidad, Kenya,

Zanzibar, Algeria, the Congo, Tanganyika, Gambia, Lesotho, Bechuanaland, Botswana, Guiana, Barbados, Mauritius, Northern Rhodesia (Zambia)

1989   fall of the Berlin Wall

1991   dissolution of the USSR

1994   Nelson Mandela becomes president of South Africa, thus ending the rule of the last settler population in Africa

1997   end of British rule in Hong Kong

1999   end of Portuguese rule in Macao

Index